The New Governance
of Addictive Substances
and Behaviours

Governance of Addictive Substances and Behaviours Series

Series Editors: Peter Anderson and Antoni Gual

Titles in the series

Governance of Addictions: European Public Policies
Tamyko Ysa, Joan Colom, Adrià Albareda, Anna Ramon, Marina Carrión, and Lidia Segura

The Impact of Addictive Substances and Behaviours on Individual and Societal Well-being
Edited by Peter Anderson, Jürgen Rehm, and Robin Room

What Determines Harm from Addictive Substances and Behaviours?
Edited by Lucy Gell, Gerhard Bühringer, Anne Lingford-Hughes, Petra Meier, John Holmes, Lucy Gell, Sarah Forberger, and Jane McLeod

Concepts of Addictive Substances and Behaviours across Time and Place
Edited by Matilda Hellman, Virginia Berridge, Karen Duke, and Alex Mold

Impact of Market Forces on Addictive Substances and Behaviours: The Web of Influence of the Addictive Industries
David Miller, Claire Harkins, Matthias Schlögl, and Brendan Montague

The New Governance of Addictive Substances and Behaviours

Peter Anderson
Fleur Braddick
Patricia Conrod
Antoni Gual
Matilda Hellman
Silvia Matrai
David Miller
David Nutt
Jürgen Rehm
Jillian Reynolds
Tamyko Ysa

OXFORD
UNIVERSITY PRESS

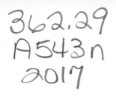

OXFORD
UNIVERSITY PRESS

Great Clarendon Street, Oxford, OX2 6DP,
United Kingdom

Oxford University Press is a department of the University of Oxford.
It furthers the University's objective of excellence in research, scholarship,
and education by publishing worldwide. Oxford is a registered trade mark of
Oxford University Press in the UK and in certain other countries

Published in the United States of America by Oxford University Press
198 Madison Avenue, New York, NY 10016, United States of America

British Library Cataloguing in Publication Data

Data available

Library of Congress Control Number: 2016955724

ISBN 978–0–19–875983–6

Printed in Great Britain by Ashford Colour Press Ltd, Gosport, Hampshire

Foreword

Consider the travel of ideas. This book, *The New Governance of Addictive Substances and Behaviours*, is a collection of contributions to the body of knowledge on the governance of addictions in Europe, based on interdisciplinary research from the European Union (EU) project Addictions and Lifestyles in Contemporary Europe—Reframing Addictions Project (ALICE RAP). With this project, the European Commission's Social Sciences and Humanities Division challenged academia to contribute to enhancing policies for addictive substances and addictive behaviors. The ALICE RAP project serves as a vehicle for the travel of ideas in transnational governance and as an actor in epistemic governance (Alasuutari and Qadir, 2014).

In what Freeman and Sturdy (2015) see as a new phenomenology of knowledge, are described embodied, inscribed, and enacted knowledge. Embodied knowledge is experience based on and expressed in people's activities; inscribed knowledge is formalized and written down in artefacts such as documents; and enacted knowledge is knowledge in action, which is also constantly monitored and regulated, and is essential when it comes to the realization of new policies.

The scientific production and dissemination of knowledge, as well as the translation of knowledge into policy practices, are central processes in the travel of ideas at the transnational level. Knowledge transfer comprises two processes: decontextualization (translation from practice in one context into abstract ideas) and contextualization (translation from abstract ideas to practice in a new context). Translation competence is a key requirement of making appropriate translations. Røvik (2011) has criticized the 'management fashion' theory, a leading theory on how management ideas, trends, and concepts travel from one sector to another, and even on a global scale, from country to country. As an alternative, Røvik (2011) introduced a virus-inspired theory that he claims offers more appropriate concepts and models with which to understand the translation and diffusion of ideas such as governance recipes.

In the broad output from the ALICE RAP project, there has been a particular focus on the conceptual frameworks of well-being, health footprint, and margin of exposure. By the finalization of the project, ALICE RAP aims to offer concepts that can provide a basis for a comprehensive future policy for the area of addiction. To do so, ALICE RAP needs to identify institutional preconditions and constraints to the social innovations represented by these concepts. In the translation from science to future governance and policies, we need to ask: how 'translationable' are these three conceptual frameworks and the three types of knowledge in the transnational decontextualization and contextualization governance processes?

From ideas to action

Governance involves 'processes and structures of public policy decision making and management that engage people constructively across the boundaries of public agencies, levels of government, and/or the public, private and civic spheres' (Emerson et al., 2012: 2). In the addiction field, we can add the aim of decreasing the negative individual, relational, and social (and cultural) consequences of addiction.

The transition from government to governance, marked by the establishment of more collaborative and knowledge-oriented modes of governance practices, represents an intensification of the interface activity between ideas and institutions. The introduction of more collaborative strategies in governance is part of a transnational trend. The interface between ideas and institutions becomes formative for the travel of ideas in multilevel governance structures. Thus, globalization becomes a changing and converging force, not just within the national state, but also taking place within the national systems in thought and action (Kettunen and Petersen, 2011).

The well-being framework grew out of transnational cooperation in the late 1970s. The framework added strength to the social and political dimensions of the work of the World Health Organization, and later became a basis for collection of information on the quality of life globally by the Organisation for Economic Co-operation and Development and other organizations. The measurement of well-being has been continuously discussed together with questions about where moral and political thought fit into it (Griffin, 1986). Thus, the idea of *social well-being* as relevant for research and policy-making has travelled in time and space. It is inscribed in governance strategies at all governance levels from local to transnational. In ALICE RAP, well-being has functioned as a source for the formulation of an ethical aim of research. In the process of knowledge translation, it contributes to the inclusion of embodied, inscribed, and enacted knowledge in ALICE RAP's approach.

The concept of a *health footprint* has borrowed inspiration from the concept of the carbon footprint (Rees and Wackernagel, 1996; Wackernagel and Rees, 1998). The development of measurements of health footprints for addictive substances could increase our capacity to make industry accountable for the health effects of the consumption of their products. Above all, the carbon footprint has been shown to be a forceful term in communication with civil society. It has become a basis for our understanding of lifestyle choices, and has in this sense become embodied. The aim of increasing industry accountability is more complicated to achieve, and we can expect the same to be the case with the health footprint as with the carbon footprint.

Measurement of the *margin of exposure* (MOE) has travelled from the area of toxicology to the addiction area. With its introduction, ALICE RAP has improved the capacity to make objective rankings of risk related to lethal doses of different substances. The model was first presented in ALICE RAP (Lachenmeier and Rehm, 2015; Lachenmeier et al., 2011) and the inscribed knowledge travelled into the scientific community and social media. In social media, MOE, originally developed as an instrument to depict *risk level* in drugs, has been inferred as a way to represent the *level of safety* in cannabis use. Consequently, the MOE and its ranking of drugs has been unintentionally reinterpreted as an argument for the liberalization of the use of cannabis. Here, the actors have regulated the practice of the knowledge. It is significant for the future governance of addictions to follow the different contextualized forms that the knowledge of MOE may take.

Knowledge translation in the making

The contribution of the AR concepts to the knowledge base could also be considered as steps in the travel of ideas. The concepts travel between thematic scientific areas and policy fields. In efforts to make knowledge and concepts relevant for future governance, we need to highlight the processes when measurements, models, or knowledge contextualize into policy and governance. By understanding these processes, we aim to promote co-production between science, policy, and civil society.

Therefore, we should pay special attention to the relationship between the scientific community and civil society in the future. It is at this interface that we find important sources for the validation of our concepts and further scientific work, and for securing the relevance of the concepts. This is in line with the elaboration by Alasuutari et al. (2015: 60) of the term epistemic governance to '... stress that ... in modern world society are all about participants attempting to influence other actors' understandings: not only what reality is but also what is desirable, virtuous and acceptable and with whom people identify themselves'.

Hopefully, with MOE, the scientific community has developed objective criteria relevant for knowledge-based decisions. However, knowledge perception and application in governance practice are normally beyond the scope and responsibility of the research community. We consider the barrier in knowledge translation to constitute a gap between science and governance, which it is possible to reveal by analysing conceptual frameworks from ALICE RAP in light of the forms of knowledge it takes (Freeman and Sturdy, 2015).

The challenge for the research community is to bridge the gaps between civil society and governance actors. It is important to try out scientific concepts on the ground in deliberative processes with people affected by addiction problems, civil society groups, organizations, and formal authorities at different governance levels. Enacted knowledge is also knowledge on the move in processes of monitoring and redefinition of concepts. Deliberative processes and co-production in governance contribute to the validation of concepts and improve the knowledge base, thereby also securing accountability and safeguarding democracy. Arguably, future governance will profit from collaborative knowledge development on an equal footing in its processes of de-contextualization and contextualization. This book is a major starting point of such a process.

Hildegunn Sagvaag
Associate Professor, Dr. PH, University of Stavanger, Norway

Svanaug Fjær
Dr. polit, Head of Department, Bergen University College, Norway
Associate Professor (political science) University of Stavanger, Norway

Jan Erik Karlsen
Professor Emeritus, Dr. Oecon
University of Stavanger, Norway

References

Alasuutari P, Raualin M, and Syväterä (2015) Organisations as epistemic capital: the case of independent children's rights institutions. *Int J Polit Cult Soc* **29**: 57–71.

Alasuutari P and Qadir A (2014) Epistemic governance: an approach to the politics of policy-making. *Eur J Cult Polit Sociol* **1**: 67–84.

Emerson K, Nabatchi T, and Balogh S (2012) An integrative framework for collaborative governance. *J Public Adm Res Theory* **22**: 1–29.

Freeman R and Sturdy S (2015) Introduction: knowledge in policy—embodied, inscribed, enacted. In: Freeman R and Sturdy S (eds) *Knowledge in Policy: Embodied, Inscribed, Enacted*. Bristol: Policy Press, pp. 1–17.

Griffin J (1986) *Well-being: Its Meaning, Measurement, and Moral Importance.* Oxford: Oxford University Press.

Kettunen P and Petersen K (2011) *Beyond Welfare State Models.* Cheltenham: Edward Elgar.

Lachenmeier DW and Rehm J (2015) Comparative risk assessment of alcohol, tobacco, cannabis and other illicit drugs using the margin of exposure approach. *Sci Rep* **5**: 8126.

Lachenmeier DW, Kanteres F, and Rehm J (2011) Epidemiology-based risk assessment using the benchmark dose/margin of exposure approach: the example of ethanol and liver cirrhosis. *Int J Epidemiol* **40**: 210–18.

Rees W and Wackernagel M (1996) Urban ecological footprints: why cities cannot be sustainable—and why they are a key to sustainability. *Environ Impact Assess Rev* **16**: 223–48.

Røvik KA (2011) From fashion to virus: an alternative theory of organization' handling of management ideas. *Organ Stud* **32**: 631–54.

Wackernagel M and Rees W (1998) *Our Ecological Footprint: Reducing Human Impact on the Earth.* Gabriola Island: New Society Publishers.

Preface

Study of evolutionary biology finds that humans have evolved to seek out and extract, among other drugs, cholinergic agents from plants in order, among other things, to combat invertebrate parasites such as helminths (Sullivan and Hagen, 2015). Present-day examples of pharmacophagy are seen with Congo basin hunter–gatherers, among whom the quantity of cannabis (Roulette et al., 2016) and nicotine (Roulette et al., 2014) consumed is titrated against intestinal worm burden—the higher the intake, the lower the worm burden. Moreover, when treated with the anti-worm drug abendazole the number of nicotine-containing cigarettes smoked is reduced (Roulette et al., 2014). This does not imply that humans evolved to consume specifically, for example. cannabis or tobacco, or that cannabis or tobacco use is beneficial in the modern world. What is novel in the modern world is the level of availability and format of consumption. With alcohol, the evolutionary evidence implies that the genomes of modern humans began adapting at least ten million years ago to dietary ethanol present in fermenting fruit— a source of ethanol that is remarkably similar in concentration and form (i.e. with food) to the low levels of ethanol consumption that might reduce the risk of ischaemic events (Dudley, 2014). Again, what is different in the modern world is novel availability through fermentative technology enabling humans to consume beverages (devoid of food bulk) with higher ethanol content than fruit fermenting in the wild.

The findings of evolutionary biology imply, on the one hand, that it is no surprise that prohibition is unlikely to work, and that with prohibition of drug use, widespread adverse side effects occur. Does it make sense to lock people up (or worse, kill them) for selling, let alone taking drugs, that, worldwide, are used by over five per cent of those aged 15–64 years in any one year (UNODC, 2015)? In the UK, lifetime use of an illicit drug reaches as high as 36 per cent (UK Focal Point on Drugs, 2014). Does it make sense to design a system of governance in which murder is so rife—do alcohol company producers and sellers murder each other with such regularity?

On the other hand, however, the findings of evolutionary biology imply that if drugs are too readily available in terms of access and price, no wonder that so many people use them heavily and thus run into problems. In this book, an outcome of the Addictions and Lifestyles in Contemporary Europe—Reframing Addictions Project (ALICE RAP) project (www.alicerap.eu), better regulation of drugs is the watch-phrase. This means better regulation of the legal market through stricter regulation, and better regulation of the illegal market through legalization, and subsequent strict regulation.

Better regulation implies better management and a management system that transfers across all drugs. This book proposes three new management tools. These management tools can help with better regulation of nicotine and alcohol. And, they can help United Nations organizations as they reconsider international drug prohibition with an eye toward policies focused on health and sustainability.

The first management tool is to use the Organisation for Economic Co-operation and Development's well-being frame (OECD, 2015) to assess the overall impact of drug policies on different domains of individual and societal well-being. This identifies both co-benefits and adverse consequences, and brings to the fore many of the negative consequences of prohibitionist policies (Stoll and Anderson, 2015).

The second management tool is to implement a standard monitoring tool across drugs. Once such tool comes from toxicology: margin of exposure analysis, which compares the ratio of the toxic dose of a drug with exposure to that drug (Lachenmeier and Rehm, 2015). There is still a lot of work to be done because, at present, the only common standard of the toxic dose across drugs is the benchmark dose of acute death. Nevertheless, this method has promise as it leads to policy changes to improve safety margins of drug taking by either manipulating the potency of drugs, or by reducing exposure.

The third management tool is to promote accountability for harm (Anderson, 2014). We are used to the carbon footprint that apportions carbon dioxide emissions to the actions of public and private sector entities, as well as sectors across society, for example agriculture and transport (Williams et al., 2012). In the same way, a health footprint, based on disability-adjusted life year metrics, can apportion harm across the actions of public and private sector entities. Annual reporting could list jurisdictional, sector, and company-based drug-related health footprints (alcohol, nicotine, and illegal drugs), with plans of how they could be reduced.

These three management tools are not panaceas to reducing the harm done by drugs, but, if well implemented, are likely to drive policies and actions in favour of reducing harm from alcohol, nicotine, and illegal drugs.

Peter Anderson

International Coordinator of the ALICE RAP project; Chief Series Editor, Governance of Addictive Substances and Behaviours; Professor, Substance Use, Policy and Practice, Newcastle University, England; Professor, Alcohol and Health, Maastricht University, Netherlands.

References

Anderson P (2014) Reframing the governance of addictions. *Sucht* **60**: 1–3.

Dudley TR (2014) *The Drunken Monkey: Why We Drink and Abuse Alcohol.* Berkeley, CA: University of California Press.

Lachenmeier DW and Rehm J (2015) Comparative risk assessment of alcohol, tobacco, cannabis and other illicit drugs using the margin of exposure approach. *Sci Rep* **5**: 8126.

OECD (2015) *How's Life? 2015* Paris: OECD.

Roulette CJ, Kazanji M, Breurec S, and Hagen EH (2016) High prevalence of cannabis use among Aka foragers of the Congo Basin and its possible relationship to helminthiasis. *Am J Hum Biol* **28**: 5–15.

Roulette CJ, Mann H, Kemp B, Remiker M, Wilcox J, Hewlett B, et al. (2014) Tobacco vs. helminths in Congo basin hunter-gatherers: self medication in humans? *Evol Hum Behav* **35**: 397–407.

Stoll L and Anderson P (2015) Well-being as a frame for understanding addictive substances. In: Anderson P, Rehm J, and Room R (eds) *The Impact of Addictive Substances and Behaviours on Individual and Societal Well-Being.* Oxford, Oxford University Press, pp. 53–76.

Sullivan RJ and Hagen EH (2015) Passive vulnerability or active agency? An evolutionarily ecological perspective of human drug use. In: Anderson P, Rehm J, and Room R (eds) *The Impact of Addictive Substances and Behaviours on Individual and Societal Well-Being.* Oxford, Oxford University Press, pp. 13–36.

UK Focal Point on Drugs (2014) United Kingdom drug situation. Available at: http://www. nta.nhs.uk/uploads/uk-focal-point-report-2014.pdf (accessed 1 January 2016).

UNODC (2015) World drug report. Available at: https://www.unodc.org/documents/ wdr2015/World_Drug_Report_2015.pdf (accessed 1 January 2016).

Williams I, Kemo S, Coello J, Turner DA, and Wright LA (2012). A beginner's guide to carbon footprinting. *Carbon Manage* **3**: 55–67.

Acknowledgements

The research leading to these results or outcomes has received funding from the European Union's Seventh Framework Programme (FP7/2007-2013), under Grant Agreement n° 266813—Addictions and Lifestyle in Contemporary Europe—Reframing Addictions Project (ALICE RAP—www.alicerap.eu).

Participant organizations in ALICE RAP can be seen at http://www.alicerap.eu/about-alice-rap/partner-institutions.html.

Disclaimer

Contents

Abbreviations

1,4-BD	1,4-butanediol
AA	Alcoholics Anonymous
ALICE RAP	Addictions and Lifestyles in Contemporary Europe-Reframing Addictions Project
APHA	American Public Health Association
ASSIST	Alcohol, Smoking and Substance Involvement Screening Test
BAT	British American Tobacco
BMD	benchmark dose
BMDL10	benchmarke dose lethal 10%
BMI	brief motivational intervention
CAADA	campaign against alcohol and drug abuse
CEO	chief executive officer
CI	confidence interval
CS	civil society
CSO	civil society organization
CSR	corporate social responsibility
DALY	disability-adjusted life years
DSM	Diagnostic and Statistical Manual of Mental Disorders
DUO	drug-user organization
EAHF	European Alcohol and Health Forum
eHealth	Internet-based health
EMA	European Medicines Agency
EMCDDA	European Monitoring Centre for Drugs and Drug Addiction
ENDS	electronic nicotine delivery system
EPC	European Policy Centre
EPIN	European Policy Institutes Network
ERT	European Roundtable of Industrialists
EU	European Union
FCTC	Framework Convention on Tobacco Control
fMRI	functional magnetic resonance imaging
GBL	gamma-butyrolactone
GCDP	Global Commission on Drug Policy
GDP	gross domestic product
GHB	gamma-hydroxybutyric acid
GHI	global health initiative
H2O	harm to others
HBSC	Health Behaviour in School-aged Children
HiAP	Health in All Policies
HUOT	heavy use over time
ICAP	International Center for Alcohol Policies
ICD	International Classification of Diseases
ICT	information and communications technologies
ILSI	International Life Sciences Institute
LCHF	low carbohydrates and high fat
LD	lethal dose
mHealth	mobile health
MNC	multinational corporation
MOE	margin of exposure
MUP	minimum unit price
NGO	non-governmental organization
NRDC	Natural Resources Defense Council
OECD	Organisation for Economic Co-operation and Development
OST	opiod substitution treatments
P4	predictive, preventive, personalized, and participatory
PFI	personal feedback interventions

PR	public relations	UN	United Nations
QALY	quality-adjusted life years	WEF	World Economic Forum
SANCA	South African National Council on Alcoholism and Drug Dependence	WHO	World Health Organization
		WTO	World Trade Organization
		YLL	years of life lost
SAPRO	social aspects/public relations organizations	ZADP	Zambia Alcohol and Drug Programme
SD	standard deviation	ZAIADA	Zanzibar Association of Information Against Drug and Alcohol
SIRC	Social Issues Research Centre		
TPN	Transatlantic Policy Network		

Chapter 1

Key elements for a new governance of addictive substances and behaviours

1.1 The background

In 2009, the European Commission, through the Social Sciences and Humanities division of the FP7 research programme, set the following challenge (European Commission, 2009):

> Addictions have become a pervasive feature of contemporary societies but at the same time they bring a lot of concern. As their number has notably increased over the last decades, they have become a focus of social, economic and political attention and polarise societies and politics more and more. In addition to the widely-acknowledged problem of various substance addictions, there is a growing problem of new addictions such as gambling, eating disorders, anxiolytics, polydrug use and the internet. The development of addictions is a concern in many public policy arenas, in particular health and various forms of social cohesion such as family and work. According to conservative estimates, one tenth of all costs in Europe's health systems flow into the treatment of various addictions. There is also the cost in terms of prevention and crime, which increasingly has a global dimension (organised crime networks, the geo-politics of drugs). At the same time though, societies often tolerate addictions quite differently. The definition and the role of professionals in dealing with addiction prevention and treatment may vary from one country to another, as may vary a lot the level of public concern for the impact of various addictions according to countries and social traditions. The challenge is thus for Europe to build balanced anti-addiction policies, endorsed by societies, that enable at the same time sufficient social integration and individual freedom.

> Reproduced with permission from Work European Commisssion. *Programme 2010—Cooperation: Theme 8—Socio-Economic Sciences and Humanities*, http://ec.europa.eu/research/participants/data/ref/fp7/89059/h_wp_201001_en.pdf, accessed 1 November 2015, Copyright © 2009 European Union.

The text continued to say that a wide variety of situations and policies are challenged:

- Policies need to balance carefully individual freedom and social responsibility, while taking into account social, economic, and ethical considerations. It is of utmost importance that European Union (EU) countries exchange their understanding and experiences of addictions in order to alleviate the worst effects of addiction, while at the same time respecting sufficient diversity of lifestyles and values.

- Addictions (especially drug use) constitute a global problem (organized crime, and impact on development of countries, health, and diseases) and demand systems of international cooperation, and at least European cooperation, which so far have failed to curb drug traffic significantly.

♦ Owing to the health impacts of addictions, preventive, as well as pathological and clinical medical, expertise is needed. Moreover, in order to understand addictive behaviours, sociological, and, in particular, psychological and cognitive insight into human behaviour is required. Europe has a long scientific tradition in the analysis of and dealing with addictions, but there is a need to confront and combine the numerous scientific disciplines in the field given the increasing trends in addiction and the social and individual costs.

♦ Owing to their vulnerability and sensitivity to social and media impact, young people are a very special group of concern and the role of education in preventing addiction and of other policies in helping young people out of addiction is of particular importance. At a time when a high number of young people may find it more difficult to find a place in society, the EU can help promote useful debates on the expectations of young people in our societies and ways to curb the worst effects of youth addiction.

The Commission invited proposals to address the challenge through a balanced combination of research work and complementary activities. Research should be interdisciplinary, allowing for cross-fertilization and innovative research. Complementary activities (such as stock-taking, foresight, dissemination, and management activities) should buttress research to enhance its relevance for current, as well as future, public policies. In particular, the Commission invited research covering five core dimensions:

1. Social, economic, and individual determinants of addiction and behavioural borderline disorders, including how cognition, learning, memory, desire, and affects are individual, social, and brain processes. The significance of the links between addictions and the focus of modern societies on individual autonomy and individual performance as a social rule deserves special attention.

2. Comparative definitions of addictions in the EU member states (given the changing social and cultural significance of addiction and drug use in different countries) and the potential development of quantitative solid data on addictions across Europe (in terms of population concerned, professionals involved, impact on health budgets, economic dependency of users, trade, and profits, for instance).

3. Comparative legal and regulatory frameworks for various new substances that are linked to addictions (for instance, those aimed, in particular, at cognitive enhancement or physical performance).

4. The trade and profits around addiction development in the case of licit drugs or other products, food, or activities linked to new forms of addiction (such as gambling, amphetamines, antidepressants, Internet gaming). The role of economic actors in supporting addictive behaviours.

5. Who defines addiction and addictive behaviours? The role of various health and medical professions and other professions in the definition and treatment of addiction in Europe in a historical perspective. The use of scientific knowledge in defining addiction.

A group of 67 scientific institutions from 24 European countries covering over 30 scientific disciplines ranging from anthropology to toxicology put together a proposal to meet the challenge and were fortunate enough to be awarded €8 million to undertake the work, co-financed by an additional €2 million from the scientific institutions themselves. We called our project ALICE RAP (Addictions and Lifestyles in Contemporary Europe—Reframing Addictions Project). Our goal, as reflected in the project website, www.alicerap.eu, was to do much more than just study the place of addictions in contemporary Europe, but, rather, reach a reframing of our understanding of addictions—elucidating where our concepts and beliefs about addictions come from, how we use them, and with what consequences for societies and individuals. With this reframing, we intended to propose a redesign of addictions governance. One of the main outcomes, a summary of the ALICE RAP work on redesigning addictions governance, is this book.

Over the course of the project, ALICE RAP has produced over five million words in its scientific reports (http://www.alicerap.eu/resources/documents). On top of that, as of the end of 2015, there have been more than 150 scientific publications in peer-reviewed journals, journal supplements, and books (http://www.alicerap.eu/resources/documents). There have been five previous books in this series (Ysa et al., 2014; Anderson et al., 2015; Hellman et al., 2016; Gell et al., 2016; Miller et al., 2016). We do not pretend that this book deals with all the scientific output from ALICE RAP—that would be an impossible task, and one that would make the book unreadable, as well as overly long. However, we believe that we have captured the main issues that result from the work of ALICE RAP. These issues are driven not only by the immense scientific output of ALICE RAP, but also by the intense formal and informal conversations that took place during the estimated 1000 hours that some or all of the 180 scientists met together while working on ALICE RAP.

In our work, we have built on two main strengths—our multidisciplinarity, and our ability to network across topics and disciplines. Our disciplines stretch across the humanities and social sciences and the biological and medical sciences, with expertise in addiction studies, anthropology, cognitive science, criminology, demography, economics, education, engineering, epidemiology, evolutionary biology, foresight management, history, journalism, law, mathematics, media, neurobiology, political science, psychiatry, psychology, psychotherapy, public health, public management, social marketing, social policy, social psychology, sociology, technology, and toxicology.

The strength of our networking during the third year of the five-year project is illustrated in Figure 1.1 with each line representing a stated collaboration between ALICE RAP scientists, clustered in the Work Areas A1–A6 of the project,[1] and the Global Science Group (GSG) of international addiction research experts. Between end of the first year and the third year of the project, network density had increased by 20 per cent, and the number of isolated participants had decreased by nearly two-fifths.

1.2 **Harm done by drugs**

That a redesign of the governance of addictions is needed is simply reflected in the harm data. Just taking drugs alone, in the EU in 2010, illegal drug use was

---

[1] Area 1: Ownership of addiction, Area 2: Counting addiction, Area 3: Determinants of addiction, Area 4: Business of addiction, Area 5: Governance of addiction, Area 6: Addicting the young, Area 7: Coordination and integration.

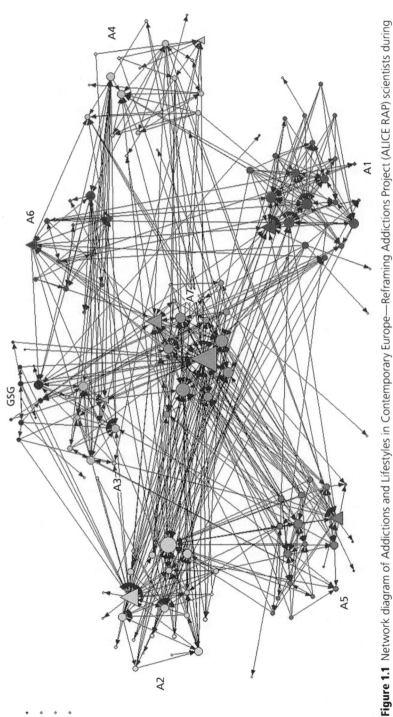

Figure 1.1 Network diagram of Addictions and Lifestyles in Contemporary Europe—Reframing Addictions Project (ALICE RAP) scientists during the third year of the five-year project.

The 'As' represent different areas of work, with groups of scientists: A1, culture and history of addictions; A2, epidemiology of addictions; A3, determinants of addictions; A4, business of addictions; A5, governance of addictions; A6, youth and addictions; A7, project coordination, evaluation and dissemination; GSG, Global Scientific Advisory Group. Reproduced with permission from Albareda A and Ysa T. *ALICE-RAP Network Evaluation: Second Wave Survey (Area 7: Work Package 20)*, Barcelona: ESADE Business School, http://www.alicerap.eu/resources/documents/doc_download/225-wp20-alice-rap-network-evaluation-report-2nd-wave.html, accessed 01 Dec. 2015. Copyright © 2015 Addiction and Lifestyles in Contemporary Europe Reframing Addictions Project (ALICE-RAP).

responsible for 0.5 million years of life lost due to premature mortality (0.7% of all years of life lost (YLL) as a result of premature mortality) and 2 million disability-adjusted life years (DALYs) lost (1.4% of all DALYs lost) (see Table 1.1). YLLs are calculated by subtracting the actual age at death from the life expectancy given that age; if somebody died aged 65 years, and the life expectancy for people his or her age would be 80 years, then YLLs would amount to 15 years. DALYs are a measure that combines years of life lost as a result of premature mortality with YLLs due to disability (Murray, 1994), with disability rated for severity between perfect health (0) and death (1) (Rehm and Frick, 2010). Alcohol consumption contributed to the burden of disease to a greater extent than illegal drug use but less than tobacco use with 5.9 million YLL (7.9% of all YLL) and 7.5 million DALYs lost (5.3% of all DALYs lost). Tobacco use in the EU contributed the most to the burden of disease of all drugs, and was responsible for 13.8 million YLL (18.5% of all YLL) and 16.2 million DALYs lost (11.4% of all DALYs lost). The burdens caused by illegal drug use, alcohol, and tobacco in the EU were greater among men than among women, with alcohol and drug burdens incurring at much younger ages than tobacco; for all drugs, the burden of disease in the EU was proportionally larger than the global burden (Institute for Health Metrics and Evaluation, 2015; Shield and Rehm, 2015), which is not surprising, as the prevalence of use and heavy use is larger in the EU than the rest of the world (for illegal drug use see Degenhardt and Hall, 2012;for alcohol see World Health Organization, 2014; for tobacco see http://gamapserver.who.int/gho/interactive_charts/tobacco/use/atlas.html).

Table 1.1 Burden of illegal drug use, alcohol consumption, and tobacco use in the European Union in 2010*

Risk factor	Sex	YLLs (1000s)	YLLs per 100,000	% of all YLLs	DALYs (1000s)	DALYs per 100,000	% of all
Illicit drug use	Men	435.9	178	1.0	1453.6	593	1.9
	Women	109.2	43	0.4	554.4	216	0.8
	Total	545.2	109	0.7	2008.0	400	1.4
Alcohol consumption	Men	4543.5	1854	10.3	6020.6	2457	7.9
	Women	1380.0	538	4.5	1508.0	588	2.2
	Total	5923.5	1181	7.9	7528.6	1501	5.3
Tobacco use	Men	10,318.6	4211	23.3	11,725.2	4785	15.4
	Women	3514.4	1369	11.4	4535.5	1767	6.8
	Total	13,832.9	2757	18.5	16,260.8	3241	11.4

YLLs, years of life lost; DALYs, disability-adjusted life years.

*Based on revised estimates.

Source: data from Institute for Health Metrics and Evaluation. *GBD Compare*, http://vizhub.healthdata.org/gbd-compare, accessed 01 Nov. 2015. Copyright © 2015 University of Washington.

Owing to this high disease burden, the EU incurs substantial social costs (Shield et al., 2015), in the magnitude of several hundred billion Euros per year. These costs are not limited to the healthcare sector but comprise the legal sector (police, court, prison), the workplace (productivity losses via absenteeism, presenteeism, disability, and mortality), and the family (see Single et al., 2003; for alcohol as an example see Rehm et al., 2012; for ALICE RAP studies, see Mielecka-Kubien et al., 2014). Social cost studies are limited as not all burdens, such as pain and suffering, can be quantified in monetary terms, so-called intangible costs (Single et al., 2003), resulting from drugs, which add to their burden to European societies. It is heavy use that makes up the substantial part of the burden and the costs of drug use (for illegal drugs see Whiteford et al., 2013; for alcohol see Rehm et al., 2013; for tobacco see Marmet et al., 2014).

1.3 Replacement concept of addiction—heavy use over time

By addictions, we meant those drugs and behaviours that can lead to addiction. ALICE RAP predominantly studied alcohol, illegal drugs and nicotine, and gambling. We did not to any great extent study other behaviours, prescription medicines, or other potentially addictive substances, including sugar. As we considered and studied the term addiction more and more, we concluded that it is a highly malleable term, whose exact meaning varies over time and place (Berridge et al. 2016; Hellman et al. 2014, 2016; Thom et al. 2015), and whose exact meaning is influenced by which stakeholder group has the ear of society and its elites at any point in time. Thus, as we develop in Chapter 2, we have gone back to the basics of epidemiology and concluded that all that is needed to define addictions is heavy use over time, a behaviour that is on a continuum, rather than an 'all-or-nothing' phenomenon. As a concept, heavy use over time has advantages over currently used medical definitions, and converges the definitions of various scientific disciplines with views of the general population. As we note in Chapter 2, heavy use over time is consistent with recent advances in basic sciences, and fits better with models of public health, bringing in health and social consequences over and above the criteria currently derived from medical classifications. Heavy use over time has the potential to reduce stigma, being based on a continuous rather than a dichotomous variable.

1.4 Well-being frame and ethical approach to drugs

Heavy use over time of addictive products is united by specific characteristics, including recognition of these behaviours as lifestyle choices, a wide variety of sectors in which the determinants and effects of heavy use over time can be found, particular effects of heavy use on an individual's decision-making abilities, and an unparalleled web of corporate and criminal interests surrounding the products themselves. As we discuss in Chapter 3, these characteristics imply that the governance of drug use in populations is subject to some very unique ethical considerations. We argue that by adopting a well-being framework for drug policy, where regulations and legislation are created with the aim of maximizing population well-being and capital, we can better ensure that citizens and societies are treated ethically with regard to their drug behaviour. Further, adopting a well-being framework immediately calls into question criminalization and incarceration penalties for the consumption of drugs, given that prison time detracts so greatly from well-being and contributes to entrenching stigma and discrimination (see Moskalewicz and Klingemann 2015; Stoll and Anderson 2015).

1.5 Drivers of drug-related harm

The wide variety of drivers of drug-related harm can be grouped into three levels. In the first level are structural elements that are immediate drivers of harm. These operate at biological and population levels. As we present in Chapter 4, there is biological evidence that human brains are hard-wired to seek out drugs, many of which are plant neurotoxins. In the presence of widespread exposure to industrially produced and increasingly potent drugs, such hard-wiring can, inevitably, drive drug use and drug-related harm. Other structural elements that can drive drug use and related harm include the genetic, sex, age, wealth, and inequality structures of populations. In the second level of drivers are a range of core factors that drive drug-related harm. These include potency of and exposure to drugs, and the technological developments that can reduce potency and exposure, and less harmful drug delivery systems. Core factors also include social networks, which can operate positively and negatively as drivers of harm, and social exclusion, social stigma, and discrimination, all of which can lead to more harm than the drugs themselves. In Chapter 4, we introduce 'margins of exposure' analyses as a toxicological tool to standardize comparative harm across different drugs. Recognizing that there are a range of potentially different outcomes, we illustrate the approach comparing the ratio of a benchmark toxic dose based on risk of death with daily exposure of a range of drugs used by European adults (see Lachenmeier and Rehm, 2015).

In the third level are policies and measures that can reduce exposure, incentivize individual behaviour, and promote research and development for less potent drugs and delivery systems and access to advice and treatment. The presence or absence of meaningful private sector rules of engagement in policy-making can drive harm, and the societal well-being frame, introduced in Chapter 3, can identify the co-benefits and adverse consequences of drug policies. In Chapter 4, we propose the concept of a health footprint as the tool to apportion harm across the different levels and drivers, similar to the carbon footprint that apportions greenhouse gas emissions across actions, industries, sectors, and jurisdictions. The health footprint can also act as the accountability and monitoring tool to drive improved health action by public and private sectors alike.

1.6 Dual approaches to reducing harm

Approaches to reducing drug-related harm are driven by the nature of risk functions between levels of exposure and outcomes. When there is an exponential relationship between exposure and adverse outcomes, greater health gain is achieved by reductions in heavy users. When the population distribution of exposure is such that the majority of the people are not at high risk and the relationship between exposure and outcome is more or less linear, then an improvement in the norm, that is the population mean, brings greatest health gain. As the risk curves between drug-related exposure and harm vary between linear and exponential, depending on the drug and the outcome of interest, then normally a combination of policies and actions that address the overall population and target heavy users is needed. Often, both groups can be addressed with the same policies and measures, and new technologies are also increasingly being employed to potentiate the reach and specificity of measures to reduce harm through e- and m-health initiatives (see Civljak et al., 2013; Kaner et al., 2015). With exponential risk curves, emphasis also needs to be placed on providing advice and treatment and closing existing treatment gaps between need and provision (Grant et al., 2015). Importantly, as we emphasize in Chapter 5, addressing the harm done by drugs in a socially equitable manner requires raising awareness of drug-related harm as whole-of-society problems, which need to be addressed with the participation of the whole population.

1.7 **Reducing drug-related harm**

A starting point of ALICE RAP was that drugs pose challenges to modern societies. The factors that influence how drugs challenge societies are multiple, with complex interactions between the factors. Yet, societal responses tend to be simple (labelling products as legal or illegal) and poorly evidence based. Legal products tend to be extensively marketed, while illegal products tend to be criminalized. Both of these approaches, as we point out in Chapter 6, fall short and fail in reducing harm. Drugs, whether legal or illegal, are not ordinary commodities, and need to be managed through effective regulation of the market that deals with price, availability, and commercial communications. In Chapter 6 we discuss how the criminalization of illegal drugs can create more problems than it solves. Evidence indicates that decriminalization does not necessarily lead to increased use, and can decrease social and health costs. Just as decriminalization can be seen as an action to empower citizens, access to treatment in appropriate settings is a fundamental need to be improved in most countries and potentiate that empowerment. Normalization of treatment settings brings an added advantage of reducing drug-related stigma. As with most health conditions, the impact of drugs on society depends not only on the products themselves, but also on the living conditions of citizens. Thus, drug policy has to be embedded in 'health in all policies' approaches involving the whole of government and whole of society.

1.8 **Youth-centred policy**

Given the multiple pathways to youth-centred drug use and drug-related harm, compounded by interacting biological, psychological, and environmental influences, youth-centred drug prevention policies need to be comprehensive and supported by sustainable, long-term investment and organizational structures. As we describe in Chapter 7, this is not the case at the moment. Investment in prevention research and delivery typically represents less than one per cent of all costs of drug use to society in a given year (see Rehm et al., 2006); surprising, given the substantial cost savings that accrue from each delayed or prevented case of drug-related harm (e.g. Hurley et al., 2004). As governments contemplate new drug policies, which include legalization and regulation, we argue that incomes from sumptuary taxes should be meaningfully reinvested into drug prevention research and delivery.

1.9 Whole-of-society approaches to wicked problems

The complexity of drug issues leaves no doubt that drugs are wicked problems (the term wicked in this context is used not in the sense of evil but rather as an issue that is highly resistant to resolution) that must be tackled by different levels of governments in collaboration with a range of stakeholders from health, justice, public order, safety, economy, and trade, and so on (see Kickbusch and Behrendt, 2013). This wide range of stakeholders, as well as the international domain of drug trafficking, makes the governance of addictions more complex. The complexity of drug issues is shaped by three main trends: decriminalization of drug use, wider introduction of harm reduction for both illegal and legal drugs, and a shift from repression to regulation. As we put forward in Chapter 8, drug governance requires a whole-of-government approach, moving from single-purpose organizations towards a more integrated approach to public service delivery (networked governance). Governments need to provide leadership for whole-of-society approaches to be able to deliver broad solutions to both individuals and society, and not only reactive partial programmes. If we would like to move drug governance from its current status to a well-being and whole-of-government approach, the challenge, as we point out in Chapter 8, is to establish the rules regarding which phase of the policy cycle and which typologies of stakeholders can provide a contribution for the public good along with the stakeholders' own interests.

1.10 Private sector unpacked

In Chapter 9, we conclude that corporations in the drug business are constitutionally bound to pursue profit, not only by economic means, but also by the conscious planning and pursuit of political strategies. Political strategies include the pursuit of downstream policies that directly relate to a corporation's products, and the design and redesign of upstream policy architecture that determines the general way in which specific decisions about their products are taken. We propose two courses of action to manage corporations. The first is regulation. Illegal drugs can be regulated through decriminalization and legalization, which will improve drug quality and potency, undermine the intrinsic harms of illegal markets, and reduce the perverse outcomes of attempts at suppression. Legalization will bring additional benefits of raising revenue through tax that can be channelled to health and social care for the most disadvantaged communities. Regulation of legal substances should be strengthened, recognizing that business regulation can be one of the most significant cutting edge policies to building a society-wide coalition to reduce drug-related harm.

The second course of action is negotiation, partnership, and coalition building. We argue that very little will be achieved if we only wait for governments to act. Society-wide coalitions to reduce harm are not only important to improve public health, but are also important to encourage government action and to make it harder for the private sector to resist positive moves.

1.11 Hearing civil society voices

As noted in Chapter 10, the potential of civil society organizations to influence drug policies and preventive actions has been very strong historically. They are still a powerful voice, representing large, voting subpopulations and their concerns about health, social issues, environment, and lifestyle. However, civil society organizations have no monopoly in claiming ethical accountability for the improvement of citizens' well-being. Besides the struggle of dealing with the forces of the business sector that profits from drugs, there is an ongoing parallel struggle of how to deal with the over-lapping claims of responsible action made by the business sector. The work required for civil society organizations to claim their own role and to profile themselves, and, often, to defend their views on effective action in relation to business actors is a tough task. In public hearings and policy consultations, civil society organizations compete for influence with representatives of the business sector; with, therefore, an in-built bias against them due to the disparity in financial resources and historical connec-tions. Civil society organizations have more chances for success in parliamentary representative processes than through executive channels, but this requires effective coalition building, something yet to be fully achieved.

1.12 Towards a policy frame

At the outset of ALICE RAP, we convened a two-day electronic scenario workshop of 20 international drug experts to provide an initial vision and a reframing as to how scientific, technological, and social advancement may impact on our under-standing of addictions and lifestyles over the next 20 years ('Vision 2030+') (Karlsen et al., 2013). The vision is summarized in four boxes, across axes of values and the nature of response. The redesign of addictions governance that we propose moves us in the direction of the bottom right-hand corner box, solidarity prevails (see Figure 1.2). ·

Thus, we conclude our book in Chapter 11 by bringing together much of its sub-stance, and by drawing on all of the work of the ALICE RAP project (www.alicerap. eu) to propose 12 governance approaches to be considered in redesigning govern-ance to reduce the individual and societal harm done by alcohol, illegal drugs, and tobacco. What binds these governance approaches together is a well-being frame-work that leads to improved outcomes across many domains, including health, edu-cation, civic engagement, and personal security, that are sustainable over time.

Of course, this book, and ALICE RAP, on which it draws, is not the end answer to better governance of drugs. We have tried to show a direction. We have also raised many ideas that are not completed, and that require further unpacking and further research. We hope, however, that some of our ideas will be put into practice. And, we

		Nature of response	
		React and mitigate	**Anticipate and prepare**
Individual res-ponsibility first		**Inequality prevails** MS2 Intense individualism and short term reactions to addiction	**Vocal player's arena** MS4 Market driven society, prepares for future challenges of addiction
Values		**Ad hoc treatment society** MS1	**Solidarity prevails** MS3
Social res-ponsibility first		Inclusive debate, challenges of addiction met when they occur	Feelings of societal vulnerability engender large scale, long term actions on addiction

Figure 1.2 The scenario axes of addiction and lifestyles in Europe 2030.
Reproduced with permission from Karlsen JE, Gual A, and Anderson P. *Foresighting Addiction and Lifestyles In Europe 2030+*, http://www.alicerap.eu/resources/documents/doc_download/78-deliverable-20-1-vision-2030-report.html, accessed 01 Dec. 2015. Copyright © 2015 Addiction and Lifestyles in Contemporary Europe Reframing Addictions Project (ALICE-RAP).

expect that, if this is the case, the lives of all of us and the lives of all of us who use drugs will be somewhat improved.

References

Anderson P, Rehm J, and Room R (eds) (2015) *The Impact of Addictive Substances and Behaviours on Individual and Societal Well-Being*. Oxford: Oxford University Press.

Berridge V, Edman J, Mold A, and Taylor S (2016) ALICE RAP deliverable 1.1: addiction through the ages: a review of the development of concepts and ideas about addiction in European countries since the nineteenth century and the role of international organisations in the process. Available at: http://www.alicerap.eu/resources/documents/doc_download/276-deliverable-01-1-addiction-through-the-ages.html) (accessed 1 January 2016).

Civljak M, Stead LF, Hartmann-Boyce J, Sheikh A, and Car J (2013) Internet-based interventions for smoking cessation. *Cochrane Database of Systematic Reviews* 7: CD007078.

Degenhardt L and Hall W (2012) Extent of illicit drug use and dependence, and their contribution to the global burden of disease. *Lancet* 379: 55–70.

European Commission (2009) SSH.2010.3.2-1 Addictions and lifestyles in contemporary European societies (p.20) In: FP7 Cooperation Work Programme: Socio-Economic Sciences and the Humanities. Available at: http://ec.europa.eu/research/participants/data/ref/fp7/89059/h_wp_201001_en.pdf (accessed 27 November 2015).

Gell L, Bühringer G, McLeod J, Forberger S, Holmes J, Lingford-Hughes A, and Meier P (eds) (2016) *What Determines Harm from Addictive Substances and Behaviours?* Oxford: Oxford University Press.

Grant BF, Goldstein RB, Saha TD, Chou SP, Jung J, Zhang H, et al. (2015) Epidemiology of DSM-5 alcohol use disorder: results from the National Epidemiologic Survey on Alcohol and Related Conditions III. *JAMA Psychiatry* 20852: 1–10.

Hellman M, Majamäki M, Beccaria F, Egerer M, Rolando S, Bujalski M, and Moskalewicz J (2014) ALICE RAP deliverable 3.2: professional images. Available at: http://www.alicerap. eu/resources/documents/doc_download/217-deliverable-03-2-professional-s-images-of-addictions.html (accessed 11 August 2015).

Hellman M, Berridge V, Duke K, and Mold A (eds) (2016) *Concepts of Addictive Substances and Behaviours across Time and Place*. Oxford: Oxford University Press.

Hurley SF, Scollo MM, Younie SJ, English DR, and Swanson MG (2004) The potential for tobacco control to reduce PBS costs for smoking-related cardiovascular disease. *Med J Aust* **181**: 252–5.

Institute for Health Metrics and Evaluation (2015) GBD Compare. Available at: http:// vizhub.healthdata.org/gbd-compare (accessed 1 November 2015).

Kaner EF, Beyer FR, Brown J, Crane D, Garnett C, Hickman M, et al. (2015) Personalised digital interventions for reducing hazardous and harmful alcohol consumption in community-dwelling populations (Protocol). *Cochrane Database Syst Rev* **1**: CD011479.

Karlsen J-E, Gual A, and Anderson P (2013) Foresighting addiction and lifestyles in Europe 2030+. *Eur J Futures Res* **1**: 19.

Kickbusch I and Behrendt T (2013) *Implementing a Health 2020 Vision: Governance for Health in the 21st Century. Making it Happen*. Copenhagen: World Health Organization Regional Office for Europe.

Lachenmeier DW and Rehm J (2015) Comparative risk assessment of alcohol, tobacco, cannabis and other illicit drugs using the margin of exposure approach. *Sci Rep* **5**: 8126.

Marmet S, Rehm J, Kraus L, Pabst A, Trapencieris M, Bloomfield K, et al. (2014) Tobacco use and dependence. In: Marmet S, Gmel G, and Rehm J (eds) *Addiction and Lifestyles in Contemporary Europe: Reframing Addictions Project (ALICE RAP)—Prevalence of Substance Use, Dependence and Problematic Gambling in Europe*. Lausanne: Addiction Switzerland, pp. 25–53.

Mielecka-Kubień Z, Okulicz-Kozaryn K, Zin-Sędek M, Oleszczuk M, Brzózka K, Colom J, et al. (2014) ALICE RAP deliverable 6.1: social costs: a report specifying the costs of addiction to societies. Available at: http://www.alicerap.eu/resources/documents/doc_ download/219-deliverable-06-1-social-costs-of-addiction.html (accessed 11 August 2015).

Miller D, Harkins C, and Schlögl M (2016) *Impact of Market Forces on Addictive Substances and Behaviours*. Oxford: Oxford University Press.

Moskalewicz J and Klingemann JI (2015) Addictive substances and behaviours and social justice. In: Anderson P, Rehm J, and Room R (eds) *The Impact of Addictive Substances and Behaviours on Individual and Societal Well-being*. Oxford: Oxford University Press, pp. 143–60.

Murray CJL (1994) Quantifying the burden of disease: the technical basis for disability-adjusted life years. *Bull World Health Organ* **72**: 429–45.

Rehm J and Frick U (2010) Valuation of health states in the U.S. study to establish disability weights: lessons from the literature. *Int J Meth Psychiatric Res* **19**: 18–33.

Rehm J, Baliunas D, Brochu S, Fischer B, Gnam W, Patra J, et al. (2006) *The Costs of Substance Abuse in Canada 2002: Highlights*. Ottawa: Canadian Centre on Substance Abuse.

Rehm J, Shield KD, Rehm MX, Gmel G, Jr, and Frick U (2012) *Alcohol Consumption, Alcohol Dependence, and Attributable Burden of Disease in Europe: Potential Gains from Effective Interventions for Alcohol Dependence*. Toronto: Centre for Addiction and Mental Health.

Rehm J, Shield KD, Rehm MX, Gmel G, and Frick U (2013) Modelling the impact of alcohol dependence on mortality burden and the effect of available treatment interventions in the European Union. *Eur Neuropsychopharmacol* **23**: 89–97.

Shield KD and Rehm J (2015) The effects of addictive substances and addictive behaviours on physical and mental health. In: Anderson P, Rehm J, and Room R (eds) *The Impact of Addictive Substances and Behaviours on Individual and Societal Well-being.* Oxford: Oxford University Press, pp. 77–118.

Shield KD, Rehm MX, and Rehm J (2015) Social costs of addiction in Europe. In: Anderson P, Rehm J, and Room R (eds) *The Impact of Addictive Substances and Behaviours on Individual and Societal Well-being.* Oxford: Oxford University Press, pp. 181–8.

Single E, Collins D, Easton B, Harwood H, Lapsley H, Kopp P, and Wilson E (2003) *International Guidelines for Estimating the Costs of Substance Abuse,* 2nd edition. Geneva: World Health Organization.

Stoll L and Anderson P (2015) Well-being as a framework for understanding addictive substances. In: Anderson P, Rehm J, and Room R (eds) *The Impact of Addictive Substances and Behaviours on Individual and Societal Well-being.* Oxford: Oxford University Press, pp. 53–76.

Thom B, Beccaria F, Bjerge B, Duke K, Eisenbach-Stangl I, Herring R, et al. (2015) ALICE RAP deliverable 2.1: stakeholder ownership: a theoretical framework for cross national understanding and analyses of stakeholder involvement in issues of substance use, problem use and addiction. Available at: http://www.alicerap.eu/resources/documents/doc_download/273-d2-1-stakeholder-ownership.html (accessed 1 January 2016).

Whiteford HA, Degenhardt L, Rehm J, Baxter AJ, Ferrari AJ, Erskine HE, et al. (2013) Global burden of disease attributable to mental and substance use disorders: findings from the Global Burden of Disease Study 2010. *Lancet* **382**: 1575–86.

World Health Organization (2014) *Global Status Report on Alcohol and Health,* Geneva: World Health Organization.

Ysa T, Colom J, Albareda A, Ramon A, Carrión M, and Segura L (2014) *Governance of Addictions: European Public Policies.* Oxford: Oxford University Press.

Chapter 2

New concepts of addiction

2.1 Definitions of addictive behaviours

Addictive behaviours have been defined differently over time (Room, 1998; Crocq, 2007; Room et al., 2015), and, as of today, there are different definitions across and within disciplines, even in those that have actively aimed at mainstreaming the use of concepts, such as psychiatry. We will start with the medical definitions. Two main definitions are currently used for addictive behaviours in medicine, the International Classification of Diseases (ICD), currently in its tenth edition (ICD-10; World Health Organization, 1992, 1993), and the Diagnostic and Statistical Manual of Mental Disorders (DSM, fifth edition (DSM-5) (American Psychiatric Association, 2013a)). Both definitions are based on the same methodology of using multiple criteria (e.g. loss of control, role failure, craving, tolerance, withdrawal, continuation of consumption despite harmful consequences) describing consequences or potential consequences of heavy consumption (Martin et al., 2014), with minimal thresholds for the number of criteria present at the same time (e.g. two or three) necessary for diagnosis. However, while criteria used in ICD and DSM are overlapping, they are not the same between diagnostic systems. For example, the minimal thresholds are different, and the concepts used differ as well (e.g. 'dependence' and 'harmful use' in ICD-10; 'substance use disorders' in DSM-5; for details see Rehm et al., 2014a).

Also, as the interpretation of consequences is, in part, culture-dependent, current assessments of substance use disorders across countries involve substantial measurement error (see Rehm et al., 2015a, 2015b; e.g. for alcohol). For instance, loss of control has negative connotations in catholic Southern European countries, and relatively positive connotations for many groups in the North of Europe (Room, 2006, 2007); and many of the consequences chosen as criteria are relatively broad and unspecific (e.g. role failure) (Rehm and Room, 2015).

Addictive behaviours are characterized differently in non-medical research traditions and contexts. For example, the United Nations System uses the term 'problem drug users' (United Nations Office on Drugs and Crime, 2014), a term that includes but is not limited to people qualifying for medical diagnoses described above. According to this definition, all people 'who engage in high risk consumption of drugs' would be considered problem users, and risk includes all types of consequences, including legal consequences, which is a circular definition as these depend on the legal situation in the respective country and its enforcement. The European Monitoring Centre for Drugs and Drug Addiction (EMCDDA) has used a similar definition of high-risk drug use, focusing on the behaviour rather than the person. This indicator, which has recently been revised mainly owing to changing drug policies across Europe, focuses on 'recurrent drug use that is causing actual harms (negative consequences) to the person (including dependence on the drug, but also other health, psychological or social problems), or is placing the person at a high probability/risk of suffering such harms' (Thanki and Vicente, 2013).

From an ecological and evolutionary scientific perspective, psychoactive substance use is thought to be explained by a broad range of psychosocial, behavioural, and neurobiological theories, which all share the notions of reward and reinforcement (Thorndike, 1911; Sullivan et al., 2008). According to these theories, recreational drugs reward and/or reinforce consumption, initially via hedonic (pleasurable or positively experienced) effects but later by avoidance of negative consequences such as withdrawal (Koob and Le Moal, 2005; Nestler, 2005). While use of psychoactive substances dates back long into history (e.g. McGovern, 2009), heavy use over time, or addiction as a general population phenomenon, is more recent. This has to do with more modern ways to produce, conserve, and apply psychoactive substances such as distillation, bottling, or applying concentrated substances via syringes (Sullivan and Hagen, 2014), which humans have yet to better adapt to.

Sociology and other social sciences stress the importance of the (natural and social) environment, both in the emergence and continuation of use, as well as in the understanding of addictive behaviours (e.g. Sulkunen, 2015). For example, consider the classic paper of Lindesmith (1938), where the author stressed that the social environment provides beliefs and interpretations about experiencing withdrawal symptoms. Accordingly, these beliefs and interpretations would determine whether an individual would continue using the drug to deal with withdrawal leading to addiction, or whether he or she would stop regular use. Based on this theory, the social environment would thus be crucial in answering the question of why some people become dependent on drugs after using them, and others do not (for recent answers from multiple perspectives see Gell et al., 2016). Another concrete example of contextual factors is the experiences of US veterans of the Vietnam conflict, where a sizeable number of US soldiers became addicted to heroin, but the vast majority stopped using after returning home (Robins, 1993). This partly contributed to a renewed interest in social determinants of addictive behaviours, as well as to some discussion on genetic vulnerability, as it had to be explained why a minority of the veterans continued their drug use (Tsuang et al., 1998). A more recent empirical study examining all the different social, psychological, and biological risk correlates of heavy drinking among adolescents using machine-learning prediction models supports this view and suggests a strong role of life events and current psychosocial environment in risk for heavy drinking (Whelan et al., 2014).

Finally, the current view of addictive behaviours is strongly influenced by the concept of addiction as a 'chronic and relapsing brain disease' (Leshner, 1997; McLellan et al., 2000; Volkow et al., 2003; Heilig 2015). We have already introduced some basic concepts of this approach in the short paragraph of the ecological and evolutionary scientific perspective above (see also Sullivan and Hagen, 2014). In short, research on addiction as a brain disease has shifted the attention to brain structures and functions (Baler and Volkow, 2006) away from other organs such as the examination of liver functions. In particular, it has turned to the reward/motivation circuitry in the brain and to neuroadaptations in that circuitry that can change sensitivity to addictive substances to try to explain the compulsive dimension of drug seeking in users (Wise, 2000; Wise and Koob, 2014). The focus on brain mechanisms of reward began with the discoveries of the brain reward circuitry in the 1950s and was accelerated by research into the opioid receptors peptides in the 1970s. More recently, with the recognition that drug users also show abnormalities in cortical regions of the brain (e.g. Goldstein and Volkow, 2002; Whelan et al., 2012), theories now focus on decision-making processes in the initiation stages of drug use, as well as the potential neurotoxic effects of early exposure on the development of higher cognitive functions involved in decision-making and behavioural regulation (Whelan et al., 2012). While demonstrating causality in neurodevelopmental studies of humans remains elusive, it remains a topic of profound interest to the addiction research community (e.g. www.imagen-europe.com; see http://addictionresearch. nih.gov/adolescent-brain-cognitive-development-study).

In survey studies concerned with beliefs about addiction among the general population, the dominant view is to blame those affected for their conditions; this holds even with those who see such disorders as a disease (Caetano, 1989; Room, 2005; Schomerus et al., 2010; Schomerus et al., 2011). As a systematic review of population studies revealed, people with addictive behaviours are held more responsible for their condition than people suffering from other mental disorders (Schomerus et al., 2011); they are also seen as unpredictable and dangerous. Psychosocial causal attributions prevail over biological explanations (Schomerus et al., 2010). This view has not changed much in recent decades (Schomerus et al., 2011, 2014a; Angermeyer et al., 2013) with the exception that treatment is now more accepted (Schomerus et al., 2014b). To summarize: even although most of the general population in many high-income countries believe that substance use disorders are a disease, a large proportion hold afflicted individuals responsible for these disorders in the sense that they see substance use disorders as uncontrolled heavy use of substances by people lacking character and willpower to control them (Caetano, 1989; Room, 2005; Schomerus et al., 2010; Schomerus et al., 2011). Therefore, a key definition of addiction, held within lay culture and (sometimes) in policy networks is one in which heavy users are understood as lacking self-control and morality.

Most of the above definitions have the problem of dichotomizing people as having, or not having, the disease, without giving sufficient weight to the fact that the underlying phenomena are continuous. The DSM-5 has begun to move in the latter direction by establishing a continuum of severity, but still the continuum is mainly among those who have the disorder (American Psychiatric Association, 2013b). This division into seemingly distinct categories has been found to increase stigmatization (Tajfel, 1982; Schomerus et al., 2013; Angermeyer et al., 2015) (see Box 2.1).

2.2 Heavy use over time as a new definition

While almost never mentioned explicitly (for exceptions see Li et al., 2007; Bradley and Rubinsky, 2013), there is one constant underlying criteria in medical conditions

Box 2.1 Definitions of addictive disorders

Addictive behaviours have been defined differently across recent decades and by different disciplines, and scientific definitions differ from the view of the general population. Even the two most widely used current medical definitions differ substantially. Current definitions are associated with problems of measurement and stigmatization.

and all alternative definitions mentioned above: heavy use over time (HUOT) (Rehm et al., 2014a, 2014b). Some of the current medical criteria are physiological consequences of heavy use of psychoactive substances over time (tolerance, withdrawal); some criteria are linked to (bio)psychological consequences (e.g. craving via brain processes); some criteria are linked to social and behavioural consequences, such as 'giving up important social, occupational, or recreational activities'; some criteria are linked to health or physical consequences (e.g. liver cirrhosis or the other 200 ICD three-level codes linked to heavy alcohol use (Rehm et al., 2010a, b) (see Rehm et al., 2010a for an overview of all alcohol-attributable health consequences, and for a recent overview of heavy use of all substances see Shield and Rehm, 2015)).

In fact, all consequences listed in current definitions have 'heavy use over time' as the major risk factor. But, as is the case for risk factors, these are probabilistic relationships (maybe with the exception of tolerance, which seems an inevitable outcome of HUOT for many drugs; for a definition of risk factor see Ezzati et al., 2004; Rothman et al., 2008; Parascandola, 2011). Heavy use over time alone is neither a necessary nor sufficient condition for negative consequences, that is, not all people with heavy substance use will have any consequence with certainty, yet most of these consequences will have heavy use alone as a necessary antecedence. Exceptions are conditions like alcoholic liver cirrhosis or opiate poisoning, that is, disease or injury conditions with substance use as part of their name (for an overview of such conditions, which are 100 per cent attributable to a substance, see Shield and Rehm, 2015).

This reasoning is very much in line with arguments made by sociologist Kettil Bruun in 1970 for excluding 'alcoholism' in the listing of factors to be included when calculating the harm caused by alcohol in populations (Bruun, 1970). Bruun argued that the harm caused by alcoholism will inevitably be included in all other categories captured as consequences of heavy and harmful use (over time). Alcoholism as a separate category would, according to Bruun, just increase the overlap between the categories (Bruun, 1970).

2.3 **Heavy use over time as a diagnostic criterion**

Heavy use over time is clearly linked to consequences articulated in the existing literature. Heavy use impacts the human brain, mostly independently of circumstances (Nutt, 2012; Nutt and Nestor, 2013). Different substances have different impacts on neurobiology (World Health Organization, 2004), but, overall, as indicated above,

Box 2.2 Heavy use over time as a new definition of substance use disorders

Heavy use over time is suggested as a new definition for what is currently subsumed under the heading of 'substance use disorders'. This definition is in line with recent scientific findings including but not limited to the neurobiological findings.

there are enough commonalities to subsume the consequences of heavy use of psychoactive substances under one unifying label of 'addictive brain disorders' (Leshner, 1997; McLellan et al., 2000; Volkow et al., 2003; Baler and Volkow, 2006). Summarizing the neurocognitive effects of substance use disorders (dependence, abuse) versus heavy use for the Dutch Medical Research Council, a group of Dutch researchers concluded that based on the current literature any such distinction is impossible to make, because there are no studies on neural effects of substance dependence without prolonged heavy use (Wiers et al., 2012). Thus, the effect of prolonged heavy use on the brain appears to be at least largely overlapping if not identical with what is called 'substance use disorders'.

How close is the link between current criteria and amount consumed? Rehm et al. (2014a) demonstrated a very close relationship for alcohol from the USA National Epidemiologic Survey on Alcohol and Related Conditions (average correlation of the four Pearson correlation coefficients by sex and treatment status > 0.9). Similarly, in a Catalonian cohort of people treated for alcohol dependence, level of use, sex, and age 'explained' 94 per cent of the variance of DSM-III-R symptoms (for a description of the cohort see Gual et al., 1999). In the German Epidemiological Survey of Substance Abuse (Kraus et al., 2013), high correlations were found for all substances but not at the same very high levels as in the above-cited studies (Rehm et al., 2014a).

In sum, level of heavy use over time and number of DSM-IV criteria correlate substantially. Given this fact, it is not surprising that the health or social effects resulting from heavy use over time seem to be similar to those that are currently labelled 'substance use disorders' (Rehm et al., 2013a; for a detailed example of alcohol, see Rehm et al., 2013b). What may be different, however, is the additional dimension of stigmatization, which has been linked to the concepts of 'addiction' and 'substance use disorders', but not necessarily to the continuum of use, or to heavy use (see Box 2.2).

2.4 **Public health implications**

How should we interpret the cases where the application of the concept 'heavy use over time' results in different conclusions than using current medical classification systems? From a public health point of view, there are good reasons to prefer HUOT over the medical or other definitions. Consider the following examples: somebody who has been smoking 20 cigarettes a day over the last year but does not qualify for nicotine dependence in ICD-10, or for tobacco use disorders in DSM-5, because the number of criteria are below the threshold. This case seems to be relatively frequent (Rehm et al., 2013a), and based on risk for mortality and hospitalization, which follows a dose–response relationship (Baliunas et al., 2007a, b), one would clearly see 20 cigarettes as more important than the medical diagnoses for starting interventions to quit or reduce smoking, because it is linked to death and other severe outcomes, independent of the diagnosis. Now consider some smokers who did not smoke daily over the past year with, on average, fewer than five cigarettes per occasion but who qualify for nicotine dependence. While this pattern of smoking may still incur risks, the risks are certainly considerably lower than the risks of somebody who smokes 20 cigarettes but does not qualify for dependence. One may argue here that tobacco is a special substance, and smoking a special addictive behaviour, which was not always included in substance use disorders in various medical classification systems (e.g. see World Health Organization, 1957, or earlier versions of the DSM or ICD). However, first, the current medical systems explicitly include tobacco and related disorders; and, second, the same can be said about many other psychoactive substances, which were not considered to be addictive in the past and thus not included in the medical systems.

Let us consider alcohol use disorders and the average level of alcohol consumption in grams. Heavy drinking has been shown to be responsible for the vast majority of alcohol-attributable harm in Europe (Rehm et al., 2013b). The dose–response curves are mostly exponential (Rehm et al., 2010a; Rehm et al., 2011; Rehm and Roerecke, 2013), leading to the following implication: the same reduction in level of consumption (e.g. 40 grams per day) leads to considerably more pronounced reductions in mortality and hospitalizations if it is taken off from a higher level of consumption than from a lower level of consumption (Rehm and Roerecke, 2013; Nutt and Rehm, 2014). For public health, it is vital to reduce consumption, especially at high levels of consumption, even if these people do not qualify for alcohol dependence or alcohol use disorders. Similarly, it is important to reduce high levels of consumption, even if the people who reduce do not change their status as having an alcohol dependence or alcohol use disorder based on the diagnostic criteria of the current medical systems. Heavy drinking over time is clearly the more meaningful criterion with respect to health consequences compared with a diagnosis of alcohol dependence or alcohol use disorders.

Similar arguments could be made for cannabis (Fischer et al., 2011). Heavy cannabis use over time has been linked to a number of health effects such as altered brain development, cognitive impairment, chronic bronchitis, psychosis and schizophrenia, and lung cancer (Hall and Degenhardt, 2009; Volkow et al., 2014; Fischer et al., 2016) and single-occasion heavy use has been linked to acute effects such as motor vehicle and other injury (Asbridge et al., 2012), independently of whether the criteria for cannabis use disorders were fulfilled or not. A definition based solely on heavy use criteria would also facilitate concentration on the public health aspects of cannabis use, independently of its legal situation, where too often one is confronted with the false dichotomy of equating policy option preferences with presumed presence or absence of consequences (i.e. 'cannabis should be legalized because it is a benign substance' vs 'cannabis is linked to considerable health harm, and thus should be prohibited' (see Box 2.3).

> ## Box 2.3 Advantages of the concept of 'heavy use over time'
>
> The concept of 'heavy use over time' has distinctive advantages over current diagnostic criteria for substance use disorders for public health.

2.5 Implications for preventive and clinical interventions

Clinically, heavy use over time can be easily measured in many settings with reliable and valid short screening instruments (such as the Alcohol, Smoking and Substance Involvement Screening Test (ASSIST; World Health Organization ASSIST Working Group, 2002); or the AUDIT C (Bush et al., 1998)); but even single questions may prove feasible (Saitz et al., 2014). Heavy use can be measured in multiple ways in primary healthcare practices or other community-based access points, such as schools; or via the Internet/self-help applications, administered either by a professional or through automated systems, with the results being fed back to healthcare workers, or into an App with very little time lag or investment (Free et al., 2013a, b).

Based on the results, the user could then be engaged in a conversation about reduction if substance use is above a certain threshold. The underlying logic could be the same as for hypertension (Nutt and Rehm, 2014) in primary healthcare settings, or for learning difficulties in school settings, where values above a threshold lead to interventions (Conrod et al., 2013; Mancia et al., 2013; Lammers et al., 2015).

To illustrate the logic further, we can look at the similarities between heavy use over time and hypertension. Both conditions mark values of one key parameter above a threshold on continua (the continuum of substance use for heavy use, and the continuum of blood pressure for hypertension); they have multiple underlying causes that could be changed (for blood pressure salt intake, cigarette smoking or alcohol consumption, see Mancia et al., 2013; for substance use stress or environmental factors, see Gell et al., in press), both conditions can be relatively asymptomatic but lead to severe health outcomes without interventions, and for both conditions there are interventions available within the primary healthcare sector, which span from lifestyle advice to brief interventions (Bien et al., 1993; World Health Organization, 2010) to formal psychotherapy (Magill and Ray, 2009; Smedslund et al., 2011) to pharmacologically based therapies for alcohol (Jonas et al., 2014), tobacco (Hughes et al., 2014), and at least some illegal drugs (Shapiro et al., 2013). It should be noted that this proposal somewhat changes the role of the primary healthcare sector to include treatment of heavy use, including, but not limited to, pharmacological treatment, instead of just referral for dependence in the classic screening, brief intervention, and referral to specialized treatment paradigm (http://www.samhsa.gov/sbirt; for alcohol, see ; Laramée et al., 2015;).

Box 2.4 Advantages of continuous disease concepts

One of the main implications of the concept of 'heavy use over time' is to put emphasis on levels of use lying on a continuum, similar to blood pressure and hypertension. For primary healthcare, this means regular check-ups for use, and a variety of interventions, including treatment for heavy use over time.

As indicated above, there are effective interventions to reduce heavy use that will result in risk reductions for morbidity and mortality (for alcohol, see, e.g., Rehm and Roerecke, 2013 and Roerecke et al., 2013). Are the effects on the brain reversible as well and what are the consequences for clinical practice? Schulte et al. (2014) conducted a recent review and found that some of the effects on the brain were, indeed, reversible, but there are others which seem to persist. Another conclusion of their review was that better measurement was needed for brain consequences. The same is true for measurement of exposure to substances: level of substances should be measured over time with multiple measures to be able to correlate the exact level of substance use over time with these consequences. Moreover, the specific risks of irregular binge use need to be taken into consideration for some substances (for alcohol, see Rehm et al., 1996 and Room et al., 2005; for illegal drugs, see Kreek, 1996 and Mitra et al., 2015).

However, as a summary, it can be stated that while some brain consequences may be irreversible, reduction of heavy use and/or abstinence lead to considerable health gains, including an increase of life expectancy (Roerecke et al., 2013; Schulte et al., 2014). While substance use disorders are currently classified a chronic relapsing brain disease (Leshner, 1997), this conceptualization neither precludes a permanent change to stable reduction nor stable abstinence with the associated health gains. As seen with Vietnam veterans, even severe opioid addictions can be reversed completely (Robins, 1993). This means that interventions to reduce heavy substance use over time are important to societies to reduce the health burden and costs associated with these conditions for both developed and developing countries (Hall et al., 2006; Jha et al., 2006; Rehm et al., 2006) (see Box 2.4).

2.6 Conclusions

Overall, the concept of heavy use over time seems to have advantages over currently used medical definitions and additionally could lead to an ultimate convergence of definitions in various scientific disciplines with the view in the general population. This concept is consistent with recent advances in basic sciences, and fits better into the reasoning of public health as it is more closely linked to health and social consequences than the currently used criteria derived from medical classifications. It is clinically applicable in primary care with easy operationalization and sufficient interventions at that level, and it promises to reduce stigmatization as it is based on a truly continuous variable. We will thus frame all conclusions in this book using the concept of heavy use over time.

References

American Psychiatric Association (2013a) Substance use and addiction-related disorders. In: *Diagnostic and Statistical Manual of Mental Disorders*, 5th edition. Arlington, VA: American Psychiatric Association, pp. 481–589.

American Psychiatric Association (2013b) *Diagnostic and Statistical Manual of Mental Disorders*, 5th edition. Philadelphia, PA: American Psychiatric Association.

Angermeyer MC, Matschinger H, and Schomerus G (2013) Attitudes towards psychiatric treatment and people with mental illness: changes over two decades. *Br J Psychiatry* **203**: 146–51.

Angermeyer MC, Millier A, Rémuzat C, Refaï T, Schomerus G, and Toumi M (2015) Continuum beliefs and attitudes towards people with mental illness: results from a national survey in France. *Int J Soc Psychiatry* **61**: 297–303.

Asbridge M, Hayden JA, and Cartwright JL (2012) Acute cannabis consumption and motor vehicle collision risk: systematic review of observational studies and meta-analysis. *BMJ* **344**: e536.

Baler RD and Volkow ND (2006) Drug addiction: the neurobiology of disrupted self-control. *Trends Mol Med* **12**: 559–66.

Baliunas D, Patra J, Rehm J, Popova S, Kaiserman M, and Taylor B (2007a) Smoking-attributable mortality and potential years of life lost in Canada 2002: conclusions for prevention and policy. *Chronic Dis Can* **27**: 152–64.

Baliunas D, Patra J, Rehm J, Popova S, and Taylor B (2007b) Smoking-attributable morbidity: acute care hospital diagnoses and days of treatment in Canada. *BMC Public Health* **7**: 247.

Bien TH, Miller WR, and Tonigan JS (1993) Brief interventions for alcohol problems: a review. *Addiction* **88**: 315–36.

Bradley KA and Rubinsky AD (2013) Why not add consumption measures to current definitions of substance use disorders? Commentary on Rehm et al. 'Defining substance use disorders: Do we really need more than heavy use?'. *Alcohol Alcoholism* **48**: 642–3.

Bruun K (1970) Skadeverkningarna så ringa som möjligt [Reducing harmful effects as much as possible]. *Alkoholpolitik* **33**: 97–103.

Bush K, Kivlahan DR, McDonell MB, Fihn SD, and Bradley KA (1998) The AUDIT alcohol consumption questions (AUDIT-C): an effective brief screening test for problem drinking. *Arch Intern Med* **158**: 1789–95.

Caetano R (1989) Concepts of alcoholism among whites, blacks and Hispanics in the United States *J Stud Alcohol* **50**: 580–2.

Conrod PJ, O'Leary-Barrett M, Newton N, Topper L, Castellanos-Ryan N, Mackie C, and Girard A (2013) Effectiveness of a selective, personality-targeted prevention program for adolescent alcohol use and misuse: a cluster randomized controlled trial. *JAMA Psychiatry* **70**: 334–42.

Crocq MA (2007) Historical and cultural aspects of man's relationship with addictive drugs. *Dialogues Clin Neurosci* **9**: 355–61.

Ezzati M, Lopez A, Rodgers A, and Murray CJL (2004) *Comparative Quantification of Health Risks. Global and Regional Burden of Disease Attributable to Selected Major Risk Factors*, Geneva: World Health Organization.

Fischer B, Jeffries V, Hall W, Room R, Goldner E, and Rehm J (2011) Lower risk cannabis use guidelines for Canada (LRCUG): a narrative review of evidence and recommendations. *Can J Public Health* **102**: 324–7.

Fischer B, Imtiaz S, Rudzinski K, and Rehm J (2016) Crude estimates of cannabis-attributable mortality and morbidity in Canada—implications for public health focused intervention priorities. *J Public Health (Oxf)* **38**: 183–8.

Free C, Phillips G, Galli L, Watson L, Felix L, Edwards P, et al. (2013a) The effectiveness of mobile-health technology-based health behaviour change or disease management interventions for health care consumers: a systematic review. *PLOS Med* **10**: e1001362.

Free C, Phillips G, Watson L, Galli L, Felix L, Edwards P, et al. (2013b) The effectiveness of mobile-health technologies to improve health care service delivery processes: a systematic review and meta-analysis. *PLOS Med* **10**: e1001363.

Gell L, Bühringer G, McLeod J, Forberger S, Holmes J, Lingford-Hughes A, and Meier PS (eds) (2016) *What Determines Harm from Addictive Substance and Behaviours?*. Oxford: Oxford University Press.

Goldstein RZ and Volkow ND (2002) Drug addiction and its underlying neurobiological basis: neuroimaging evidence for the involvement of the frontal cortex. *Am J Psychiatry* **159**: 1642–52.

Gual A, Lligoña A, and Colom J (1999) Five-year outcome in alcohol dependence. A naturalistic study of 850 patients in Catalonia. *Alcohol Alcoholism* **34**: 183–92.

Hall W and Degenhardt L (2009) Adverse health effects of non-medical cannabis use. *Lancet* **374**: 1383–91.

Hall W, Doran C, Degenhardt L, and Shepard D (2006) Illicit opiate abuse. In: Jamison DT, Breman JG, Measham AR, Alleyne G, Claeson M, Evans DB, et al. (eds.) *Disease Control Priorities in Developing Countries*, 2nd edition. Washington, DC: Oxford University Press and World Bank, pp. 907–32.

Heilig M (2015) *The Thirteenth Step. Addiction in the Age of Brain Science.* New York: Columbia University Press, 2015.

Hughes JR, Stead LF, Hartmann-Boyce J, Cahill K, and Lancaster T (2014) Antidepressants for smoking cessation. *Cochrane Database Syst Rev* **8**: CD000031.

Jha P, Chaloupka FJ, Moore J, Gajalakshmi V, Gupta PC, Peck R, et al. (2006) Tobacco addiction. In: Jamison DT, Breman J, Measham A, Alleyne G, Claeson M, Evans D, et al. (eds.) *Disease Control Priorities in Developing Countries*, 2nd edition. Oxford and New York: Oxford University Press, pp 869–86.

Jonas DE, Amick HR, Feltner C, Bobashev G, Thomas K, Wines R, et al. (2014) *AHRQ Comparative Effectiveness Reviews. Pharmacotherapy for Adults With Alcohol-Use Disorders in Outpatient Settings.* Rockville, MD: Agency for Healthcare Research and Quality (US).

Koob GF and Le Moal M (2005) Plasticity of reward neurocircuitry and the 'dark side' of drug addiction. *Nat Neurosci* **8**: 1442–4.

Kraus L, Piontek D, Pabst A, and Gomes De Matos E (2013) Studiendesign und Methodik des Epidemiologischen Suchtsurveys 2012 [Study design and methodology of the 2012 Epidemiological Survey of Substance Abuse]. *Sucht* **59**: 309–20.

Kreek MJ (1996) Cocaine, dopamine and the endogenous opioid system. *J Addict Dis* **15**: 73–96.

Lammers J, Goossens F, Conrod P, Engels R, Wiers RW, and Kleinjan M (2015) Effectiveness of a selective intervention program targeting personality risk factors for alcohol misuse among young adolescents: results of a cluster randomized controlled trial. *Addiction* **110**: 1101–9.

Laramée P, Leonard S, Buchanan-Hughes A, Warnakula S, Daeppen J-B, and Rehm J (2015) Alcohol dependence and mortality: implications for treatment—authors' reply. *EBioMedicine* **2**: 1283.

Leshner AI (1997) Addiction is a brain disease, and it matters. *Science* **278**: 45–7.

Li TK, Hewitt BG, and Grant BF (2007) Is there a future for quantifying drinking in the diagnosis, treatment, and prevention of alcohol use disorders? *Alcohol Alcoholism* **41**: 57–63.

Lindesmith AR (1938) A sociological theory of drug addiction. *Am J Sociol* **43**: 593–613.

McGovern P (2009) *Uncorking the Past: The Quest for Wine, Beer, and Other Alcoholic Beverages.* Berkley, CA; Los Angeles, CA; London: The Regents of the University of California.

McLellan AT, Lewis D, O'Brien C, and Kleber H (2000) Drug dependence, a chronic medical illness: implications for treatment, insurance, and outcomes evaluation. *JAMA* **284**: 1689–95.

Magill M and Ray LA (2009) Cognitive-behavioral treatment with adult alcohol and illicit drug users: a meta-analysis of randomized controlled trials. *J Stud Alcohol Drugs* **70**: 516–27.

Mancia G, Fagard R, Narkiewicz K, Redon J, Zanchetti A, Bohm M, et al. (2013) 2013 ESH/ESC Guidelines for the management of arterial hypertension: the Task Force for the management of arterial hypertension of the European Society of Hypertension (ESH) and of the European Society of Cardiology (ESC). *J Hypertension* **31**: 1281–357.

Martin CS, Langenbucher JW, Chung T, and Sher KJ (2014) Truth or consequences in the diagnosis of substance use disorders. *Addiction* **109**: 1773–8.

Mitra G, Wood E, Nguyen P, Kerr T, and DeBeck K (2015) Drug use patterns predict risk of non-fatal overdose among street-involved youth in a Canadian setting. *Drug Alcohol Depend,* **153**: 135–9.

Nestler EJ (2005) Is there a common molecular pathway for addiction? *Nat Neurosci* **8**: 1445–9.

Nutt D (2012) *Drugs Without the Hot Air.* Cambridge: UIT Cambridge Ltd.

Nutt DJ and Nestor LJ (2013) *Addiction.* Oxford: Oxford University Press.

Nutt DJ and Rehm J (2014) Doing it by numbers: a simple approach to reducing the harms of alcohol. *J Psychopharmacol* **28**: 3–7.

Parascandola M (2011) Causes, risks, and probabilities: probabilistic concepts of causation in chronic disease epidemiology. *Prev Med* **53**: 232–4.

Rehm J and Roerecke M (2013) Reduction of drinking in problem drinkers and all-cause mortality. *Alcohol Alcoholism* **48**: 509–13.

Rehm J and Room R (2015) Cultural specificity in alcohol use disorders. *Lancet* [Epub ahead of print 3 September 2015].

Rehm J, Ashley MJ, Room R, Single E, Bondy S, Ferrence R, and Giesbrecht N (1996) On the emerging paradigm of drinking patterns and their social and health consequences. *Addiction* **91**: 1615–21.

Rehm J, Chisholm D, Room R, and Lopez A (2006) Alcohol. In: Jamison DT, Breman JG, Measham AR, Alleyne G, Claeson M, Evans DB, et al. (eds) *Disease Control Priorities in Developing Countries.* Washington, DC: Oxford University Press and World Bank, pp. 887–906.

Rehm J, Baliunas D, Borges GL, Graham K, Irving HM, Kehoe T, et al. (2010a) The relation between different dimensions of alcohol consumption and burden of disease—an overview. *Addiction* **105**: 817–43.

Rehm J, Taylor B, Mohapatra S, Irving H, Baliunas D, Patra J, and Roerecke M (2010b) Alcohol as a risk factor for liver cirrhosis—a systematic review and meta-analysis. *Drug Alcohol Rev* **29**: 437–45.

Rehm J, Zatonski W, Taylor B, and Anderson P (2011) Epidemiology and alcohol policy in Europe. *Addiction* **106**: 11–19.

Rehm J, Marmet S, Anderson P, Gual A, Kraus L, Nutt DJ, et al. (2013a) Defining substance use disorders: do we really need more than heavy use? *Alcohol Alcoholism* **48**: 633–40.

Rehm J, Shield KD, Rehm MX, Gmel G, and Frick U (2013b) Modelling the impact of alcohol dependence on mortality burden and the effect of available treatment interventions in the European Union. *Eur Neuropsychopharmacol* **23**: 89–97.

Rehm J, Probst C, Kraus L, and Lev-Ran S (2014a) The addiction concept revisited. In: Anderson P, Bühringer G, and Colom J (eds) *Reframing Addiction: Policies, Processes and Pressures*. Barcelona: ALICE RAP, pp. 103–17.

Rehm J, Anderson P, Gual A, Kraus L, Marmet S, Room R, et al. (2014b) The tangible common denominator of substance use disorders: a reply to commentaries to Rehm et al. (2013). *Alcohol Alcoholism* **49**: pp. 118–22.

Rehm J, Allamani A, Elekes Z, Jakubczyk A, Landsmane I, Manthey J, et al. (2015a) General practitioners recognizing alcohol dependence: a large cross-sectional study in six European countries. *Ann Fam Med* **131**: 28–32.

Rehm J, Anderson P, Barry J, Dimitrov P, Elekes Z, Feijão F, et al. (2015b) Prevalence of and potential influencing factors for alcohol dependence in Europe. *Eur Addict Res* **21**: 6–18.

Robins LN (1993) The sixth Thomas James Okey Memorial Lecture. Vietnam veterans' rapid recovery from heroin addiction: a fluke or normal expectation? *Addiction* **88**: 1041–54.

Roerecke M, Gual A, and Rehm J (2013) Reduction of alcohol consumption and subsequent mortality in alcohol use disorders: systematic review and meta-analysis. *J Clin Psychiatry* **74**: e1181–9.

Room R (1998) Alcohol and drug disorders in the International Classification of Diseases: a shifting kaleidoscope. *Drug Alcohol Rev* **17**: 305–17.

Room R (2005) Stigma, social inequality and alcohol and drug use. *Drug Alcohol Rev* **24**: 143–55.

Room R (2006) Taking account of cultural and societal influences on substance use diagnoses and criteria. *Addiction* **101**: 31–9.

Room R (2007) Understanding cultural differences in young people's drinking. In: Järvinen M and Room R (eds) *Youth Drinking Cultures: European Experiences*. Burlington, VT: Ashgate Publishing, pp. 17–40.

Room R, Babor T, and Rehm J (2005) Alcohol and public health: a review. *Lancet* **365**: 519–30.

Room R, Hellman M, and Stenius K (2015) Addiction: the dance between concept and terms. *Int J Alcohol Drug Res* **4**: 27–35.

Rothman KJ, Greenland S, and Lash TL (2008) *Modern Epidemiology,* 3rd edition. Philadelphia, PA: Lippincott Williams & Wilkins.

Saitz R, Cheng DM, Allensworth-Davies D, Winter MR, and Smith PC (2014) The ability of single screening questions for unhealthy alcohol and other drug use to identify substance dependence in primary care. *J Stud Alcohol Drugs* **75**: 153–7.

Schomerus G, Lucht M, Holzinger A, Matschinger H, Carta MG, Angermeyer MC (2011) The stigma of alcohol dependence compared with other mental disorders: a review of population studies. *Alcohol Alcohol* **46**:105–12.

Schomerus G, Holzinger A, Matschinger H, Lucht M, and Angermeyer MC (2010) Public attitudes towards alcohol dependence. An overview. *Psychiatrische Praxis* 37: 111–18.

Schomerus G, Matschinger H, and Angermeyer MC (2013) Continuum beliefs and stigmatizing attitudes towards persons with schizophrenia, depression and alcohol dependence. *Psychiatry Res* 209: S0165–1781.

Schomerus G, Matschinger H, and Angermeyer MC (2014a) Attitudes towards alcohol dependence and affected individuals: persistence of negative stereotypes and illness beliefs between 1990 and 2011. *Eur Addict Res* 20: 293–9.

Schomerus G, Matschinger H, Lucht MJ, and Angermeyer MC (2014b) Changes in the perception of alcohol-related stigma in Germany over the last two decades. *Drug Alcohol Depend* 1: 225–31.

Schulte MHJ, Cousijn J, Den Uyl TE, Goudriaan AE, Van Den Brink W, Veltman DJ, et al. (2014) Recovery of neurocognitive functions following sustained abstinence after substance dependence and implications for treatment. *Clin Psychol Rev* 34: 531–50.

Shapiro B, Coffa D, and McCance-Katz EF (2013) A primary care approach to substance misuse. *Am Fam Physician* 88: 113–21.

Shield KD and Rehm J (2015) The effects of addictive substances and addictive behaviours on physical and mental health. In: Anderson P, Rehm J, and Room R (eds) *The Impact of Addictive Substances and Behaviours on Individual and Societal Well-being.* Oxford: Oxford University Press, pp. 77–118.

Smedslund G, Berg RC, Hammerstrom KT, Steiro A, Leiknes KA, Dahl HM, and Karlsen K (2011) Motivational interviewing for substance abuse. *Cochrane Database Syst Rev* 5: CD008063.

Sulkunen P (2015) The images theory of addiction. *Int J Alcohol Drug Res* 4P 5–11.

Sullivan RJ, Hagen EH, and Hammerstein P (2008) Revealing the paradox of drug reward in human evolution. *Proc R Soc B Biol Sci* 275: 1231–41.

Sullivan RJ and Hagen EH (2014) Passive vulnerability or active agency? An ecological and evolutionary perspective on human drug use. In: Anderson P, Rehm J, and Room R (eds) *The Impact of Addictive Substances and Behaviours on Inidvidual and Societal Well-being.* Oxford: Oxford University Press, pp. 13–35.

Tajfel H (1982) *Social Identity and Intergroup Relations*, Cambridge: Cambridge University Press.

Thanki D and Vicente J (2013) *PDU (Problem Drug Use) Revision Summary.* Lisbon: European Monitoring Centre for Drugs and Drug Addiction.

Thorndike EL (1911) *Animal Intelligence: Experimental Studies*, New York: Hafner.

Tsuang MT, Lyons MJ, Meyer JM, Doyle T, Eisen SA, Goldberg J, et al. (1998) Co-occurrence of abuse of different drugs in men: the role of drug-specific and shared vulnerabilities. *Arch Gen Psychiatry* 55: 967–72.

Volkow ND, Fowler JS, and Wang GJ (2003) The addicted human brain: insights from imaging studies. *J Clin Invest* 111: 1444–51.

Volkow ND, Baler RD, Compton WM, and Weiss SR (2014) Adverse health effects of marijuana use. *N Engl J Med* 370: 2219–27.

Whelan R, Conrod PJ, Poline JB, Lourdusamy A, Banaschewski T, Barker GJ, et al. (2012) Adolescent impulsivity phenotypes characterized by distinct brain networks. *Nat Neurosci* 15: 920–5.

Whelan R, Watts R, Orr CA, Althoff RR, Artiges E, Banaschewski T, et al. (2014) Neuropsychosocial profiles of current and future adolescent alcohol misusers. *Nature* **512**: 185–9.

Wiers RW, Cousijn J, Ter Mors-Schulte M, Den Uyl T, Goudriaan AE, Schilt T, et al. (2012) State of the art: neurocognitieve effecten van verslaving [Neurocognitive effects of addiction]. Den Haag: ZonMw—Programma Risicogedrag en Afhankelijkheid.

Wise RA (2000) Addiction becomes a brain disease. *Neuron* **26**: 27–33.

Wise RA and Koob GF (2014) The development and maintenance of drug addiction. *Neuropsychopharmacology* **39**: 254–62.

World Health Organization (1957) *WHO Expert Committee on Addiction-Producing Drugs, Seventh Report*. Geneva: World Health Organization.

World Health Organization (1992) *International Statistical Classification of Diseases and Related Health Problems, 10th Revision (ICD-10). Tabular List*. Geneva: World Health Organization.

World Health Organization (1993) *The ICD-10 Classification of Mental and Behavioural Disorders: Diagnostic Criteria for Research*. Geneva: World Health Organization.

World Health Organization (2004) *Neuroscience of Psychoactive Substance Use and Dependence*. Geneva: World Health Organization, 2004.

World Health Organization (2010) *Brief Intervention. The ASSIST-linked Brief Intervention for Hazardous and Harmful Substance Use. Manual for Use in Primary Care*. Geneva: World Health Organization.

World Health Organization Assist Working Group (2002) The Alcohol, Smoking and Substance Involvement Screening Test (ASSIST): development, reliability and feasibility. *Addiction* **97**: 1183–94.

United Nations Office on Drugs and Crime (2014). *World Drug Report 2014*. New York: United Nations.

Chapter 3

The ethical basis for preventing harm from heavy use of addictive products

3.1 Introduction

Chapter 2 laid out a proposal for redefining the conceptualization of addiction or substance use disorder as heavy use over time, and mechanisms by which this could be beneficial in minimizing confusion and stigma and maximizing population well-being. In this chapter we turn to the value that a study of ethics can bring to the planning of approaches (on small or large scale) to reduce harm from heavy use of addictive products, and a proposal for such an ethical framework; subsequent chapters will examine the determinants, approaches, and actors involved in a new governance of addiction

3.2 Ethics vs morals

Philosophers, and those applying philosophical ideas to many different fields, have attempted to define succinctly ethics and morals and the relationship between the two. For our purposes here, from the standpoint of considering issues in public health, we will adopt a simplified version of the distinction.

Morals define personal character and rules for behaviour, and are determined by an individual's upbringing, secular guidelines or religious beliefs on what is right and wrong, while ethics comprises a consensual social system in which those morals are weighed and applied, or rejected. In this view, ethics is an overall framework for making decisions that balances the multitude of factors in a given scenario, and morality is but one of the pillars upon which this framework is based. Put another way, ethics is an analytical methodology, while morality is a personal code. Both can be (and currently are) employed as decision-making tools in governance and policy-making for health and behaviour. In this chapter, we will examine the appropriateness (or not) of ethics and morals as a basis for approaches to preventing harm in public health, and specifically in relation to harms that arise from the heavy use of addictive products. We will consider the components of an ethical framework for handling these problems, and instances in the domain of addictive behaviour that may challenge points in such a framework.

As discussed in Chapter 2 and elsewhere (Rehm et al., 2013), 'addictions' or 'substance dependence' have proven particularly elusive in terms of universal definition, and there are persuasive arguments for adopting a definition of heavy use over time (HUOT), with regard to harmful addictive substances, as the parameter that represents the best fit with the epidemiological and social data on harm. From here on, then, we refer, where possible, to HUOT of addictive products, rather than 'addiction' or 'dependence'.

3.3 Why do we need an ethical basis for preventing harm from addictive products?

Policy decisions and action in relation to the provision, selling, and marketing of addictive substances or activities—are typically plagued by moral overtones ('Taking drugs is wrong'; 'Intoxication is irresponsible'; 'Why should taxpayers' money be spent on treatment for people who just want to get high?'; 'It is wrong to interfere in lifestyle choices', etc.). While moral opinions are an inescapable part of human nature, in the policy context, these can cloud the vision of decision makers and contribute to the development of policies and overall governance approaches that may not only be ineffective in reducing harms, but also exacerbate harm in the most vulnerable populations and contribute to growing social and economic inequalities.

An ethical approach, unlike a moral approach, utilizes a socially shared system of principles to reach decisions that will maximize the common good. An ethical system will necessarily incorporate a moral principle, the objective being to achieve a 'good' rather than 'bad' outcome, but the definitions of 'good' and 'bad' are, de facto, the result of a consensus and the product of informed common debate, rather than individuals' subjective beliefs (see Box 3.1).

It is worth noting that while moral opinions are one component of an ethical decision making framework, the widespread acceptance and adoption of such a framework imbues it with a moral character, which, in time, can mean it becomes incorporated into personal moral values (Thomas et al., 2002), potentially bringing ethics and morals in line with each other. In particular, the need to accept a common societal framework and abide by its decisions (even if not concurrent with one's own moral viewpoints) is itself a moral demand and one that is important in order for individuals to live within a democratic and consensual social order.

Box 3.1 Ethics as a basis for policy making

The application of ethics is necessarily more objective and impartial than moral reasoning, and based on validated evidence and agreed social goals, it clearly provides a more adequate basis for policy making, where the common good of the population should be the driving objective of the whole process and institutions of governance.

3.4 **Philosophical ideas behind ethical governance**

Petrini and Gainotti (2008) discuss the difficulties in defining ethical principles for public health that can also be applied to this area of policy to shape approaches to addictive products. They point out that, at first sight, the utilitarian or consequentialist schools of thought seem to be a good fit with the requirements of ethical practice of public health. In this framework, decisions are judged by their consequent outcomes for well-being and thus policies should maximize the greatest good for the greatest number of citizens. They note, however, that there are attendant problems in adopting this standpoint—first the difficulty of measuring well-being objectively; second, the free rein that such a philosophical stance appears to give to unfairly compromise the individual's rights and freedoms in the name of public utility (in particular, the risk of excessively punishing or repressing those at the extremes of continua of behaviour to maximize the common good).

Regarding this first difficulty, well-being has typically been defined with reference to more objective and measurable components, for example disability-adjusted life years (DALYs) or quality-adjusted life years (QALYs) in epidemiology and in public health arenas, although it can be argued that this misses a critical dimension, relating to personal, non-medical experiences over those years. Furthermore, as will be discussed in section 3.11, significant advances have been made (e.g. by the OECD, 2012) and the New Economic Foundation (n.d.) towards measuring and objectively quantifying societal well-being, which can be brought to bear on the indicators of relative success of policy decisions and approaches.

The second concern (that individual freedom could be compromised) was the basic driving force of liberalism, the world view based on the ideas of personal liberty and equality, arguably founded on the ideas of the seventeenth-century philosopher John Locke (Locke, 1700). The political philosophy of liberalism has had an enormous influence on the public health policies of governments in modern societies, but in strikingly contradictory directions, depending on the differing interpretations that have been made of the concept of *individual freedom* and the emphasis (or not) placed on the connected principle of *equality*.

The social liberalist school of thought posited a legitimate role of the government was to intervene to address economic and social issues such as poverty, healthcare, and education, believing that there was no virtue in individual freedom of choice without the practical means to enact such choices, thus placing a high measure of importance on the principle of equality in society.

This school of political thought, dating back to the mid-nineteenth century can be encapsulated in John Stuart Mill's 1879 definition of social justice as equal treatment for all citizens, with the important caveat that only *virtuous* citizens deserve equal treatment. Moving into the last century, Lloyd George's redistributive budgets of the 1900s in the UK and Roosevelt's 1930s New Deal in the USA developed the idea of a 'welfare state'—that is, the idea that government has a responsibility to ensure universal welfare, including the support of those who find themselves in economic or social difficulties. Another famous example is the 1942 Beveridge Report, towards the end of the Second World War, which laid out social welfare measures that should be introduced in peace time, and which were then taken up by the subsequent Labour government in the UK between 1945 and 1950 (including the creation of the National Health Service). Such measures have become a feature of social and economic policy in most economically advanced nations, notably in Nordic and Western Europe, and countries such as Australia and New Zealand. They imply an egalitarian motivation, in that the state should attempt to iron out some of the harmful consequences of differences in personal wealth. This motivation may arise from a genuine philosophical belief in human equality, or from a concern among those more privileged and powerful that relative deprivation may lead to damaging social unrest, thus adopting measures of social justice as a means to maintain the hierarchical status quo.

Economic liberalism, in contrast, has its origins in the rise of merchant and entrepreneurial classes in the nineteenth century and their struggle against restrictive domination of economic activity by the formerly dominant aristocratic and royalist elite. In recent decades it has been revived in the form of neoliberalism, as a reaction against the egalitarian doctrine of social liberalism, and fuelled by the tenets of economic growth and globalization. Neoliberals and economic liberals hold an ideological belief in organizing the economy on individualist lines, meaning that the greatest possible number of economic decisions be made by individuals and not by collective institutions or organizations (Duménil and Lévy 2004). This position stems from the belief that market forces maximize the efficiency and productivity of society as a whole, but the ideologies also treat individuals' freedom of choice as an over-riding principle. This school of thought, which has shaped governance in the capitalist societies of many developed countries since the 1980s, stands strongly against the intervention of governments, particularly in the free market. It also almost completely negates the principle of equality, except in terms of individuals possessing an equal right to freedom of choice. The arguments of both opposing liberalist branches are especially relevant to the governance of lifestyle behaviours, such as consumption of addictive products, and have been used in the political and economic negotiations around the governance and determination of this consumption, as we shall see subsequently.

As Petrini and Gainotti (2008) point out, all these philosophical standpoints neglect two key aspects: that of the communal nature of human societies and the inherent and inalienable value of humans as persons. They propose a personalist approach which is based upon our common shared human nature. This approach takes as its primary ethical principle that all human beings deserve respect (on the grounds of being the only animal capable of self-reflection and comprehension of the meaning of life). The principles of ontologically based personalism in bioethics can be summed up in four points:

- the defence of human life as sacred, and of intangible value;
- the therapeutic principle—intervention on life is justified only for therapeutic purpose;
- the freedom and responsibility principle—freedom has primacy but can be limited where respect for life is at stake;

◆ the sociality and subsidiarity principle—the achievement of common good through individual well-being.

Petrini and Gainotti (2008) claim that personalism is not opposed to other ethical theories but has points in common with them and also divergences from them. In a personalist view, for example, the consequentialist–utilitarian approach can certainly be part of a public health policy as long as the lives and well-being of individuals are preserved. With regard to individual freedom, so important to the liberalist view, a moderate form of restriction is justified both in serious or emergency circumstances (e.g. isolation to prevent the spread of an epidemic disease), and in routine conditions where the subject may not be in full charge of the situation and hence it becomes necessary to oblige certain behaviours (such as limits on blood alcohol levels when driving).

3.5 What components make up an ethical framework for public health?

Some authors have suggested the application of the principles of North American bioethics (autonomy, beneficence, non-maleficence, justice) (Neiburg and Shannon, 1999) to public health ethics. However, as they stand, the four principles are not sufficient for ethical guidance of public health action, referring as they do to concepts that are relative and changeable in different subsections of society or for different stakeholders affected by any public health action.

There have been several attempts to develop an ethical framework for public health, most notably by the American Public Health Association (APHA) and the Nuffield Council on Bioethics. As both organizations acknowledge, the key challenge in public health ethics is attaining a balance between the need for intervention (or the exercise of power, as the APHA term it), on one hand, and safeguarding against excessive coercion (or abuses of such power) on the other. Both also mention the shift in focus in addressing public health rather than traditional medical ethics: from the individual to the population; from cure to prevention (and therefore, from 'sick' people to 'healthy' people); and, critically for our discussion of addictive products, from the health service sector to an intersection of multiple sectors (e.g. health, criminal justice, economic regulation, education, social services), in which many different players have roles, reactions, and responsibilities.

The APHA Code, in its simplest form, consists of 12 ethical principles (Thomas et al., 2002), which are further supported by a series of documents providing further details on each and information on their public health context and values. While the 12 APHA principles cover a great many valuable considerations, they also contain a number of elements that are open to fairly flexible interpretation, not being of a concrete nature, resulting in their ethical integrity being less robust. For example, one recommendation is that 'Public health institutions should act in a timely manner on the information they have' ('timely' being a relative term). The final principle: '12. Public health institutions and their employees should engage in collaborations and affiliations in ways that build the public's trust and the institution's effectiveness' clearly leaves the door open for academic and industry collaborations, as described in volume 5 of this book series

(Miller et al., 2016), which could be very effective at gaining public trust and increasing the institutions' influence with little public health benefit.

The Nuffield report puts forward a 'stewardship model' of the role of the state in relation to public health, a series of non-hierarchical positive goals and negative constraints, according to which the state should not coerce people or restrict their freedoms unnecessarily, but has a responsibility to provide the conditions for healthy lives (see Exhibit 3.1).

The authors note that the implementation of the principles may lead to conflicting directions in policy decisions, and for this reason they propose a ladder of intervention, ranking options in terms of limitations on individual freedom, which should be used to resolve such conflicts by opting for maximum individual freedoms (see Exhibit 3.2).

It is important to note here that the option 'do nothing' also represents an active policy decision; a point that is particularly salient when doing nothing can actively

---

Exhibit 3.1 **The stewardship model**

Concerning goals, public health programmes should:

- aim to reduce the risks of ill health that people might impose on each other;
- aim to reduce causes of ill health by regulations that ensure environmental conditions that sustain good health, such as the provision of clean air and water, safe food, and appropriate housing;
- pay special attention to the health of children and other vulnerable people;
- promote health not only by providing information and advice, but also by programmes to help people overcome addictions and other unhealthy behaviours;
- aim to ensure that it is easy for people to lead a healthy life, for example by providing convenient and safe opportunities for exercise;
- ensure that people have appropriate access to medical services;
- aim to reduce health inequalities.

In terms of constraints, such programmes should:

- not attempt to coerce adults to lead healthy lives;
- minimize interventions that are introduced without the individual consent of those affected, or without procedural justice arrangements (e.g. democratic decision-making procedures), which provide adequate mandate;
- seek to minimize interventions that are perceived as unduly intrusive and in conflict with important personal values.

Exhibit 3.2 **The ladder of possible government actions**

+ *Eliminate choice.* Regulate in such a way as to eliminate choice entirely, for example through compulsory isolation of patients with infectious diseases.

+ *Restrict choice.* Regulate in such a way as to restrict the options available to people with the aim of protecting them, for example removing unhealthy ingredients from foods, or unhealthy foods from shops or restaurants.

+ *Guide choice through disincentives.* Fiscal and other disincentives can be put in place to influence people not to pursue certain activities, for example through taxes on cigarettes, or by discouraging the use of cars in inner cities through charging schemes or limitations on parking spaces.

+ *Guide choices through incentives.* Regulations can be offered that guide choices by fiscal and other incentives, for example offering tax breaks for the purchase of bicycles that are used as a means of travelling to work.

+ *Guide choices through changing the default policy.* For example, in a restaurant, instead of providing chips as a standard side dish (with healthier options available), menus could be changed to provide a more healthy option as standard (with chips as an option available).

+ *Enable choice.* Enable individuals to change their behaviours, for example by offering participation in a National Health Service 'stop smoking' programme, building cycle lanes, or providing free fruit in schools.

+ *Provide information.* Inform and educate the public, for example as part of campaigns to encourage people to walk more or eat five portions of fruit and vegetables per day.

+ *Do nothing or simply monitor the current situation.*

Reproduced with permission from Nuffield Council on Bioethics. *Public Health: Ethical Issues.* London: Nuffield Council on Bioethics, Copyright © 2007 Nuffield Council on Bioethics, http://nuffieldbioethics. org/wp-content/uploads/2014/07/Public-health-ethical-issues.pdf, accessed 01 Nov. 2015.

---

permit the intervention on individual freedoms of non-governmental actors (such as corporations acting through incentives, disincentives, or restrictions in choice).

3.6 What is the special case of public health ethics in the area of heavy use over time of addictive products?

There is robust evidence for the high level of population harm caused by heavy use of addictive products (Shield and Rehm, 2015). These harms span health and social dimensions and clearly warrant attention, with the intent to reduce the resulting costs to society and individual human suffering brought about by their HUOT.

Yet there are several features of HUOT that makes it stand out among other public health issues and complicate the application of ethical codes to the regulation of this behaviour at the population level. These characteristics are summarized in Box 3.2:

Box 3.2 Characteristics of heavy use over time which influence ethical considerations

- HUOT is one of several *lifestyle choices*.
- Because of concurrent intoxication, HUOT has been the subject of *extreme levels of social control*.
- Because of compulsive nature of the behaviour, HUOT has a parallel *impact on individual freedom of choice*.
- Economic returns on the sales of addictive products result in a *high degree of influence from the corporate sector* in policy to address HUOT.

These characteristics, although interlinked, will be dealt with in the subsequent sections.

3.7 Lifestyle choices—beyond the medical sector and in the private realm

As with other lifestyle choices with health implications, such as physical activity, diet, sexual protection, car driving, place of dwelling (city/country), hobbies (such as dangerous sports), or occupation, certain factors come into play around government intervention to promote or protect health that are not necessarily relevant to policy decisions in other areas of public health. These factors are more pronounced with the governance of HUOT of addictive products than with the other lifestyle choices mentioned above. Lifestyle choices have also been held up by many political and philosophical thinkers as sacred and to be defended against intervention or manipulation, especially where the consequences of the choice are primarily seen as affecting only the individual, and not third parties. This dates back to James Stuart Mill's anti-paternalist injunction that 'his own good, either physical or moral, is not a sufficient warrant' for the state to impose an intervention to make a person healthier (Mill, 1859).

Many areas of public health decision making are strongly rooted within the institutions of medical practice, for example immunization programmes or restrictions on the transmission of epidemic diseases. These areas may require legislative enforcement and so ultimately invoke the coercive power of the state, but such legislation basically gives medical and paramedical practitioners the authority of state power to request or require strongly certain behaviours (childhood vaccinations or isolation to prevent infection), without intruding much on other aspects of the individual's relation with the state. In facing the problems of HUOT of addictive products, a much wider range of the machinery of government is necessarily involved. These include:

♦ *The healthcare system at all levels.* Because of the high level of comorbidity of HUOT with other diseases, patients with heavy use may present to primary healthcare providers or to those in emergency hospital facilities for treatment of other injuries or diseases but unwilling to recognize or are unaware of HUOT as their primary problem. This implies, first, that ethical principles for intervention on HUOT (or other lifestyle factors) in medical settings have to encompass a wide range of medical situations; and, second, that the importance of addressing HUOT as significant risk factors in the development or prognosis of comorbid conditions may be accepted by health professionals as justifying intervention even when the problem is not recognized by patients themselves. More specialist levels of medical care have to face ethical issues such as whether it is justified to prioritize a liver transplant for an alcohol-using patient given the risk this lifestyle factor poses to his or her new liver. Healthcare professionals in non-medical settings (e.g. schools, prisons, or workplaces) are also brought into play in public health measures to reduce harm from HUOT.

♦ *The criminal justice system.* If a substance is legally banned (as a number of addictive and intoxicating drugs are in different countries), then police, courts, and prison and probation systems become heavily involved, with attendant consequences for ethical considerations around human rights, civil liberties, and equality. As a method of (extreme) social control, the ethical considerations of working at this intersection between public health and criminal justice, i.e. depriving those who use addictive products (majorly, those whose behaviour constitutes HUOT) of their liberty or exacting fines, are further explored in Section 3.8.)

♦ *The regulation of commerce.* Some addictive products (tobacco, alcohol) are legally traded in many parts of the world, but in almost all countries these products are subject to various degrees of special regulation (only sold on licensed premises, restrictions on sale to minors or proximity to schools, restrictions on sales hours, limitations on advertising, etc.) Historically, restrictions may have been set in place on grounds of acknowledged social goals (e.g. restrictions on the strength and hours for the sale of alcohol were introduced in the UK during the First World War because it was thought that lunchtime drinking was damaging the productivity of munitions workers (Berridge, 2014)). More recently, the justification for these restrictions are framed in terms of the high costs to society of HUOT and a growing awareness of the psychological processes and mechanisms that lead to greater and greater consumption of these products (which will be further addressed in Section 3.8).

♦ *The tax system.* In many countries, the most important intervention in the commerce of legal addictive products is heavy taxation on their sale. Like many other taxes, this has two purposes which may sometimes be in conflict: to raise the maximum amount of revenue to support government activities (including health and social services needed to address the consequences of HUOT of such products), and to discourage behaviours that the government wishes to reduce (in this case, substance use). Another policy that has been proposed is to set a minimum unit price (MUP) for alcohol (Holmes et al., 2014), which would have similar effects on the consumer to taxation (raising the price relative to other goods) but with the difference that the increased income goes to the traders or producers rather than to the government. Despite this, the alcohol industry has actively opposed and successfully lobbied against the introduction of MUP in several countries that have considered the measure to reduce alcohol-related harm (Gornall, 2014).

◆ *The role of corporations.* The manufacture and supply of legal addictive products (alcohol and tobacco) is very big business, indeed, controlled primarily by large and powerful multinational companies. These companies have strong interests which they vigorously pursue against the restriction of their trade, and against public health initiatives which alert the public to the damaging effects of their products (see Chapter 9). Ethical considerations include the role of government to protect citizens from corporate manipulation through marketing and policy interference, which will be discussed further in Section 3.9.

3.8 **Extreme levels of social control**

Addictive products have played significant, varied, and sometimes contradictory roles in policies and movements related to social justice (or injustice) and control throughout history. Since the mid-nineteenth century and up until recent times, alcohol and other drugs have been used by those struggling for social justice to assert the moral standing of their cause, as well as by those looking to discredit egalitarian movements by calling into question the 'virtue' of those demanding social justice (Moskalewicz and Klingemann, 2015). Among other historical examples, in early nineteenth-century Poland (at the time divided between Prussia, the Russian Empire, and Austria), and cited in several other historical cases, high availability of alcohol and ownership of the points of sale of alcohol by the landed gentry meant the recirculation of working-class incomes into the pockets of the ruling classes. Indeed, in Prussia at this time, certain financial transactions with workers (signing contracts and receiving wages) have been documented as taking place in inns or public houses, where many were tempted to stay and drink. At the same time, intoxication of the same workers was held up as proof of their irresponsible or undeserving character, justifying low resources for working classes and leading to further disempowerment (and arguably to greater disillusionment and escapism through intoxication). Consequently, temperance ideas have entered into the doctrines of egalitarian political movements, with 'alcoholism' viewed as a tool of capitalist oppression, and temperance gatherings used as a cover for socialist meetings where such movements were prohibited. However, temperance has also been held up as acting against the interests of working classes by vilifying a substance (alcohol) that promoted solidarity with co-workers; and pubs in late nineteenth-century Germany became a place for social activists to meet. More recently, and famously, alcohol prohibition in America was ostensibly introduced to reduce social harms from the substance, but could be interpreted as an attempt to legitimize political force over immigrants from heavy-drinking European populations at that time (Gusfield, 1986).

Moving away from alcohol, there have been multiple instances of drug prohibition resulting in control and stigmatizing marginal segments of societies, seen most

> ## Box 3.3 Influence of social control on heavy use over time
>
> HUOT is subject to high levels of social control, for example as a basis for incarceration, which, it has been argued here and elsewhere, has been used as a tool of social injustice and perpetuates inequalities in societies.

strongly in the USA and Russia but adopted widely throughout the world. The prohibition of recreational opiate use was a means of criminalizing Chinese migrant workers and justifying their poor labour conditions; it has been argued that cannabis prohibition was the tool for subjecting black South Africans in South Africa and Afro-Americans and Latin Americans in the USA; the anti-crack campaign in the 1980s that spread from America to Europe in effect stigmatized subpopulations of poor ethnic minorities, who were able to purchase this cheaper and faster acting form of cocaine but not the more expensive, and less adulterated, powder cocaine (cocaine hydrochloride) that was widely used among some wealthier segments of society (Reinarman and Levine, 1997).

Arguably, then, drug prohibition increases the criminalization of groups who are already stigmatized (e.g. young people, ethnic minorities), whereas 'drug offenses' (particularly possession) within the more 'respectable' segments of society may be much less frequently penalized (Eastwood et al., 2013). As well as the criminalization of users, prohibition leads to an active illegal trade, both within and between nations, with potentially very high rewards and inevitable criminal activity such as violence in the protection of markets. Overall, use and illegal trading of addictive substances becomes one of the major demands on the time and resources of all parts of the criminal justice system, raising ethical questions around the justification for directing resources at such enforcement activities, particularly in times of economic austerity. For example, it is estimated that in 2010, 18.5 per cent of sentenced prisoners in 25 European Union countries (excluding Austria and Poland) were sentenced for a drug-law offence, ranging from less than five per cent (in Romania, Hungary, and Lithuania) to as high as 50 per cent in Greece (EMCDDA, 2014) (nearly as high as the 51% of prisoners reported as incarcerated in the USA between 2009 and 2013 on drug-related offences (Carson, 2014)). Furthermore, the fact that a large majority of these are from ethnic minority backgrounds is both a result and a cause of the marginalization of these groups within societies, which reduces their opportunities for legal economic activity. Given all this, and the readiness with which concern about crime can be stimulated among voters, it is not surprising that the contribution of addictive substances to crime and its control is a major and enduring concern of many governments (see Box 3.3).

3.9 Impact on individual freedom of choice

Ethical philosophy on freedom of choice has a clear and direct bearing on issues of criminalization of drug use. Apart from corporal or capital punishment, there is really no stronger expression of restricting individual choice than prohibiting an action on pain of imprisonment and loss of the right to freedom of movement. The UK philosopher A.C. Grayling (2002) writes that 'One measure of a good society is whether its individual members have the autonomy to do as they choose in respects that principally concern only them' and that 'a society in which such substances are legal and available is a good society not because drugs are in themselves good, but because the autonomy of those who wish to use them is respected'. In this view, in line with a personalist viewpoint, as can be adopted in the arena of public health, to deny an adult human the right to take into his or her body a substance of his or her choosing is to deny an integral part of their personhood, namely their autonomy. This is certainly in line with the respect for autonomy and need to balance it against public benefit which is inherent in the American code of ethics for public health and Nuffield intervention ladder (Thomas et al., 2002; Nuffield Council on Bioethics, 2007).

Supporters of drug prohibition could take up Grayling's modifying clause, arguing that the effects of drug use do not 'principally only concern' the user. Indeed, it is true that the costs of drug use (legal and illegal) for society, including costs incurred by those other than the user, is a field of research at the intersection of economics, epidemiology, and sociology which is rapidly gaining in its evidence base and impact. The clear financial and psychological impacts of HUOT on the family members, and impacts on workplaces (e.g. through reduced productivity or poor decision making) and societies mean that we have to acknowledge that HUOT of addictive substances is not only of concern to the user. However, two further ethical questions then arise: (1) whether the negative impact of incarceration on family members, friends, and co-workers is less or more than that of living with an individual suffering under HUOT; and (2) what the overall objective of incarceration is and whether it is achieved through these means.

From a socioeconomic perspective, we might be able to compare the relative negative impact of incarceration on families, friends, or colleagues of a heavy user against those of living with the heavy user. It is conceivable that the loss of income, lost potential from any training received, and stigma associated with incarceration would be balanced by possible reductions in stress or relief from the threat of violence or accident. Without concrete data, it is not possible to make a convincing comparison. However, any such comparison would not take into account the alternatives to incarceration that might be available, such as treatment or preventive services, and several have argued that the savings the state could make by abolishing the prohibitive drug laws and freeing up resources currently spent on drug offense prisoners (estimated in European countries as between 0.03 and 0.05 per cent of gross domestic product (GDP), on average (EMCDDA, 2014)) could improve provision and access to these services beyond recognition (Transform, 2015).

Regarding the objective of incarcerating people for use of certain psychoactive substances, and accepting that we would require a more egalitarian or inclusive motivation than the suppression of subpopulations in society (as explored in Section 3.8) to justify these prohibitive policies, incarceration has multiple but sometimes muddled purposes. Most straightforwardly, it removes individuals from the social context in which they can harm others. It purportedly aims to provide a deterrent or disincentive to the behaviour for which it is inflicted. It may, optimistically, reduce the opportunities for individuals to harm themselves, and generally has a goal of rehabilitation or therapy (although, in practice, the availability and use of addictive substances is often more widespread *in* prisons than outside, and individuals often leave prisons with heavier habits of use than they had initially).

A less concrete purpose is that incarceration serves as a statement by social authorities, on behalf of society as a whole, of strong public disapproval of the use of certain substances; this 'statement' is presumed to deter the use of these drugs and thereby reduce consumption and consequent harm. The mechanism posited as deterrent is to 'send a message' to potential drug users that the societal system is intolerant of intoxication through these substances (Jenkins, 2014). However, a growing number of political analysts have highlighted evidence that the incarceration of users is not effective in reducing drug use or drug-related harms (Room et al., 2009; Apfel, 2014). In particular, the experience in Portugal, where all drug use was decriminalized in July 2001, illustrates that overall drug-related harms have not increased in the absence of prison sentences for drug use (despite an indication of an increase in cannabis use), and that, indeed, drug market violence appears to have decreased (Hughes and Stevens, 2010; Werb et al., 2011). Some authors argue that as many as 80 per cent of deaths related to drug use can be shown to be caused by prohibition (not including deaths from HIV contracted through risky behaviour in pursuit of drug use) (Ostrowski, 1989) (see Box 3.4).

A major countervailing argument against many potential public health interventions is that they constrain the choices available to individuals. As discussed earlier, alternative social and political stances place different values on the primacy of freedom of choice relative to values of social justice, equality, and other aspects of individual well-being. However, most current systems of social and political philosophy (apart from extreme libertarianism on one hand and some forms of authoritarianism based on claims of divine revelation on the other) would accept that while individual freedom of choice is a major ethical priority, there are some circumstances in which it is justifiable for social authorities to constrain, or seek to direct, individuals' choices.

The ethical arguments surrounding the popular public health approach of 'nudging' (sometimes also called 'stealth' health policy) have been explored by Saghai (2013), following on from the work of Thaler and Sunstein (2008). A typical example of nudging health policy could be placing healthy food options in a cafeteria more within reach or in a more flattering light than unhealthy options. Subtle pricing policies can also be used to nudge consumer choices. Saghai defines the concept of 'nudge' as actions 'designed to pick up efficacious influences that preserve freedom of choice, yet bypass the deliberative capacities of those influenced'; and he clarifies

Box 3.4 Prohibition from an ethical standpoint

From an ethical standpoint, the prohibition of certain drugs and criminalization of users seems not to fulfill any of the requirements in protection of the rights of individuals to freedom of choice, reducing risks, or promoting well-being of communities freedom of choice being preserved only if the choice set is unaltered or expanded compared with baseline (before nudging), and the influence is substantially or fully non-controlling (i.e. can be resisted without effort). One question is how ethical an action that does not explicitly gain the consent of the person influenced by it (by engaging unconscious or automatic cognitive processes) can be—that is, influences that bypass deliberation. Saghai supports the employment of nudges (of benefit to either the one nudging or being nudged, both, or a third party) which involve such unconscious decision making, or, at least, 'shallow cognitive processes', on the condition that they are 'easily resistible', given a normal capacity for attention, decision, and inhibition in the subject (Saghai, 2013).

In considering freedom of choice and HUOT, another set of factors that contribute to ethical discussions, deserves mention; these are the biological and environmental contexts that frame human decision making and necessarily provide a background to any 'free choice' a human being makes.

As will be mentioned in Chapter 4, as organisms we are shaped by evolution to be active agents in our relationship with addictive products; hard wired with preferences for the natural components or sources of drugs, with neurotransmitters that mirror and respond to their active chemical forms. Viewed in this light, freedom of choice faced with addictive products is a little like the freedom of choice an individual has to save their own child or a stranger's in the face of danger.

However, it would require the adoption of an extreme view of biological determinism to argue that this evolutionary predisposition should render individuals incapable of rational free choice in the face of addictive products. A further version of the argument of evolutionary predisposition is that it may apply differently to different individuals, as there is evidence for genetic variability in the propensity to addictive behaviour. Again, this is an argument whose scope may become disturbingly extended as genetic knowledge increases (or a general belief in genetic determinism increases, even on the basis of inadequate evidence).

As discussed in Chapter 2, HUOT of addictive products results in changes in brain function, including decision-making facilities, along with other cognitive and emotional brain functions, which could be said to impact on an individual's capacity to choose freely and without prejudice. In terms of public health ethics, this adds an imperative to the duty of governing bodies to protect citizens who use addictive substances from the increased number of risk factors implied by these brain changes. The selective attention brought about addictive substances in those who use them early in development or heavily over time also means that the marketing techniques routinely employed by corporate actors can dramatically increase desire, availability, and use of these substances, to the extent that exposure to marketing can be identified as a leading risk factor for increased use and harm, warranting state intervention to protect health (see Box 3.5).

Similarly, fashion (social and peer pressure) in this domain (especially in the direction of increasing use) has a strong determining effect, and can be seen as a risk factor to be addressed and reduced through public health measures in social settings (such as school programmes, public campaigns, and interventions to reduce intergenerational transfer of HUOT habits).

> ## Box 3.5 'Nudging' and freedom of choice
>
> Individuals' right to freedom of choice is similarly affected by private producing and retailer companies' marketing techniques, as well as 'nudging' public health policies.

3.10 **Influence from the corporate sector**

Grayling is on record as calling for governments to 'legalise currently illegal substances under the same kinds of regime that govern nicotine and alcohol' (Grayling, 2002). It should be pointed out, however, that the current regimes for regulating tobacco and alcohol have some shortfalls in terms of effectiveness in reducing harm, often owing to a strong degree of influence from the corporate sector on policy; and which is, in part, owing to the revenue that governments receive from taxes on these legal addictive products.

Significant lobbying efforts are made by corporate actors on behalf of their organizations and industry as a whole to reduce the restrictive legislation put into place by governments and push instead for self-governance or voluntary guidelines, sometimes in the frame of so called 'public–private partnership' approaches. In terms of ethics, the primary problem we can see with such partnerships and self-regulation is that the overarching goals of public health and private enterprise are fundamentally and profoundly misaligned, with incentives for each pulling in contrary directions. While the duty of public health organizations is to the well-being if its population, the corporations have a duty to maximize profits for their shareholders (that, in some countries, e.g. Sweden, can include the government). In the case of those industries producing harmful addictive products, maximizing profits has the side effect of damaging the well-being of large swathes of society (Moodie et al., 2013).

One of the nominal harm prevention approaches of the private sector has been the development of corporate social responsibility (CSR) strategies. In business terms, these exist to raise the profile of the company and enhance trust among consumers. Therefore, it has been argued that there is an inherent ethical conflict in CSR activities as to whether raising the profile with the aim of selling more of a harmful product could ever be justified as 'socially responsible'. One exception could be eliminating harmful components of the products or enhancing sales of less addictive alternatives, but there are scarce examples of this. It is notable that the CSR initiatives undertaken by enterprises are hardly ever robustly evaluated, and where convincing studies on effectiveness exist, have never been shown to reduce use or harm from products (Baumberg et al., 2014).

Finally, it is worth noting that the corporate interests in addictive products reach far beyond the production of products themselves. For instance, it has been highlighted that the arms industry and prison services and supplies are the main sectors that profit from the large number of people incarcerated on drug-related charges,

Box 3.6 Corporate interest and influence

A web of corporate entities are supported by different aspects of the heavy use of addictive products over time and affected by public policy on these in different sectors (health, economy, trade, and others), and there are considerable financial interests at stake. Consequently, these companies act to exert a great deal of influence on public policy and preserve their interests.

with a very significant financial interest in the growth of the prison industry and increasing number of prisoners (Harcourt, 2012) (see Box 3.6).

3.11 Stigma and discrimination

Inequalities are important in that they impact on well-being (Stiglitz, 2002; Wilkinson and Picket, 2011), in particular where stigma is attached to the disadvantaged groups. We have already indicated how drug and alcohol policy can contribute to inequalities, and therefore to social injustice and to reduced well-being. Although it is widely agreed that stigma and discrimination have a negative net value on population well-being, there is a possible ethical tension. Stigma can contribute to the positive effect of a policy intervention by making HUOT of addictive products a less desirable behaviour (acting as a disincentive), while at the same time it also clearly detracts from the individual well-being of those suffering the stigma and discrimination (in both psychological and practical terms—reduced self-esteem, poorer provision of and access to services, and lesser financial and occupational opportunities). Stigmatization also contributes to under-presenting of HUOT problems to healthcare and counselling, and to reduced help-seeking behaviour by those who could benefit from assistance to reduce their heavy use (Wallhed Finn et al., 2014).

3.12 A well-being framework as an ethical basis for prevention of harm

For over a decade, there has been a growing sense that the reliance on GDP as measure of progress for societies is neither comprehensive nor ethically valid, placing too much emphasis on the material wealth at the expense of recognition of the damaging effects of inequalities and other non-material aspects. Well-being has been proposed as an alternative indicator of progress, but, until recently, the concept remained unclear at the societal level (Seaford, 2011). An objective and considered framework for evaluating the effects of public health measures requires us to consider the components of societal well-being in its broadest sense.

Figure 3.1 illustrates a framework put forward by the Organisation for Economic Co-operation and Development (OECD)—How's Life? (OECD, 2011). The OECD framework considers societal well-being as a state with three different dimensions. Two of the dimensions—quality of life and material living conditions—relate to

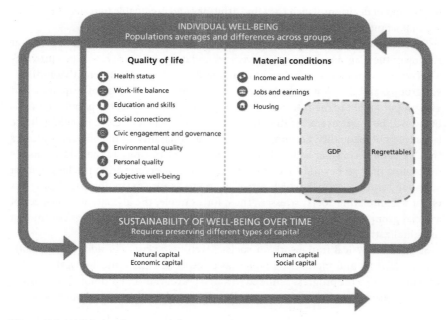

Figure 3.1 Well-being framework for measuring progress.
GDP: gross domestic product. Reproduced with permission from OECD, 'Measuring Well-being and Progress: Well-being Research', Copyright © 2011 Organisation for Economic Co-operation and Development, http://www.oecd.org/statistics/measuring-well-being-and-progress.htm, accessed 01 Nov. 2015.

human well-being, and the third dimension—preserving different types of capital—relates to sustainability of well-being over time. Within each dimension, there are a number of different elements. Within the dimension quality of life is the element subjective well-being, which can be measured by a number of validated instruments. Finally, as the OECD frame illustrates, there is not only an overlap between material living conditions and GDP, but also an area, termed *regrettables*, which, while contributing to GDP does not enhance well-being. While this model does not stipulate the relative weight of various components, the online tool allows these weights to be set according to individual preference. However, in its static form, the model is valuable in highlighting the range of elements that must be considered. It is notable that the 'quality of life' variables are more numerous and more diverse than the material indicators that are most readily quantified by economists. The authors of the framework define societal progress as occurring when 'there is an improvement in the "sustainable and equitable well-being of a society"' (OECD, 2012).

In our discussions here we have placed considerable emphasis on 'freedom of choice' and 'autonomy' as important individual elements in well-being. They do not appear under these names in the OECD scheme. Nonetheless 'Civic Engagement and Governance' may be considered as involving people's sense that they have a role in decisions which affect them and are satisfied with their relationship with law and government; and 'Personal Security' must include people's protection from the imposition of decisions which they find arbitrary and are unable to resist. Both these are important components of autonomy and freedom.

Two other elements in the OECD scheme should be noted. First, the caption at the top of the diagram ('Population averages and difference across groups') provides a necessary reminder that factors affecting well-being will act differently on different groups, and decision making needs to be aware of this range of responses and give proper weight to their diversity, while also recognizing that the population well-being will be lower overall if the differences in components across groups indicate large levels of inequality. Second, the box on 'Sustainability' at the bottom expresses that we cannot consider well-being at a single point in time. Rather, decisions we make now may go beyond their immediate effects in determining the longer-term social and human capital, which serves as the basis for continuing social progress or for accumulating social stresses. Thus, for example, the alienation or neglect of a social group may be transmitted inter-generationally to determine its continuing marginalization in the future.

Such an analytical framework for societal well-being could be adopted by public health planners and monitoring bodies as a respectful and ethically tactical value system by which the progress achieved through prevention and promotion initiatives can be measured, and also adjusted to allow for variable contexts and political value systems.

3.13 Maximizing well-being: an inverted U-shaped curve

The discussion in this chapter makes clear that the range of governmental health interventions do not have a simple linear relation to the outcome in terms of well-being. Greater intervention does not simply translate into greater population effects and reductions of harm. The fact that a particular measure may improve well-being through reduced HUOT does not necessarily mean that stronger application of the same principle would be ethically justified. Nor does the fact that a public health measure may reduce a positive value, such as individual autonomy, provide an inevitable argument against establishing or extending such a measure. Rather, almost any measure is likely to have opposing effects on different aspects of well-being for different groups of society, and the balance of these effects provides a difficult problem for ethical calculus.

The knowledge base and level of evidence on public health measures in relation to any particular addictive product interacts with ethical tenets in policy decision making. This can be seen quite clearly in recent scientific and political debates around decisions of how to regulate and whether to allow the sale of electronic nicotine delivery systems (ENDS) in different countries around the world. Hall et al. (2015) argue that in considering basic principles of autonomy, beneficence, non-maleficence and justice, there is little ethical basis for a ban on ENDS. Their main points centre on the rights of smokers to switch to a less harmful alternative to tobacco, lack of demonstrable protection from ENDS as a result of bans on sales, and international inequalities between those countries where ENDS sales are permitted and those where they are prohibited. Respondents to these arguments point out the paucity of evidence for ENDS as an effective means to reducing tobacco use or cessation, and the fact that a great deal of further research is needed to identify and quantify potential harm from ENDS. The potential of ENDS to act as a gateway behavior to smoking is also important to ethical considerations of legislation and regulation of their sales (Chapman and Daube, 2015). This is also an area where corporate interests and influence is unclear, with ENDS representing both a potential competing market and emerging market for tobacco companies and all those who stand to benefit from their sales (Chapman and Daube, 2015) (see Box 3.7).

At the other end of the intervention ladder from incarceration, where the regulatory powers of the state are minimized (because of the dominance of corporate interests and the free market, for example), the effect must be the increase of harm through an increase of HUOT of addictive products, particularly among those who are most vulnerable, while any benefits of increased autonomy at this limit will be minimal. Thus, the function relating well-being to the level of intervention is an inverted U-shaped curve, with a maximum outcome of well-being at some intermediate point (see Figure 3.2).

The position of the optimal point of maximum societal well-being (the top of the arc) depends on the relative value placed on different components of well-being, a balance that will vary with cultural and historical factors that will surely differ between societies and vary over time. Ethical decisions are further complicated by the fact that societies are not homogeneous; it is likely that the benefits and penalties of any given intervention will accrue differently to different social and demographic groups. This problem is exacerbated by the fact that the interests of the marginalized and stigmatized groups, who suffer much of the harm associated with HUOT, are unlikely to be expressed loudest or most forcefully, or most readily appreciated by those actively engaged in governance and decision making. Nonetheless, it would be damaging to see the problems as ones of competing interest groups. The harms of HUOT, and the benefits of effective interventions, should be seen as applying to society as a whole, as what is at stake is the cohesion and common purpose of a society based on mutual respect and equal rights for all its members.

Box 3.7 Questioning criminalization

If we adopt a well-being framework, we immediately have to call into question the criminalization of activity arising from HUOT (i.e. taking illicit drugs), for the reason that prison time detracts so greatly from individual and population well-being and contributes so strongly to entrenching stigma and discrimination, leading to a negative iterative cycle (stigma detracting from well-being, which, in turn, detracts from emotional/social/economic capital, leading to increased drug use, etc.).

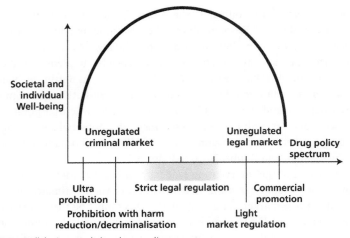
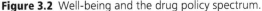

Figure 3.2 Well-being and the drug policy spectrum.
Adapted with permission from Transform: Getting drugs under control. *How to regulate Cannabis: A practical guide.* Bristol, UK: Transform Drug Policy Foundation, Copyright © 2014 Transform Drug Policy Foundation, http://www.tdpf.org.uk/resources/publications/how-regulate-cannabis-practical-guide, accessed 01 Nov. 2015.

3.14 **Conclusions**

Specific characteristics of the heavy use over time of addictive products, such as the recognition of this behaviour as a lifestyle choice, the wide variety of sectors in which the determinants and impacts of HUOT can be found, the particular effects of heavy use on an individual's decision-making faculties, and the unparalleled web of corporate and criminal interests that surround the products themselves, mean that the regulation of this behaviour in the population is subject to some very unique ethical considerations. Adopting a well-being framework for drug policy, where regulations and legislation are created with the aim of maximizing population well-being and capital, can be seen as an effort to ensure that citizens and societies are treated ethically with regard to this behaviour.

However, if we adopt a well-being framework, we immediately have to call into question criminalization and incarceration penalties for the consumption of psychoactive drugs which lead to their heavy use, given that prison time detracts so greatly from well-being and contributes to entrenching stigma and discrimination.

References

Apfel F (2014) AR Policy Brief 5—Cannabis—From Prohibition to Regulation 'When the Music Changes so Does the Dance'. ALICE RAP Policy Paper Series. Available at: http://www.alicerap.eu/resources/documents/doc_download/185-policy-paper-5-cannabis-from-prohibition-to-regulation.html (accessed 2 July 2015).

Baumberg B, Cuzzocrea V, Morini S, Ortoleva P, Disley E, Tzvetkova M, et al. (2014) ALICE RAP deliverable 11.2: corporate social responsibility. Available at: http://www.alicerap.eu/resources/documents/doc_download/209-deliverable-11-2-corporate-social-responsibility.html (accessed 6 September 2016).

Berridge V (2014) Drugs, alcohol, and the First World War. *Lancet* **384**: 1840–1.

Carson EA (2014) *Prisoners in 2013*. NCJ247282. Washington, DC: US Dept of Justice Bureau of Justice Statistics.

Chapman S and Daube M (2015) Ethical imperatives assuming ENDS effectiveness and safety are fragile. *Addiction* **110**: 1068–9.

Duménil G and Lévy D (2004). *Capital Resurgent: Roots of the Neoliberal Revolution*. Boston, MA: Harvard University Press.

Eastwood N, Shiner M, and Bear D (2013) The Numbers in Black and White: Ethnic Disparities in the Policing and Prosecution of Drug Offences in England and Wales. Available at: http://www.release.org.uk/sites/default/files/pdf/publications/Release%20-%20Race%20Disparity%20Report%20final%20version.pdf (accessed 8 June 2015).

EMCDDA (2014) *Estimating Public Expenditure on Drug-law Offenders in Prison in Europe*. EMCDDA Papers. Luxembourg: Publications Office of the European Union.

Gornall J (2014) Alcohol and public health. Under the influence. *BMJ* **348**: f7646.

Grayling AC (2002) Why a high society is a free society. Available at: https://www.theguardian.com/observer/drugs/story/0,,718157,00.html (accessed 8 June 2015).

Gusfield JR (1986) *Symbolic Crusade. Status Politics and the American Temperance Movement*, 2nd edition. Urbana and Chicago, IL: University of Illinois Press.

Hall W, Gartner C, and Forlini C (2015) Ethical issues raised by a ban on the sale of electronic nicotine devices. *Addiction* **110**: 1061–7.

Harcourt B (2012) *The Illusion of Free Markets: Punishment and the Myth of Natural Order*. Boston, MA: Harvard University Press.

Holmes J, Meng Y, Meier PS, Brennan A, Angus C, Campbell-Burton A, and Purshouse RC (2014) Effects of minimum unit pricing for alcohol on different income and socioeconomic groups: a modelling study. *Lancet* **383**: 1655–64.

Hughes CE and Stevens A (2010) What can we learn from the Portuguese decriminalization of illicit drugs? *Br J Criminol* **50**: 999–1022.

Jenkins S (2014) Ministers high on their war on drugs need a speedy cure. Available at: http://www.theguardian.com/commentisfree/2014/nov/01/ministers-war-on-drugs-policy-british (accessed 7 July 2015).

Locke J (1700) *An Essay Concerning Human Understanding*. London: Elizabeth Holt.

Mill JS (1859) On liberty. In: Collini S (ed.) *On Liberty and Other Essays* (1989). Cambridge: Cambridge University Press, pp. 5–91.

Moodie R, Stuckler D, Monteiro C, Sheron N, Neal B, Thamarangsi T, and Lancet NCD Action Group (2013) Profits and pandemics: prevention of harmful effects of tobacco, alcohol, and ultra-processed food and drink industries. *Lancet* **381**: 670–9.

Moskalewicz J and Klingemann JI (2015) Addictive substances and behaviours and social justice. In: Anderson P, Rehm J, and Room R (eds) *The Impact of Addictive Substances and Behaviours on Individual and Societal Well-being*. Volume 2 in series: Governance of Addictive Substances and Behaviours. Oxford: Oxford University Press, pp. 143–60

Neiburg TS and Shannon DR (1999) Entry: Principle. In: *Encyclopedia of Ethics*. New York: Facts on File, pp. 218–20.

New Economics Foundation (NEF). (n.d.) Our work: wellbeing. Available at: http://www.neweconomics.org/issues/entry/well-being (accessed 7 July 2015).

Nuffield Council on Bioethics (2007) *Public Health: Ethical Issues*. London: Nuffield Council on Bioethics.

OECD (2011) *How's Life?: Measuring Well-being*. Paris: OECD Publishing.

OECD Better Life Index (2012) How's life? Available at: http://www.oecdbetterlifeindex.org/ (accessed 7 July 20150.

Ostrowski J (1989) The moral and practical case for drug legalization. *Hofstra L Rev* **18**: 607.

Petrini C and Gainotti S (2008) A personalist approach to public health ethics. *Bull World Health Organ* **86**: 624–9.

Rehm J, Marmet S, Anderson P, Gual A, Kraus L, Nutt DJ, et al. (2013) Defining substance use disorders: do we really need more than heavy use? *Alcohol Alcohol* **48**: 633–40.

Reinarman C and Levine HG (1997). *Crack in America: Demon Drugs and Social Justice*. Berkeley, CA: University of California Press.

Room R, Hall W, Reuter P, Fischer B, and Lenton S (2009) Global Cannabis Commission Report. Beckley Foundation. Available at: http://www.beckleyfoundation.org/2012/01/ global-cannabis-commission-report/ (accessed 7 July 2015).

Saghai Y (2013) Salvaging the concept of nudge. *J Med Ethics* **38**: 487–93.

Seaford C (2011) Policy: time to legislate for the good life. *Nature* **477**: 532–3.

Shield KD and Rehm J (2015) The effects of addictive substances and addictive behaviours on physical and mental health. In: Anderson P, Rehm J, and Room R (eds) *The Impact of Addictive Substances and Behaviours on Individual and Societal Well-being*. Oxford: Oxford University Press, pp. 77–118.

Stiglitz JE (2002) Employment, social justice and societal well-being. *Int Labour Rev* **141**: 9–29.

Thaler RH and Sunstein CR (2008) *Nudge: Improving Decisions About Health, Wealth, and Happiness*. New Haven, CT: Yale University Press.

Thomas JC, Sage M, Dillenberg J, and Guillory VJ (2002) A code of ethics for public health. *Am J Public Health* **92**: 1057–9.

Transform (2014) *How to Regulate Cannabis: A Practical Guide*. Bristol: Transform Drug Policy Foundation.

Transform (2015) The benefits of legal regulation. Available at: http://www.tdpf.org.uk/ resources/benefits-legal-regulation (accessed 7 July 2015).

Wallhed Finn S, Bakshi AS, and Andréasson S (2014) Alcohol consumption, dependence, and treatment barriers: perceptions among nontreatment seekers with alcohol dependence. *Subst Use Misuse* **49**: 762–9.

Werb D, Rowell G, Guyatt G, Kerr T, Montaner J, and Wood E (2011) Effect of drug law enforcement on drug market violence: a systematic review. *Int J Drug Policy* **22**: 87–94.

Wilkinson R and Pickett K (2011) *The Spirit Level: Why Greater Equality Makes Societies Stronger*. New York: Bloomsbury Publishing USA.

Chapter 4

Drivers of the harm done by drugs

4.1 Introduction

In this chapter, we describe the main drivers of the harm done by drugs, and give some illustrations. The drivers are grouped at three levels: structural drivers of harm, core drivers of harm, and the policies and measures that can influence the core drivers. We will introduce the health footprint as a concept and metric that apportions harm across the structural and core drivers and the policies and measures that affect them. The molecular, individual, and societal determinants of risky drug use, harmful drug use, and transitions out of heavy use over time have been recently reviewed (Gell et al., 2016).

Structural drivers of harm include biological attributes and functions, population size and structure, and levels of wealth and income disparities within jurisdictions (see Figure 4.1). The harm done by psychoactive substances, captured by the health footprint, can be decomposed by population size (e.g. countries), population structure (e.g. age), gross domestic product (GDP; high- and low-income countries), and income disparities (inequalities indices). The structural drivers all determine the size of the health footprint, which, in turn, is influenced by biological attributes and functions (e.g. genes and 'hard-wiring' in the brain).

Core drivers refer to the processes, mechanisms, and characteristics that influence harm, sometimes through the structural drivers, and sometimes not. Core drivers include drug potency and drug exposure, and the technological developments that might influence them, and social influences and attitudes. Included in the policies and measures level are policies that reduce drug exposure, actions that promote research and development to reduce drug potency, co-benefits, and adverse side effects of policies and measures, incentivizing healthy individual behaviour, and defining and applying rules of engagement of the private sector under regulating the private sector. Policies and measures affect the core drivers. The structural and core drivers may, in turn, influence policies and measures.

At the centre of the interconnections is the health footprint, the accounting system for identifying the determinants of drug-related harm and the management tool to evaluate opportunities by the public and private sectors and civil society to reduce harm. The health footprint can measure the impact of a range of structural and core drivers of impaired health and the policies and measures that impact upon them, thus accounting for who and what causes the harm done by drugs.

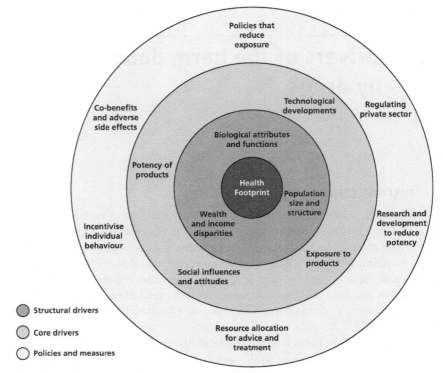

Figure 4.1 Drivers of harm done by drugs.

4.2 **Structural drivers of harm**

In this section, we give some illustrations of the impact of biological attributes and functions, population size and structure, and levels of wealth and income disparities within jurisdictions.

4.2.1 **Biological attributes and functions**

4.2.1.1 Hard-wiring that seeks out nicotine and other neurotoxins

There is archaeological and anthropological evidence of ubiquitous use of drugs throughout human prehistory, including nicotine from tobacco and pituri plants, cocaine from coca plants, arecoline from betel nut, and ephedrine from khat (Sullivan and Hagen, 2015). Biological evidence also points to a long-time co-evolutionary relationship of these neurotoxins between plants and animals. Most plant species have evolved defensive strategies that punish herbivores that feed on them. Among these strategies are psychoactive plant-based drugs that have evolved to interfere with signalling in the central and peripheral nervous systems. These drugs interfere with neurotransmitter synthesis, storage, release, binding, and re-uptake; receptor activation and function; and key enzymes involved in signal transduction (see Sullivan and Hagen, 2015).

In response to the evolution of chemical defences in plants, plant-eating animals have co-evolved a number of countermeasures and beneficial adaptations to the plant toxins. One example is nicotine, where there is evidence for plant-eating animals to exploit actively nicotine for defence mechanisms against their own parasites. For example, whereas hornworm caterpillars non-parasitized by wasp larvae survive better on a nicotine-free than a nicotine-containing diet, caterpillars parasitized by wasp larvae survive better on a nicotine-containing than a nicotine-free diet (see Ode, 2006). The ability of animals to exploit plant toxins as a beneficial adaptation does not imply positive or good attributes of the toxin. In the above example, the toxin remains poisonous to the caterpillar, and the cost-benefit ratio of the effects of toxicity becomes positive only when the caterpillar is itself parasitized. The neurotoxin is exploited because it is toxic.

A present-day example is illustrated by Congo basin hunter–gatherers, among whom the quantity of cigarettes smoked is titrated against intestinal worm burden— the higher the worm burden, the greater the number of cigarettes smoked. Further, when treated with the anti-worm drug, abendazole, the number of cigarettes smoked is reduced (Roulette et al., 2014).

4.2.1.2 Hard-wiring that seeks out ethanol

There is also evidence to suggest that humans are hard-wired to seek out ethanol. The presence of ethanol within ripe fruit suggests low-level but chronic dietary exposure for all fruit-eating animals, with volatilized alcohols from fruit potentially serving in olfactory localization of nutritional resources (Dudley, 2014). The same seems to apply to humans, also fruit-eating animals, as, whereas primate ancestors living 16–21 million years ago could not effectively metabolize consumed ethanol, by 6–12 million years ago, human's last common ancestor with gorillas and chimpanzees had evolved a digestion fully capable of metabolizing consumed ethanol, at levels found in fermenting fruits (Benner, 2013).

Ecological analyses thus suggest that we humans are active and functional in relation to the drugs that we take, rather than being passive and vulnerable. Despite their toxicity, we are hard-wired to seek them out. This implies, on the one hand, that prohibition is likely to fail, because drug use is not 'caused' by biological frailty in people in general; and, in the context of this chapter implies, on the other hand, that, at the individual level, potency and exposure are likely to be prime drivers of drug use and related harm.

4.2.1.3 An example of genetic influence: *ADH1B* rs1229984

A genetic variant in a gene (*ADH1B* rs1229984) affects an enzyme that metabolizes alcohol in the body, and is associated with lower levels of alcohol consumption and risks of heavy drinking. As variants in the *ADH1B* gene lead to increased levels of the carcinogen acetaldehyde, heavy drinkers who carry the variant have increased risk of gastrointestinal cancers (see Shield and Rehm, 2015). However, at the same time, there is evidence that variants in the gene can protect against cardiovascular disease. A large study of 260,000 European individuals compared the cardiovascular health outcomes of people with the genetic variant gene with those without (Holmes et al.,

2014). One in 14 Europeans carry the altered gene. Across all levels of alcohol consumption, drinkers with the variant consumed, on average, 17 per cent less alcohol than drinkers without the variant.

Compared with drinkers who did not have the gene variant, drinkers who had the gene variant were less likely to have high blood pressure, coronary heart disease, and ischaemic stroke. The analyses called into question alcohol's effect in reducing the risk of coronary heart diseases. From the J-shaped association between alcohol consumption and risk of coronary heart disease seen in observational studies, one would expect that for drinkers below the nadir (20 grams of alcohol daily), a reduction of 17.2 per cent in alcohol consumption corresponding to rs1229984 A-allele carriage would lead to a small increase in the risk of coronary heart disease, whereas for those with alcohol consumption above the nadir, a similar reduction in alcohol consumption would lead to a decrease in coronary heart disease risk. Contrary to these expectations, individuals drinking below the nadir with a genetic predisposition to consume less alcohol had lower odds of developing coronary heart disease at all categories of alcohol consumption (see Box 4.1).

4.2.2 Population size and structure

As an illustration of the impact of population size and structure as drivers of harm, we give examples of disability-adjusted life years (DALYs) due to tobacco and alcohol (Lim et al., 2012). Between 1990 and 2010, the absolute worldwide number of tobacco-related DALYs increased from 151.8 million to 156.8 million, and alcohol-related DALYs from 73.7 million to 97.2 million. However, when correcting for changes in population size and structure, the global burden of tobacco use decreased from 3379 DALYs per 100,000 people in 1990 to 2385 DALYs per 100,000 people in 2010, and the burden of alcohol use decreased from 1636 DALYs per 100,000 people in 1990 to 1444 DALYs per 100,000 people in 2010. These data illustrate that when correcting for changes in population structure between 1990 and 2010, DALYs per 100,000 people decreased between 1990 and 2010. However, overall, because population structures changed over this time, the absolute burden of ill health and premature death from tobacco and alcohol increased.

4.2.3 Levels of wealth and income disparities

On the one hand, as sociodemographic status improves in lower-income countries, so do years lived with disability increase from mental and substance use disorders

Box 4.1 Structural drivers of harm

The genetic make-up, and the size, structure, and wealth of populations are all structural drivers of harm that need to be taken into account when considering the impact of the underlying drivers of harm done by drugs, and the policies and measures that impact on them.

(GBD 2013 DALYs and HALE Collaborators, 2015); on the other hand, between and within countries people with lower incomes suffer more from the harm done by drugs than people with higher incomes (Room et al., 2015).

For example, as GDP increases, per capita adult alcohol consumption increases, at least up to a GDP of US$10,000 (adjusted by purchasing power parity), largely driven by abstainers starting to drink (Schmidt et al., 2010). For the same amount of alcohol consumed, people who live in lower-income regions of the world have higher alcohol-related deaths and DALYs than people who live in higher-income regions of the world (Room et al., 2015). The same applies within countries; for the same amount of alcohol consumed, people with lower incomes have higher alcohol-related deaths than people with higher incomes (Room et al., 2015). Similarly, smoking prevalence is expected to increase in low-income countries (Bilano et al., 2015), and, within countries, poorer people tend to smoke more than richer people and are more likely to die from smoking than richer people (see Hosseinpoor et al., 2012).

4.3 **Core drivers of harm**

In this section, we describe the potency and exposure of products, technological developments to reduce potency, and social influences and attitudes as drivers of exposure and harm.

4.3.1 **Drug potency**

One way to express potency, used by toxicologists and those who assess safety of consumed products, is the benchmark dose (BMD) (Crump, 1984; World Health Organization 2009). BMD10 is the benchmark dose in which an adverse event (commonly death) occurs in ten per cent of subjects (commonly animals) given a one-off dose of the drug. BMD10 is normally calculated from LD_{50} (lethal dose), the amount of a material, given all at once, that causes the death of 50 per cent (one-half) of a group of test animals, by dividing LD_{50} by 10.2. BMD10 is expressed as a mean with 95 per cent confidence interval (CI). The 'L' in BMDL10 indicates that the chosen value is the lower level of the 95% CI. The lower dose is taken for precautionary reasons. Thus, BMDL10 is the dose at the lower level of the 95% CI at which ten per cent of animals taking that dose in one go die.

The BMDL10 has been estimated for a range of drugs and is summarized in Table 4.1 (Lachenmeier and Rehm , 2015).

For an adult weighing 70 kg, the BMDL10 works out at 0.14 grams for heroin, 0.21 grams for nicotine, and 37.3 grams for alcohol. Thus, the quantity of drug in a standard unit of consumption (injection volume of heroin, nicotine content of an e-cigarette, or standard package of alcohol (beer can)) is a powerful, but modifiable, driver of harm.

4.3.2 **Drug exposure**

The harm from consuming drugs is a combination of potency and exposure. Exposures have been calculated for daily doses among European adult users and are summarized in Table 4.2 (Lachenmeier et al., 2015).

Table 4.1 Average BMDL10 for a range of drugs*

Drug	Average BMDL10 extrapolated from LD50 (mg/kg body weight)
Heroin	2
Cocaine	2
Nicotine	3
Amphetamine	7
Methadone	8
Methamphetamine	8
Diazepam	27
MDMA	32
THC	56
Alcohol	531

MDMA: 3,4-methylenedioxymethamphetamine;
THC: tetrahydrocannabinol.

*BMD10 is the benchmark dose in which an adverse event (commonly death) occurs in ten per cent of subjects (commonly animals) given a one-off dose of the drug.

Adapted with permission from Macmillan Publishers Ltd: *Scientific Reports*, Volume 5, Article 8126, Lachenmeier DW and Rehm J. Comparative risk assessment of alcohol, tobacco, cannabis and other illicit drugs using the margin of exposure approach, Copyright © 2015 Macmillan Publishers Limited.

Table 4.2 Estimates of daily drug exposure among European adults

Drug	Range (low–high) of individual daily dosage (mg)
Heroin	5–300
Cocaine	20–100
Nicotine	1.65–1.89 mg/cigarette 10–20 cigarretes/smoker/day
Amphetamine	5–50
Methadone	10–40
Methamphetamine	5–150
Diazepam	5–40
MDMA	50–700
THC	10–60
Alcohol	13.6–54.4 g (1–4 standard drinks)

MDMA: 3,4-methylenedioxymethamphetamine; THC: tetrahydrocannabinol.

Adapted with permission from Macmillan Publishers Ltd: *Scientific Reports*, Volume 5, Article 8126, Lachenmeier DW and Rehm J. Comparative risk assessment of alcohol, tobacco, cannabis and other illicit drugs using the margin of exposure approach, Copyright © 2015 Macmillan Publishers Limited.

Knowing both the potency through the benchmark dose and the exposure estimated from surveys, the margin of exposure (MOE) can be calculated as follows:

$$\text{Margin of exposure} \ (\text{MOE}) = \frac{\text{Benchmark dose}}{\text{Exposure}}$$

The MOE is the ratio of the benchmark dose divided by the exposure dose. A MOE of 100 means that an individual is consuming 1/100th of the benchmark dose (defined in Section 4.3.1 the dose that kills 10% of animals when taken in one go). A MOE of 1 means that the individual is consuming the benchmark dose. Toxicology-based risk assessment uses different MOE thresholds as guidelines, depending on whether the benchmark dose is derived from animal or human studies. For example, for carcinogens in food products, when derived from animal studies, MOEs should be higher than 10,000, whereas when derived from human studies they should be higher than 1000 (EFSA, 2005). Differing MOEs are often set for differing health outcomes, with lower MOEs for non-cancer outcomes than for cancer outcomes.

According to the typical interpretation of MOEs derived from animal experiments (i.e. as in Table 4.1), MOE < 10 is judged to pose 'high risk', while MOE < 100 are judged as 'risk'. MOEs above 100 are often judged as acceptable because the value of 100 corresponds to the default 100-fold uncertainty factor, which has been historically used in regulatory toxicology. The factor of 100 is based on scientific judgement and represents the product of two separate tenfold factors that allow for interspecies differences and human variability (EFSA, 2005; WHO, 2009). When the toxicological endpoint is based on human data and not on animal experiments as has been done for alcohol in relation to liver cirrhosis (Lachenmeier et al., 2011), MOEs above 10 would be judged acceptable and MOEs below 1 as 'high risk'.

MOEs have been estimated for European populations and are summarized in Figure 4.2 for individuals based on mean daily intake of users (Lachenmeier et al., 2015).

For individual European users, nicotine has a margin of exposure of 7.5 (95% CI 2.7–14.0), heroin 2.2 (95% CI 0.5–8.2), and alcohol 1.3 (95% CI 0.6–2.7). In other words, nicotine users are using the drug at a level of 7.5 times the benchmark dose, heroin users twice, and alcohol users just over the benchmark dose. That alcohol has a lower MOE (and thus more risky) than heroin is simply owing to the high dose that individual alcohol users take on average (see Box 4.2).

Drug policies could thus be evaluated for their impact on MOE, with a target that all policies should achieve MOEs of 100 or 10, depending on the BMDL10 data source (animal or human). Policies could achieve their result by either reducing exposure or the potency of the consumed product through technological development of less potent drugs or less amount of the drug in the standard ingestion unit.

An alternative metric is simply risk of death, and this has been considered for alcohol, where the risk of dying from alcohol before the age of 70 years increases for both men and women with increasing levels of grams of alcohol consumed per day, such that the risk of death reaches 1 in 100 just after a consumption of 20 grams per day (Rehm et al., 2014). Many involuntary risks, such as unsafe water provided to a

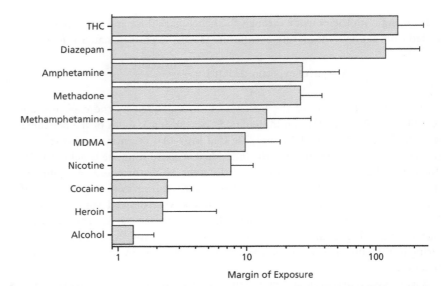

Figure 4.2 Margin of exposure for daily drug use estimated using probabilistic analysis. THC: tetrahydrocannabinol; MDMA: 3,4-methylenedioxymethamphetamine. Reproduced with permission from Lachenmeier DW and Rehm J. Comparative risk assessment of alcohol, tobacco, cannabis and other illicit drugs using the margin of exposure approach. *Scientific Reports*, Volume 5, Article 8126, Copyright © 2015 Macmillan Publishers Limited.

household, have risk thresholds set at 1 in 1 million (e.g. Hunter and Fewtrell, 2001). For voluntary risks, the public seems willing to accept voluntary risks roughly 1000 times greater than involuntary risks (Starr, 1969). By this standard, an acceptable risk for voluntary risks experienced by drug users is 1 in 1000 deaths for the pattern of behaviour over a lifetime. For alcohol this would be about 2 grams a day, similar to a MOE of 10, which for European drinkers is about 3 grams a day, in other words 10–15 times less than current exposure.

Box 4.2 Potency and exposure to drugs

Both the potency of and the exposure to drugs are powerful underlying drivers of harm. They are related to each other through margins of exposure (MOE) that measures the ratio of the benchmark dose that causes harm divided by the exposure dose of the drug. It is suggested that no drug policy should result in an MOE of less than 10, when the benchmark dose is based on human data. This implies that European adults should not consume more than 3.9 g of alcohol per day (less than three drinks a week), 16 mg of heroin per day, or 12 mg of cocaine a day. These dosages are still in a risk category but would exclude a high risk of mortality.

4.3.3 **Technological developments**

Harm from psychoactive drugs can also result for modes of drug delivery. The classic example here is nicotine—while nicotine itself is not a harm-free drug, over the last 100 years the harm has largely derived from its mode of delivery, smoked tobacco. Nicotine replacement therapies (gums, patches, etc.) have been used as treatment products to quit smoking rather than replacement products to smoked tobacco. Technological developments have now led to electronic nicotine delivery systems (ENDS; e-cigarettes) as widespread alternative delivery systems to smoked tobacco, with best estimates showing e-cigarettes to be 95 per cent less harmful to health than smoked cigarettes (see McNeill et al., 2015). There is much debate over their regulatory framework, bordering between regulations for medicinal products, tobacco products, or general product safety rules (see McNeill et al., 2015).

Margins of exposure analyses can be used to clarify the approach. For example, analyses of German e-cigarette liquids found that tobacco-specific toxicants and trace nicotine impurities were below levels likely to cause harm, suggesting that at least, from this perspective, e-cigarettes are likely to be less harmful than smoked tobacco (Hahn et al., 2014). Analyses of nicotine, glycerol, 1,2-propanediol, ethylene glycol, 1,3-propanediol, thujone, and ethyl vanillin found that nicotine was the only compound for which the complete distribution was below a MOE of 10, and on average below 0.1. From all other compounds, only ethylene glycol may have reached MOEs below 100 in about 50 per cent of cases and 1,2-propanediol in worst cases. This indicates that it is nicotine that is the toxic drug in e-cigarettes. Nicotine levels can be set, regulated, and monitored (see Box 4.3).

Opponents of ENDS are worried that ENDS are additive or gateway products to smoked tobacco, rather than replacement products (see discussion in Chapter 3). However, the evidence does not support this (see McNeill et al., 2015). And, in any case, incentives can be set (e.g. through price and availability) that steer use towards ENDS and away from smoked tobacco.

4.3.4 **Social influences and attitudes**

Social influences and attitudes are drivers of drug-related harm. Humans are hardwired social animals (Wilson, 2014). We are unusual in that we form longstanding, non-reproductive unions with unrelated individuals—friends (Christakis and Fowler, 2014). Cooperation is a defining feature of these friendships (Apicella et al.

Box 4.3 Technological developments

Technological developments can reduce both potency and exposure, as well as safer drug delivery systems. Were beer drinkers to switch from 5.5 per cent strength beer to 1.5 per cent strength beer, margins of exposure would increase at least fourfold to safer levels. While not harm free, electronic nicotine delivery systems are estimated to be 95 per cent less harmful than smoked tobacco products.

2012; Bowles and Gintis, 2011). We also learn from and influence each other, leading to an exceptional reliance on cultural transmission (Pagel, 2012). We form social networks which have a significant effect on individual behaviours, such as tobacco use (Christakis and Fowler, 2008), alcohol intake (Rosenquist et al., 2010) obesity (Christakis and Fowler, 2007), loneliness (Cacioppo et al., 2009), happiness (Fowler and Christakis, 2008), and cooperative social behaviour (Fowler and Christakis, 2010). With alcohol, for each additional heavy drinker in his or her network, the likelihood that an individual drinks heavily in the future increases by 18 per cent and decreases the likelihood of abstaining by seven per cent (Rosenquist et al., 2010). Each additional abstainer in the network significantly reduces the likelihood that an individual principal drinks heavily in the future by ten per cent and increases the likelihood of abstaining by 22 per cent.

The opposite consequence of social networks is social exclusion. Also hard-wired, possibly to avoid poor social exchange partners and risk of contact with communicable pathogens, are drivers of stigma and social isolation (Kurzban and Leary, 2001; Oaten et al., 2011), themselves independent risk factors for poorer health (Hawkley and Capitanio, 2015).

As introduced in Chapter 3, in addition to threats posed by negative societal reactions, societal norms may influence societal responses to drugs, and the harm experienced from them. Drugs can be highly moralized and are often subject to prohibitory or strict regulatory frameworks which vary from place to place and from time to time (see Hellman et al., 2016). Engagement with drugs can convey strong social meaning and may lead to stigma, which can be particularly focused on the marginalized 'misusers' as opposed to the supposedly more responsible mainstream users (Room, 2011). This can lead to punitive societal responses which are potentially harmful to well-being in themselves and, conversely, a lack of intervention into mainstream behaviour which allows harms to occur unchecked. For example, if caught using drugs in a country with a zero-tolerance approach to illegal drugs, individuals may be subject to criminal sanctions with potential negative implications for quality of life and material living conditions (see Stoll and Anderson, 2015). Countries may also change drug laws or law enforcements' response to drug use over time, perhaps resulting in the reclassification of a drug or a law enforcement crackdown, with implications for the experience of harm for those individuals continuing to use particular drugs.

Drug control policy also frames and influences drug users' health, for example through laws around the provision or lack of access to clean needles and syringes (Campbell and Shaw, 2008). Lack of access to clean needles is one example of how it may not be drug use in itself that causes health problems but a lack of services that societies offer to drug users that would enable people to take drugs in less harmful ways (Bourgois et al., 1997). The extent to which harm reduction is pursued as a policy objective in a given society thus influences the experience of negative well-being consequences resulting from the use of a drug (see Box 4.4).

Deprivation, poverty, and social exclusion are all forms of social and economic marginalization. Individuals and groups may be marginalized along such divisions as economic status, ethnicity, and education, with engagement in harmful drug use

Box 4.4 Social exclusion and stigma

Social exclusion and stigma, often the side effects of drug policies, can bring more harm than drug use itself. Analysing the impact of drug policies through the lens of societal well-being brings to the fore the co-benefits, as well as the adverse side effects, of policies.

often, although not always, seen to occur along similar societal divisions. Indicators of social marginalization such as not being in the workforce and not being stably housed are strong predictors for harmful drug use. Premature death from drug use is associated with indicators of marginalization; lower education, lower income, and lower housing stability all contribute significantly to predicting death from an alcohol-specific condition (Makela, 1999). Reasons for the social class gradient in mortality and other negative consequences might be owing to higher socioeconomic status groups having more resources to protect themselves. Additionally, people in higher socioeconomic groups are usually advantaged in terms of having a family, which may be a motivating factor in the decision to do something about a drug-use problem before severe consequences occur. Different drug using and the clustering of risk factors (such as malnutrition, poor access to health services, and low income) in some populations (Schmidt et al., 2010) may also explain why some groups suffer harm from drugs while others do not.

4.4 **Policies and measures**

Policies and measures (and their lack of them) that act on the core drivers are themselves drivers of harm.

4.4.1 **Policies that reduce exposure**

Policies that reduce exposure to drugs are essentially those that limit availability through economic (price) and physical (actual) availability. Price is purposefully controlled by governments through product-specific taxes, sales taxes, and setting a minimum price per gram of the drug. Availability is purposefully controlled by governments through a wide range of measures from prohibition ('illegal' drugs and, historically and in some jurisdictions, for alcohol), through limits on days and hours of sale, numbers and types (private or government controlled) of outlets, and minimum purchase ages. There is a wealth of evidence that such limits reduce harms to health (Babor et al., 2010; Anderson et al., 2013; Bettcher and da Costa e Silva, 2013) (see Chapters 6 and 7). Thus, the absence of evidence-based policies is an important driver of harm. As explained in Section 4.4.5 limits to availability bring a range of co-benefits (to educational achievement, and productivity, for example), but they can also bring adverse side effects—for example, the well-documented violence, corruption, and loss of public income associated with existing prohibitive 'illegal' drug policies (see Stoll and Anderson, 2015).

4.4.2 **Incentivizing individual behaviour**

Individual choices and behaviour that drive harm from drug use are determined by the environment in which those choices and behaviours operate. Given brain hard-wiring to seek out drugs, and the influence of social networks, it is no wonder that when drugs are highly marketed, cheap, and readily accessible, a greater amount of drugs are used, and a greater amount of harm ensues. Thus, banning commercial communications, increasing price, and reducing availability are all incentives that affect individual behaviour (see Chapters 6 and 7). Incentives can operate in more subtle ways—including by providing the right information and the right context aware prompts at the right times (Anderson et al., 2011; Barnett et al., 2014; Vooght et al., 2014).

4.4.3 **Research and development to reduce potency**

Research and development can be promoted to reduce the potency of existing drugs. The molecules themselves could be manipulated to less harmful variants (Nutt, 2014). The potency of standard drug delivery packages could be manipulated by reducing drug concentration (Hahn et al., 2014). Where delivery systems (e.g. smoked tobacco as the nicotine delivery system) themselves cause harm, safer delivery systems could be identified and developed (as has happened with ENDS) (McNeill et al., 2015).

4.4.4 **Resource allocation for advice and treatment**

No matter what policy or measure is in place to act on the underlying drivers, there will be many individuals who are heavy users and who find it difficult to reduce use on their own. Unfortunately, all too often there are enormous gaps between need and delivery of evidence-based self-management and talk and pharmacological therapies. These gaps cost lives (Rehm et al., 2012). It is all the more remarkable that they are not closed, as closing the gaps brings many co-benefits to society, including reduced social costs and increased productivity (OECD, 2015).

4.4.5 **Co-benefits and adverse side effects**

Assessing drug policy within the OECD societal well-being frame, as mentioned in Chapter 2, brings to the fore the many potential co-benefits of drug policy to other sectors (Stoll and Anderson, 2015), an issue brought up again in Chapter 8. The societal well-being frame also brings to the fore the many adverse side effects that can result from drug policies—social exclusion, criminalization, loss of personal security, and diminished sustainability of well-being over time consequent to policies that illegalize drugs, adverse side effects that have been well-documented (Kleiman et al., 2015).

4.4.6 **Private sector engagement**

There is considerable evidence that the private sector can shape drugs policies (Miller et al., 2016) (as well as broader health) and climate change policies (Klein, 2015), what has been termed 'vetocracy' (Fukuyama, 2015), that lead to

Box 4.5 Accountability for health

Whole-of-government and whole-of-society approaches to drug policy should define the relation with private sector stakeholders and establish the rules of the game for stakeholder engagement in the policy cycle through *accountability for health*, where private sector stakeholders contribute to the public health good, simultaneously to their own interests.

more drug-related deaths. As Chapters 8 and 9 note, managing 'wicked problems' requires clear rules of private sector engagement in policy making. As the *Economist* wrote in 2005, 'partnership between business and governments should always arouse intense suspicion' (Crook, 2005). An important implication of this is the need for a redesign of governance systems that move away from the present short-term fast-scale economic and political systems in favour of longer time scale systems that promote sustainable health and well-being. Political change in difficult areas, such as drug policies, is highly dependent on collective behaviour decisions (Granovetter, 1978), and influenced by what has been termed specular interaction (Cochet, 2015), in which a politician's acts may be less determined by his or her own conviction (which may be in favour of de-criminalization of illegal drugs) than by his or her evaluation of the strength of the belief among rivals and friends. Sometimes change requires action by players completely outside of the system (Werner, 2012) (see Box 4.5).

4.5 Health Footprint

At the centre of the interconnections of Figure 4.1 is the health footprint, the accounting system for identifying the determinants of drug-related health and the management tool used to evaluate opportunities by the public and private sectors and civil society to reduce harm.

Footprints were developed in the ecological field as a measure of human demand on ecosystems (Rees, 1992). They have since developed in a range of areas, including water footprints that measure water utilization (Hoekstra, 2013), and carbon footprints that apportion greenhouse gas emissions (normally carbon dioxide and methane) to a certain activity, product, or population (Wright et al., 2011). The central reason for estimating a carbon footprint is to help reduce the risk of climate change through enabling targeted and effective reductions of greenhouse gas emissions (Williams et al., 2012). We define the health footprint as a measure of the total amount of risk factor-attributable DALYs (Ezzati et al., 2004) of a defined population, sector, or action within the spatial (e.g. jurisdiction) and temporal boundary (e.g. stated year, such as 2012) of the population, sector, or action of interest. It can be calculated using standard risk factor-related DALY methodologies of the Global Burden of Disease Study (GBD 2013 DALYs and Hale Collaborators, 2015) and of the World Health Organization (Ezzati et al., 2004).

4.5.1 **Nations, regions, cities**

Jurisdictions at differing levels—supranational, national, regional, and city level—can influence drug exposure through the policies and programmes implemented or not. For example, the introduction of smoke-free public places, as happened in the 2000s, led to reductions in smoking, harm to the smoker, and harm to those surrounding the smoker (Bettcher and da Costa e Silva, 2013). Reducing taxes on alcohol, as happened in Finland in 2004, led to an increase in alcohol consumption, alcohol-related deaths, and health inequalities, which subsequently reversed when taxes were increased in 2008 (Österberg, 2012).

Jurisdictional entities can be ranked according to their overall health footprint, in order to identify the countries that contribute most to drug-attributable ill health and premature death and therefore where best health gain could be achieved for groupings of countries as a whole. This could be supplemented with health footprint estimates per capita, to ensure that targeted country approaches can be implemented so as to reduce health inequalities between countries. Apportioning health footprints by country and by per capita will enable jurisdictions to facilitate policy planning, to consider the need for strengthened policy for a particular population (e.g. those with younger vs older populations, those with gender disparities, or those with specific genetic profiles), and to monitor the outcomes of policies and programmes over time. Table 4.3 gives an example ranking European Union (EU) countries by an alcohol-attributable health footprint for the population up to the age of 65 years. To improve EU health as a whole, with associated productivity gains (OECD, 2015), Europe-wide policy could target the top five contributing countries (Germany, France, UK, Poland, and Romania), considering how to reduce these countries' alcohol-attributable footprint to the level (=DALY rate) of Italy. Were this to be achieved, EU alcohol-attributable DALYs could be reduced from 4.8 million to 2.7 million.

Jurisdictional footprints could be developed to what might be termed 'policy-attributable health footprints' which estimate the health footprint between current policy and ideal health policy. This would address the question: 'were the country to implement strengthened or new policies compared with present policies, what would be the improvement in the health footprint?' (see OECD, 2015). Conversely, failure to implement the evidence-based policy apportions accountability for the failure (see Box 4.6).

4.5.2 **Sectors**

A range of sectors are involved in drug-related risk factors that the health footprint encompasses. Sectors include producer organizations, retail organizations, such as large supermarket chains, and service provider companies, such as the advertising and marketing industries. There is considerable overlap between sectors, and estimates will need to determine appropriate boundaries for health footprint calculations. For the sector and company calculations, a counterfactual scenario could be constructed in which a hypothetical situation is taken for comparison where the products and services to evaluate do not exist. For example, Table 4.4 estimates the health

Table 4.3 Ranking of European Union countries by alcohol health footprint

	Total DALYs (2004)	DALYs/100,000 women	DALYs/100,000 men
Malta	1222	63	537
Cyprus	2173	No net harm	632
Luxembourg	4278	366	1573
Slovenia	29,739	464	2487
Ireland	33,781	353	1292
Estonia	43,790	860	6006
Denmark	49,615	368	1533
Finland	62,002	347	2099
Greece	62,296	209	894
Belgium	69,468	330	1045
Sweden	73,963	392	1313
Austria	74,993	324	1508
Bulgaria	77,400	239	1763
Latvia	80,890	1035	6254
Slovakia	101,221	429	3438
Netherlands	108,256	252	1129
Lithuania	113,236	788	6146
Portugal	120,922	490	1847
Czech Republic	136,523	348	2318
Italy	179,757	146	457
Hungary	264,255	767	4649
Spain	268,247	274	954
Romania	484,007	907	3734
Poland	521,557	380	2425
United Kingdom	543,377	374	1501
France	597,597	359	1694
Germany	704,462	259	1483
European Union	4,809,027	343	1649

DALY: disability-adjusted life years.

Source: data from Shield KD, Kehoe T, Gmel G, Rehm MX, and Rehm J. Societal burden of alcohol. In: Anderson P, Møller L and Galea G (Eds.), *Alcohol in the European Union: Consumption, harm and policy approaches* (pp. 10–28). Copenhagen, Denmark: World Health Organization Regional Office for Europe, Copyright © 2012 WHO.

Box 4.6 Health footprint

The health footprint is the accountability tool driving reductions in drug-related harm. It is an accounting system that identifies drivers of drug-related health and a management tool that monitors and evaluates actions by public and private sectors and entities and civil society to reduce harm.

---

footprint of a major beer producer. For the year 2012, it is estimated to have contributed 3.34 million alcohol-attributable DALYs, 3.4 per cent of all alcohol-attributable DALYs, and 0.13 per cent of all DALYs. The company could choose to commit to reducing its health footprint by ten per cent to 3 million alcohol-attributable DALYs over the next five years. One way to achieve this is by removing alcohol from the market through lower alcohol concentration products. Our own calculations show that were beers to be produced and consumed with no changes in volume, with 1.5 per cent alcohol concentration as opposed to 5.5 per cent alcohol concentration, MOEs could be increased more than fourfold.

Table 4.4 Health footprint of a major beer producer

Regions	Production in 2012 in thousand hectolitres	Attributable DALYs*
North America	125,129	749,338
Latin America North	126,189	1,645,115
Latin America South	34,292	428,060
Western Europe	2931	15,113
Central and Eastern Europe	2278	48,776
Asia Pacific	57,667	411,601
Global export and holding	7030	41,869
Globally	402,631	3,339,873
	0.13% of all DALYs, 3.4% of all alcohol-attributable DALYs	

*Author's own calculations, based on 2010 Global Burden of Disease disability-adjusted life year (DALY) values for regions, combined with adult alcohol *per capita* consumption data for 2010 from WHO Global Information System for Alcohol and Health.

Source: data from WHO, 'Health statistics and information systems: Global Burden of Disease (GBD)', Copyright © 2016 World Health Organization, http://www.who.int/healthinfo/global_burden_disease/gbd/en/, accessed 01 Nov. 2015; WHO, 'Management of substance abuse: Global Information System on Alcohol and Health (GISAH)', Copyright © 2016 World Health Organization, http://www.who.int/substance_abuse/activities/gisah/en/, accessed 01 Nov. 2015.

4.6 **Conclusion**

In this chapter, we have shown that there are structural elements that are immediate drivers of drug-related harm. These operate at biological and population levels; that human brains seem hard-wired to seek out drugs inevitably drives drug use and drug-related harm when there is widespread exposure to industrially produced potent drugs. The genetic, sex, age, wealth, and inequality structures of populations drive harm. For any given level of drug use, impoverished people suffer disproportionate harm.

We have shown that a range of core factors drive harm. We have described the importance of potency and exposure and how their ratio (margin of exposure) can be used as a policy benchmark, with a policy outcome of an MOE of 10 being an appropriate goal, when potency is assessed with human studies. We have noted how technological developments can reduce potency and exposure and reduce less harmful drug delivery systems to individual users. Social networks operate positively and negatively as drivers of harm. Social exclusion, social stigma, discrimination, and prejudice are rife in drug policy, all often causing more harm to people than the drugs themselves.

We have shown that the presence and absence of policies and measures can drive harm. Policies and measures that reduce exposure, incentivize individual behaviour, promote research and development for less potent drugs and delivery systems, and ensure universal access to advice and treatment can all reduce harm (conversely, absence of these policies increases harm). The presence or absence of meaningful private sector rules of engagement in policy-making drive harm. The societal well-being frame identifies co-benefits and adverse consequences of drug policies.

Finally, we propose a health footprint (which can be universal across all health issues) as the accountability and monitoring tool to drive improved health action by public and private sectors alike.

References

Anderson P, Harrison O, Cooper C, and Jané-Llopis E. (2011) Incentives for health. *J Health Commun* 16: 107–33.

Anderson P, Casswell S, Parry C, and Rehm J (2013) Alcohol. In: Leppo K, Ollola E, Pena S, Wismar M and Cook S (eds) *Health in All Policies*. Helsinki: Ministry of Social Affairs and Health.

Apicella CL, Marlowe FW, Fowler JH, and Christakis NA (2012) Social networks and cooperation in hunter-gatherers. *Nature* 481: 497–501.

Babor T, Caetano R, Casswell S, Edwards G, Giesbrecht N, Graham K, et al. (2010) *Alcohol: No Ordinary Commodity. Research and Public Policy*, 2nd edition. Oxford and London: Oxford University Press.

Barnett NP, Meade EB and Glynn TR (2014) Predictors of detection of alcohol use episodes using a transdermal alcohol sensor. *Exp Clin Psychopharmacol* 22: 86.

Benner S (2013) Paleogenetics and the history of alcohol in primates. American Association for the Advancement of Science Annual Meeting. Presented February 15, 2013. Available at: https://aaas.confex.com/aaas/2013/webprogram/Paper8851.html (last accessed 12 November 2014).

Bettcher D and da Costa e Silva VL (2013) Tobacco or health. In: Leppo K, Ollola E, Pena S, Wismar M and Cook S (eds) *Health in All Policies*. Helsinki: Ministry of Social Affairs and Health.

Bilano V, Gilmour S, Moffiet T, Tursan d'Espaignet E, Stevens GA, Commar A, et al. (2015) Global trends and projections for tobacco use, 1990–2025: an analysis of smoking indicators from the WHO Comprehensive Information Systems for Tobacco Control. *Lancet* 385: 966–76.

Bourgois P, Lettiere M, and Quesada J (1997) Social misery and the sanctions of substance abuse: confronting HIV risk among homeless heroin addicts in San Francisco. *Soc Probl* 44: 155–73.

Bowles S and Gintis H (2011) *A Cooperative Species*. Princeton, NJ: Princeton University Press.

Cacioppo JT, Fowler JH, and Christakis NA (2009) Alone in the crowd: The structure and spread of loneliness in a large social network. *J Pers Soc Psychol* 97: 977–91.

Campbell N and Shaw S (2008) Incitements to discourse: Illicit drugs, harm reduction and the production of ethnographic subjects. *Cult Antropol* 23: 21–39.

Christakis NA and Fowler JH (2007) The spread of obesity in a large social network over 32 years. *N Engl J Med* 357: 370–9.

Christakis NA and Fowler JH (2008) The collective dynamics of smoking in a large social network. *N Engl J Med* 358: 2249–58.

Christakis NA and Fowler JH (2014) Friendship and natural selection. *Proc Natl Acad Sci U S A* 111(Suppl. 3): 10796–801.

Cochet Y (2015) Green eschatology. In: Hamilton C, Bonneuil C, and Gemenne F (eds) *The Anthropocene and the Global Environmental Crisis*. London: Routledge, pp. 112–20.

Crook C (2005) The good company. *Economist*, 22 January 2005.

Crump KS (1984) A new method for determining allowable daily intakes. *Fundam Appl Toxicol* 4: 854–71.

Dudley TR (2014) *The Drunken Monkey: Why We Drink and Abuse Alcohol*. Berkeley, CA: University of California Press.

EFSA (2005) Opinion of the Scientific Committee on a request from EFSA related to a harmonised approach for risk assessment of substances which are both genotoxic and carcinogenic. *EFSA J* 282: 1–31.

Ezzati M, Lopez A, Rodgers A, and Murray CJL (2004) *Comparative Quantification of Health Risks. Global and Regional Burden of Disease Attributable to Selected Major Risk Factors*. Geneva: World Health Organization.

Fowler JH and Christakis NA (2008) Dynamic spread of happiness in a large social network: longitudinal analysis over 20 years in the Framingham Heart Study. *BMJ* 337: 1–9.

Fowler JH and Christakis NA (2010) Cooperative behaviour cascades in human social networks. *Proc Natl Acad Sci U S A* 107: 5334–8.

Fukuyama F (2015) *Political Order and Political Decay: From the Industrial Revolution to the Globalisation of Democracy*. London: Profile Books.

GBD 2013 DALYs and HALE Collaborators (2015) Global, regional and national disability-adjusted life years (DALYs) for 306 diseases and injuries and healthy life expectancy

(HALE) for 188 countries, 1990–2013: quantifying the epidemiological transition. *Lancet* **386**: 2145–91.

Gell L, Bühringer G, McLeod J, Forberger S, Holmes J, Lingford-Hughes A, and Meier P (eds) (2016) *What Determines Harm from Addictive Substances and Behaviours?* Oxford: Oxford University Press.

Granovetter M (1978) Threshold models of collective behaviour. *Am J Sociol* **83**: 14209–43.

Hahn J, Monakhova YB, Hengen J, Kohl-Himmelseher M, Schussler J, Hahn H, et al. (2014) Electronic cigarettes: overview of chemical composition and exposure estimation. Tob Induc Dis **12**: 23–35.

Hawkley LC and Capitanio JP (2015) Perceived social isolation, evolutionary fitness and health outcomes: a lifespan approach. *Phil Trans R Soc B* **370**: 20140114.

Hellman M, Berridge V, Duke K, and Mold A (eds) (2016) *Concepts of Addictive Substances and Behaviours across Time and Place.* Oxford: Oxford University Press.

Hoekstra AY (2013) *The water footprint of modern consumer society.* London: Routledge.

Holmes MV, Dale CE, Zuccolo L, Silverwood RJ, Guo Y, Ye Z, et al. (2014) Association between alcohol and cardiovascular disease: Mendelian randomisation analysis based on individual participant data. *BMJ* **349**: g4164.

Hosseinpoor AR, Parker LA, Tursan d'Espaignet E, and Chatterji S (2012) Socioeconomic inequality in smoking in low-income and middle-income countries: results from the World Health Survey. *PLOS ONE* **7**: e42843.

Hunter PR and Fewtrell L (2001) Acceptable risk. In: Fewtrel L and Bartram J (eds) *Water Quality: Guidelines, Standards and Health.* London: IWA Publishing, pp. 207–27.

Kleiman MAR, Caulkins JP, Jacobson T, and Rowe B (2015) Violence and drug control policy. In: Donnelly PD and Ward CL (eds) *Oxford Textbook of Violence Prevention.* Oxford: Oxford University Press, pp. 297–302

Klein N (2015) *This Changes Everything.* London: Penguin Books.

Kurzban R and Leary M (2001) Evolutionary origins of stigma: the functions of social exclusion. *Psychol Bull* **127**: 187–208.

Lachenmeier DW and Rehm J (2015) Comparative risk assessment of alcohol, tobacco, cannabis and other illicit drugs using the margin of exposure approach. *Sci Rep* **5**: 8126.

Lim SS, Vos T, Flaxman AD, Danaei G, Shibuya K, Adair-Rohani H, et al. (2012) A comparative risk assessment of burden of disease and injury attributable to 67 risk factors and risk factor clusters in 21 regions, 1990-2010: a systematic analysis for the Global Burden of Disease Study 2010. *Lancet* **380**: 2224–60.

McNeill A, Brose LS, Calder R, Hitchman SC Hajek P, and McRobbie H (2015) E-cigarettes: an evidence update. Public Health England. Available at: https://www.gov.uk/government/publications/e-cigarettes-an-evidence-update (accessed 1 January 2016).

Mäkelä P (1999) Alcohol-related mortality as a function of socio-economic status. *Addiction* **94**: 867–86.

Miller D, Harkins C, and Schlögl M (2016) *Impact of Market Forces on Addictive Substances and Behaviours.* Oxford: Oxford University Press.

Nutt D (2014) The dangerous professor. *Science* **343**: 478–81.

Oaten M, Stevenson RJ, and Case TI (2011) Disease avoidance as a functional basis for stigmatization. *Phil Trans R Soc B* **366**: 3433–52.

Ode PJ (2006). Plant chemistry and natural enemy fitness: effects on herbivore and natural enemy interactions. *Annu Rev Entomol* **51**: 163–85.

OECD (2015) *Tackling Harmful Alcohol Use: Economics and Public Health Policy.* Paris: OECD Publishing.

Österberg E (2012) Pricing of alcohol. In: Anderson P, Møller L, and Galea G (2012) *Alcohol in the European Union: Consumption, Harm and Policy Approaches.* Copenhagen: World Health Organization, pp. 96–102.

Pagel M (2012) *Wired for Culture.* London: Allen Lane.

Rees WE (1992) Ecological footprints and appropriated carrying capacity: what urban economics leaves out. *Environ Urban* **4**: 121–30.

Rehm J, Shield K, Rehm M, Gmel G, and Frick U. (2012) *Alcohol Consumption, Alcohol Dependence, and Attributable Burden of Diseasen in Europe: Potential Gains from Effective Interventions for Alcohol Dependence.* Toronto: Health, C. F. a. a. M.

Rehm J, Lachenmeier DW, and Room R (2014) Why does society accept a higher risk for alcohol than for other voluntary or involuntary risks? *BMC Med* **12**: 189–91.

Room R (2011) Addiction and personal responsibility as solutions to the contradictions of neoliberal consumerism. *Crit Public Health* **21**: 141–51.

Room R, Sankaran S, Schmidt LA, Mäkelä P, and Rehm J (2015) Addictive substances and socioeconomic development. In: Anderson P, Rehm J, and Room R (eds) *The Impact of Addictive Substances and Behaviours on Individual and Societal Well-Being.* Oxford: Oxford University Press, pp. 189–214.

Rosenquist JN, Murabito J, Fowler JH, and Christakis NA (2010) The spread of alcohol consumption behaviour in a large social network. *Ann Intern Med* **152**: 426–33.

Roulette CJ, Mann H, Kemp B, Remiker M, Wilcox J, Hewlett B, et al. (2014) Tobacco vs. helminths in Congo basin hunter-gatherers: self medication in humans? *Evol Hum Behav* **35**: 397–407.

Schmidt L, Mäkelä P, Rehm J, and Room R (2010) Alcohol: equity and social determinants. In: Blas E and Sivasankara Kurup A (eds) *Equity, Social Determinants and Public Health Programmes.* Geneva: World Health Organization, pp. 11–29.

Shield KD and Rehm J (2015) The effects of addictive substances and addictive behaviours on physical and mental health. In: Anderson P, Rehm J, and Room R (eds) *The Impact of Addictive Substances and Behaviours on Individual and Societal Well-Being.* Oxford: Oxford University Press, pp 77–118.

Shield KD, Kehoe T, Gmel G, Rehm MX, and Rehm J (2012) Societal burden of alcohol. In: Anderson P, Møller L, and Galea G (eds) *Alcohol in the European Union. Consumption, Harm and Policy Approaches.* Copenhagen: World Health Organization Regional Office for Europe, pp. 10–28.

Starr C (1969) Social benefit versus technological risk. *Science* **165**:1232–8.

Stoll L and Anderson P (2015) Well-being as a frame for understanding addictive substances. In: Anderson P, Rehm J, and Room R (eds) *The Impact of Addictive Substances and Behaviours on Individual and Societal Well-Being.* Oxford: Oxford University Press, pp. 53–76.

Sullivan RJ and Hagen EH (2015) Passive vulnerability or active agency? An evolutionarily ecological perspective of human drug use. In: Anderson P, Rehm J, and Room R (eds) *The Impact of Addictive Substances and Behaviours on Individual and Societal Well-Being.* Oxford: Oxford University Press, pp 13–36.

Vooght CV, Kuntsche E, Kleinjan M, and Engels RC (2014) The effect of the 'What Do You Drink'web-based brief alcohol intervention on self-efficacy to better understand changes in alcohol use over time: randomized controlled trial using ecological momentary assessment. *Drug Alcohol Depend* **138**: 89–97.

Werner BT (2012) Is Earth f**ked? Dynamical futility of global environmental management and possibilities for sustainability via direct action activism. American Geophysical Union Fall 2012 Meeting. Available at: http://abstractsearch.agu.org/meetings/2012/FM/sections/EP/sessions/EP32B/abstracts/EP32B-04.html (accessed 12 November 2014).

Williams I, Kemo S, Coello J, Turner DA, and Wright LA (2012) A beginner's guide to carbon footprinting. *Carbon Manage* **3**: 55–67.

Wilson EO (2014) *The Meaning of Human Existence*. New York: Norton.

World Health Organization (2009) Principles and Methods for the Risk Assessment of Chemicals in Food Environmental Health Criteria 240. Geneva: World Health Organization.

Wright LA, Kemp S, and Williams I (2011) Carbon footprinting: towards a universally accepted definition. *Carbon Manage* **2**: 61–72

Chapter 5

Approaches to reducing the harm done by addictive substances and behaviours should be comprehensive and address the whole population

5.1 Introduction

In this chapter, we first revisit Rose's conceptualization of the two ends of public health prevention strategies, that is, the population strategy aimed at shifting the distribution of a risk factor in the entire population, and the high-risk strategy targeting high-risk groups of individuals who are expected to benefit most from prevention. We propose to consider the potential and capacity of public health prevention strategies throughout a continuum, starting from whole-population approaches, risk factor-based population stratification, targeting high-risk groups of individuals, and ending at the mostly genetics-based personalized medicine. We argue for adopting mixed approaches in order to optimize the benefit of interventions to the population as a whole, while also ensuring equal opportunities to reach optimal health and social well-being to population groups in unfavourable socioeconomic situations. We understand that different behavioural and cultural patterns and diverse social and physical environmental conditions and settings require ecological models that use adapted, evidence-based comprehensive mixed intervention approaches when targeting addictive substance use and behaviours. The potential of digital health to implement and evaluate interventions throughout the prevention continuum is then explored. We end this chapter by introducing the concept of Culture of Health aimed at achieving massive and sustainable improvement in well-being through establishing health as a cultural norm over generations, and long-term, population-centred structural changes.

5.2 Re-thinking the prevention paradox

A population-centred focus has been argued to be more practical and effective from an epidemiological perspective than strategies based on individual risk identification, communication, and prevention (Rockhill, 2005). Population-level strategies are based on the seemingly paradoxical situation, where the majority of cases of a

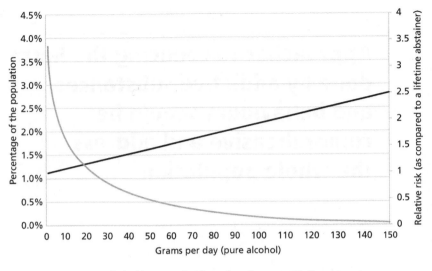

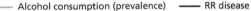

Figure 5.1 Population distribution of average level of alcohol consumption in g/day and a linear risk for disease (own calculations; alcohol distribution based on the distribution for German men for 2010; linear risk increase for fictive disorder).
RR: relative risk.
Source: data from Rehm J, Taylor B, Mohapatra S, Irving H, Baliunas D, Patra J, and Roerecke M. Alcohol as a risk factor for liver cirrhosis—a systematic review and meta-analysis. *Drug and Alcohol Review*, Volume 29, Issue 4, pp. 437–445, Copyright © 2010 Australasian Professional Society on Alcohol and other Drugs (APSAD).

disease come from a population at low or moderate risk of that disease, and only a minority of cases come from the high-risk population of the same disease (Rose, 1985). Thus, for many diseases with a single strong risk factor, the majority of sick people would come from people at low-to-moderate risk, simply because there are so many more people at low-to-moderate risk than there are at high risk (see Figure 5.1). This has been labelled the prevention paradox. This prevention paradox has been applied to alcohol, where it was found that for many alcohol-attributable outcomes (such as self-reported health or financial problems), the majority of the cases in the general population were, in fact, in groups of low-to-moderate risk (Kreitman, 1986). The underlying risk relations were almost linear increasing with increasing levels of consumption, and the population distributions of alcohol consumption were such that most drinkers in the population examined were drinking low-to-moderate quantities. It was concluded, that in such a situation for prevention, it was best to move the whole population to lower levels of drinking, as this strategy was linked to prevention of more diseases than the strategy of focusing on high-risk drinkers only (Rose, 1985; Kreitman, 1986; prevention for alcohol specifically: Bruun et al., 1975) (see Box 5.1).

Box 5.1 The prevention paradox

Population-focused prevention aims at implementing structural and environmental changes in order to shift favourably the exposure to disease risk factors in the entire population. This approach assumes that preventing disease in a large number of individuals, even at small risk, will result in greater gains than focusing on small numbers of individuals at high risk. This is known as the *prevention paradox*, as individuals at low risk are usually poorly motivated to change, and the benefit to individuals is quite low, whereas the population as a whole benefits from significant positive consequences

However, the above-described situation applies only if two assumptions hold true:

◆ the population distribution of exposure (in our example, alcohol consumption) is such that the majority of the people are not at high risk;

◆ the relative risk function between level of drinking and outcomes is linear, or otherwise in a function, that the risk differences between people with low-to-moderate risk, and with high risk levels, are not too large.

In many cases, including for most diseases associated with use of psychotropic substances, the first assumption is true, but the assumption about linearity of risks for increasing levels of consumption is not always the case (Skog, 1999; Rehm et al., 2014). For instance, as shown in Chapter 2, heavy drinking over time was related to the majority of premature alcohol-attributable adult deaths (before the age of 65 years) in Europe (Rehm et al., 2013). The reason for this is that the majority of causes of deaths attributable to alcohol (World Health Organization, 2014) show an exponential risk relationship (e.g. Rehm et al., 2011; Shield et al., 2013; see also illustration in Figure 5.2). The risk curve between specific outcomes (e.g. injury) and average drinking level per day may be more linear, or linearity may also be the case for specific age groups (i.e. the elderly), so without empirically evaluating the distribution of the risk factor in the respective population and the risk relations for different levels of exposure, one cannot assume whether the described prevention paradox applies or not.

What are the specific implications for prevention and treatment policy? In the first example, where the majority of the resulting sick people are in the low-to-moderate drinking categories, all of the prevention efforts should be within a population framework, with the respective best buys (Anderson et al., 2013). Identification of people at high risk would not yield many additional cases, and would thus be cost-ineffective, and would potentially contribute to stigmatization of people with heavy drinking. In the second case, a mixed strategy for prevention seems justified. First, because of the overall high liver burden attributable to alcohol (Rehm et al., 2010, 2013; for Europe, Shield et al., 2013), population-based measures such as increase of taxation or availability reduction seem necessary. In addition, as indicated above screening and treatment interventions for the

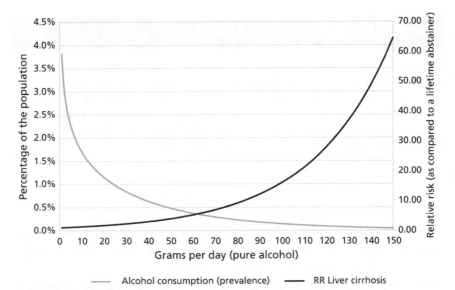

Figure 5.2 Population distribution of average level of alcohol consumption in g/day and risk for liver cirrhosis mortality (own calculations; alcohol distribution based on the distribution for German men for 2010).
RR: relative risk.
Source: data from Rehm J, Taylor B, Mohapatra S, Irving H, Baliunas D, Patra J, and Roerecke M. Alcohol as a risk factor for liver cirrhosis—a systematic review and meta-analysis. *Drug and Alcohol Review*, Volume 29, Issue 4, pp. 437–445, Copyright © 2010 Australasian Professional Society on Alcohol and other Drugs (APSAD).

high-risk users seem justified, as most of the damage for liver cirrhosis mortality can be found in high-risk users.

5.3 High-risk groups approaches and population stratification

The high-risk approach is based on establishing a cut-off point for one or multiple risk factors, and then focusing on the people at greatest risk of a condition, although the contribution of this group of people to the overall population burden of the condition may, in fact, be little. This may, however, not be case if the high-risk group includes people with established disease who contribute a large fraction to the overall burden of a disease. High-risk individuals, in particular those diagnosed with a condition, are usually motivated to change and also rely on the immediate motivation of health professionals.

The high-risk strategy is expected to be more efficient when targeting people at high overall risk rather than focusing on high risk in terms of single risk factors. Interventions in addictive substance use need to account for a number of determinants in addition to the amount of substance intake, including variables such as age, gender, cultural context, socioeconomic situation, and so on (see also Chapter 4 on drivers of harm) that influence substance use patterns in individuals and consumption trends in the population (see Box 5.2).

Box 5.2 Risk function and prevention strategies

The validity of the prevention paradox depends on the shape of the risk function; therefore, the contribution of moderate drinkers to the overall burden of alcohol is expected to vary across the spectrum of alcohol-attributable disabilities. If the risk function for a given disability is linear (Figure 5.1), moderate drinkers contribute the largest fraction to population-level harm. For disabilities with a threshold-like shape, the prevention paradox does not seem to apply, such as the case of alcohol-attributable liver cirrhosis. In contrast, alcohol-related accidents have been found to show a smoother and less convex risk curve, and can mostly be related to occasional intoxication rather than to overall annual intake of alcohol; hence the contribution of moderate drinkers to this set of problems is expected to be more significant (Skog, 1999). Identifying the underlying causes of the population distribution of a risk factor, and *combining the population strategy with a high-risk strategy* is the most efficient approach in most situations.

Segmenting the population into different strata according to the level of exposure to predictive risk factors is increasingly being considered as a 'third way' between high-risk and whole-population approaches (Burton et al., 2012; Garcia-Closas et al., 2014). A stratified approach is expected to optimize the potential of preventive interventions at whole-population level and to moderate the stigmatization of high-risk groups (see Figure 5.3). It assumes that the population can be divided into multiple

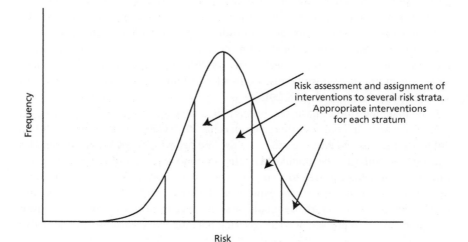

Figure 5.3 Stratified prevention strategies.
Reproduced with permission from Burton H, Sagoo GS, Pharoah P, and Zimmern RL. Time to revisit Geoffrey Rose: strategies for prevention in the genomic era?. *Italian Journal of Public Health*, Volume 9, Issue 4, Copyright © 2012 Epidemiology, Biostatistics and Public Health.

Box 5.3 The potential of a stratified approach for risk profile-specific prevention

The *stratified approach* is based on the assumption that the population can be divided into multiple groups based on the identification, measurement, and stratification of risk determinants for a given condition. This approach is applicable to the entire population and allows for the identification of specific preventive strategies throughout the continuum of risk for addictive substance use and behaviours, in addition to the traditional high risk vs. whole-population dichotomy (Burton et al., 2012).

---

groups based on the identification, measurement, and stratification of risk determinants for a given condition (see Box 5.3).

Genome-wide association studies have contributed to a better understanding of the genetic predisposition and biological pathways to complex diseases. It is also recognized that the onset of common chronic disorders results from a combination of genetic, environmental, and lifestyle factors. It is known that populations and individuals with the same genetic profile show varying prevalence rates of a disease under different environmental conditions. The variations in gene expression may be explained by the variations in exposure to specific environmental factors and in lifestyle behaviours; hence, it is crucial to identify those factors and behaviours determining the population's overall risk exposure. Determinants used for stratification should optimally include the three types of factors. One core assumption of the current conceptualization of the stratified approach is that the associations between genetic and environmental factors are multiplicative (Garcia-Closas et al., 2014). The use of genetic screening at population level is considered as a tool for risk stratification across the whole population in order to provide differentiated prevention programmes to each population stratum (Burton et al., 2012). However, the implementation of genetic testing in healthcare is still facing a number of relevant challenges, including false-positive results, incidental findings, and ethical, legal, and social implications (van El et al., 2013).

Gene mapping studies have also been applied to identify risk genes for nicotine, alcohol, cocaine, and opiates (Thorgeirsson et al., 2008; Gelernter et al., 2014a, 2014b, 2014c). In the case of addictive substance use and behaviours, the impact of genetics has been recognized to be modulated by the environmental exposure, indicating, for instance, that being exposed to a context where availability is being controlled and use is being supervised lowers the expression of genetic predisposition to alcohol use (Dick et al., 2009). Substance use should be seen as occuring along a continuum from non-problematic to problematic use covering potentially harmful use and addictive substance use, where transition, both back and forth, along the continuum is possible. Initiation in use is more influenced by environmental factors, while transition to problem use is more influenced by individual and genetic factors (Gell et al., 2016). Thus, it can be argued that measures targeting socioenvironmental changes,

---

Box 5.4 Environmental and lifestyle exposure impact on gene expression

The variations in gene expression may be explained by the variations in exposure to specific environmental factors and in lifestyle behaviours that determine the overall risk exposure. Although genetic screening is considered as an effective tool for population-level risk stratification, it is yet to overcome a number of relevant technological and implementation challenges, including overlapping genetic influences across a variety of addictive substances, false-positive results, incidental findings, and ethical, legal, and social implications.

---

including monitoring of use, urban planning, and leisure and peer group alternatives, are expected to have a harm-preventive impact at the population level. The use of genetic testing may not actually increase the impact of such measures, while it would certainly result in relevant additional costs and raise relevant ethical and social issues.

Stratification of the population according to meso- and macro-level variables such as socioeconomic conditions, social and physical environmental contexts, and access to welfare resources may result in effective and cost-effective differentiated prevention strategies in addictive substance use. The need for contextualizing population strategies at meso- and macro-levels is supported by evidence showing that the social welfare system and gender equity of a country seems to determine to a large extent how education, employment, and family roles are associated with, for instance, heavy drinking (Kuntsche et al., 2006), and that consequences of similar drinking patterns are more severe for those with lower socioeconomic status (Mäkelä and Paljärvi, 2008) (see Box 5.4).

5.4 Genetics and personalized medicine

On the other extreme of the health strategy continuum, the most escalated level of personalized medicine is linked to the human genome mapping that is expected to result in a substantially enhanced ability to assess health risk and damage of individuals based on their exposure to risk agents and their differential susceptibility and resilience to such agents (Kumar et al., 2015). However, human genome sequencing still faces some relevant scientific challenges for real-world medical applications such as those related to the number of DNA sequence variants and the delineation of the novel molecular pathways involved in the pathogenesis of the phenotype (Marian, 2012). Also, a number of moral and ethical issues have been raised from a variety of scientific, medical, and social sectors, regarding, for example, data sharing and protection of DNA databases, the potential genetic manipulation for non-medical reasons, the regulation on the acquisition and use of genetic information, mandatory genetic screening, and genotype-based discrimination in health insurance (Carroll and Ciaffa, 2003). Another issue is that the identified causal mechanisms or pathways are not homogeneous across individuals, and their average profile may not be actually representative for any individual; also, in the case of non-infectious diseases, most risk factors are associated with rather low positive predictive values (Rockhill, 2005).

The challenges faced by the P4–predictive, preventive, personalized, and participatory–medicine seem to be both economic and related to the integration of the population approach into science, practice, and health policies addressing the four components. The current practice of medicine is already conducted in a personalized manner, in most cases for the differential gender, age, and race characteristics, and some other clinical factors, and practice is also expected to be evidence based, yet P4 medicine could provide and implement novel personalized diagnostic and therapeutic applications. Although a large variety of challenges of scientific nature related, for example, to the understanding of underlying biological pathways and molecular networks, and the identification of biomarkers still remain, the operational and the economic aspects of the implementation of personalized medicine seem to be equally challenging. Major issues include addressing the balance between the patient's clinical merit for and benefit from biomarker-based diagnostics and treatment and the assessment of the aggregate population cost; establishing healthcare standards; and data security and mining. The participatory component of personalization requires understanding and integrating the social and behavioural elements involved in individual decision making already during the development of a new application.

Regarding the potential to integrate genetic variations into the prevention strategies for addictive substance use and behaviours, one issue is that genes that potentially modulate the variation in the risk for addictive substance use are not substance-specific (Li & Burmeister, 2009). Relevant evidence indicates that many genetic factors influencing addiction to different substances are shared, and these shared genetic pathways seem to be also involved in other psychological constructs such as impulsivity and compulsivity (Koob & Volkow, 2010). Genetic influences significantly overlap across alcohol, nicotine, and illegal drugs, and also across addictive substance use and other externalizing behaviour conditions (Agrawal et al., 2012). As for illegal substances, significant proportions of genetic influence on addiction to a variety of these substances could be attributed to a common genetic vulnerability (Kendler et al., 2003). In addition, comorbidity across addictions and also between addictions and other mental illnesses is partially owing to genetic factors (see Box 5.5).

Box 5.5 Genetic research is essential for high-risk approaches

Despite the current difficulties to integrate findings on genetic susceptibility to addictive substances and behaviours into an optimised delivery of effective preventive interventions in public health, genetic research is essential to improve treatment approaches for the group of high-risk individuals whose substance use and behaviour problems persist despite the environmental and structural changes, and even specialized treatment.

5.5 **Mixed approaches: the inverted intervention pyramid**

The forces modulating behaviour change should also include a mainstream and upstream perspective (i.e. the relationship of individuals with larger groups of population, and social and economic structures and policies), in addition to down-stream focus on individuals and their behaviours. Evidence-based approaches for drug use prevention and treatment should be identified both at individual and population levels. Interventions aimed at improving overall health and socioeconomic conditions may be expected to contribute to a better control of drug use at the population level, although this type of interventions needs to be tested through appropriate designs.

Interventions and measures related not only to individual drug use prevention and treatment provision, but also to the meso- and macro-level determinants of substance use over the life course should be implemented, such as the regulation of legal drug marketing, labelling, sale, taxation, and pricing; urban architecture design; and affordable community infrastructure provision facilitating drug-free choices and physical activity. It has been argued that most health-related behaviours, including smoking and alcohol use, result from routine daily activities and common patterns of everyday social life in a society or a social group (Mechanic, 1997) (see Box 5.6).

However, the translation of health-promotion messages into actual practice by the population towards a healthier lifestyle is rather scarce, although most people are actually able to recall adequately health risk-reducing behaviours. As health promotion postulates that illness can be anticipated based on certain risk determinants, and therefore can be prevented or mitigated by positively impacting on some of the determinants through individual behaviour, adopting proactive healthier behaviours is closely linked to the capacity of the individual to envisage the future ill health. It has been found that the embodied experience of ill health is a pre-requisite for anticipating ill-health in the future; this finding also supports the general observation that lifestyle changes resulting from professional advice tend to be reactive (Lawton, 2002).

Box 5.6 **Social and environmental interventions impact on risk determinants in population strategies**

Societies and communities can actually modulate harmful health behaviours by creating or remodelling environments, infrastructures, and activities in order to enable individuals to easily and readily engage in promoting and maintaining their health. In this sense, effective changes in social, economic, and political structures and processes may be seen as the most effective way to integrate evidence on risk determinants in population-level strategies.

Remedial measures in the high-risk groups are necessary, but, over the long run, the improvement of the norm, that is, the population mean, is indispensable for the improvement of the prevalence of a condition. This does not only seem to apply to medical conditions, but also to the prevalence of highly performing individuals in domains such as education, sport, and research, where a long-lasting positive improvement only seems achievable through a large-scale upgrade of standards at the whole-population level. Hence, population-focused healthcare addresses the needs of the general population rather than individuals, although it also takes into account the specific scope of services and resources to meet the particular needs of clinically or socially vulnerable high-risk groups.

The World Health Organization acknowledges that the social determinants of health, that is, 'conditions in which people are born, grow, live, work and age', are to be held accountable for avoidable inequities in health status and well-being, and thus an impaired ability of individuals to achieve good health. These circumstances are conditioned by the distribution of money, power, and resources resulting in systematic and historic socioeconomic and/or environmental disadvantages and discrimination for groups of people owing to their race or ethnicity, religion, sexual orientation, gender identity, age, intellectual or physical disability, mental status, socioeconomic status, and geographic location (World Health Organization, 2003). The impact of social determinants on the health outcomes and well-being of specific population groups needs to be part of the population-centred approach, bearing in mind that abilities, vulnerabilities, and needs vary throughout the human life course.

Social cohesion may be defined as the attitudes, behaviours, and relational, institutional, and structural dimensions tied to the factors of equality, inclusion, development, capital (i.e. norms and trust across social networks, social participation, and solidarity), and diversity. Social inclusion, capital, and diversity have been found to be positively associated with individual health after controlling for other individual characteristics (Chuang et al., 2013). Societies with high levels of tolerance towards social diversity and inclusive of all citizens into welfare structures are likely to promote the individuals' perception that they have control over their access to health and socioeconomic services that are respectful of individual differences and preferences, and thus have a positive impact on self-rated health and the society's level of tolerance of behaviours, including also those associated with addictive substance use and behaviours (see Box 5.7).

Box 5.7 We all play a role in preventing harm

Social welfare and healthcare systems should not only ensure universal access, but also serve the special needs of population subgroups. Putting the blame on substance users and those presenting with addictive behaviours is inappropriate, and there is a need to achieve a socially shared understanding of the universal impact of addictive problems and a *joint social accountability* for health promotion and addressing addiction-related harm.

Population strategies need to consider and address the full range of health determinants, including also politically controllable structural conditions related to housing, education, employment, community leisure and play facilities (Green and Allegrante, 2011), provision of health services, and availability, affordability, and marketing of legal drugs. Health-promotion strategies targeting structural changes are meant to reach and benefit a wider variety of population segments and are less resource intensive (Frieden, 2010). However, designing and implementing structural interventions not only requires identifying the conditions to change, but also understanding their determining processes (Solar and Irwin, 2007).

Both the design and the implementation of structural measures and decision-making face complex economic, social, and political challenges, and require aligning the divergent interests of a variety of stakeholders. As a result, the real-word performance of structural initiatives to achieve policy and environmental changes is quite often disappointing if not counterproductive. The role of the participatory approach in health has long been acknowledged: drugs policy planning and practice is expected to be paralleled or preceded by an inclusive public deliberative process.

However, it is also crucial to study carefully the existing and projected contextual macro-conditions and sociopolitical environments within which health-promoting policies and structures are to be shaped and implemented. Economically powerful stakeholders, whose interests may be compromised in the process, should be promptly identified in order to modulate their influence on the expected legal regulations, and to ensure that the process is informed by the best available evidence base and driven both by socially and individually meaningful values and incentives (see Chapter 9). The alcohol industry has been funding research as a means to foster their image as a socially responsible sector, and campaigning against the implementation of evidence-based effective measures such as minimum unit pricing and higher taxation on alcohol (Miller et al., 2011; Gornall, 2014).

Even in the case of tobacco control where structural actions have actually resulted in a change in social norms regarding where smoking is considered appropriate and a shared acknowledgement of the harmful effects of smoking on health, the specific population of individuals with a substance use and/or mental health disorder did not fully benefit from these gains and were not actually encouraged to quit smoking by addiction treatment services and recovery communities, even though the prevalence of tobacco use is much higher in this specific group than in the general population (Perka, 2011). This has identified the need for a change in the norms of tobacco use in addiction treatment facilities and for a specific training in effective tobacco cessation practices in addiction professionals in order to overcome this health disparity in a high-risk population group.

Some authors advocate for the P5 medicine concept (Khoury et al., 2012) that integrates the population perspective into all elements of P4, that is, predictive, preventive, personalized, and participatory, and aims at achieving a balance between individual and population health interventions and assessing their comparative effectiveness (see Box 5.8).

Actions targeting addictive substance use and behaviours may be grouped in accordance to the level of intervention, that is, intrapersonal, interpersonal, organization/

Box 5.8 The population mean of the exposure to risk factors needs to be improved

A favourable shift in the population mean of the exposure to risk factors is indispensable for the long-term improvement of the prevalence of a condition in a population. It is reasonable to assume that the higher the number and the broader the range of beneficiary groups reached by evidence-based effective prevention and guaranteed universal access to sustainable infrastructural, environmental, and social resources, in particular to healthcare and education, the more the benefit for the population as a whole.

---

community, and macro-political level, and represented in an *inverted intervention pyramid* (Figure 5.4) showing the population reach of the different levels (adapted from Healthy Minds, Healthy People, 2010). From top to bottom, each intervention level of the inverted pyramid targets a decreasing number of potential beneficiaries with an increasing perceived impact of the addictions-related problems on their life. As explained above, the improvement of the norm, that is, the population mean of the exposure to risk factors, is indispensable for the long-term improvement of the

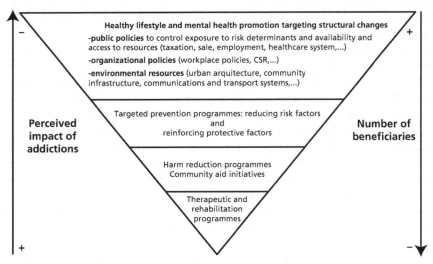

Figure 5.4 Inverted intervention pyramid.
CSR: corporate social responsibility.
Adapted from Ministry of Health Services and Ministry of Children and Family Development of British Columbia, *Healthy minds, healthy people: a 10-year plan to address mental health and substance use in British Columbia*. Ministry of Health Services and Ministry of Children and Family Development of British Columbia, Copyright © 2010 Ministry of Health Services and Ministry of Children and Family Development of British Columbia, http://www.health.gov.bc.ca/library/publications/year/2010/healthy_minds_healthy_people.pdf, accessed 01 Nov. 2015.

prevalence of a condition in a population. It is reasonable to assume that the higher the number and the broader the range of beneficiary groups reached by an evidence-based effective intervention and guaranteed universal access to sustainable infrastructural, environmental, and social resources, in particular to healthcare and education, the more the population mean will improve. This argument does not, of course, advocate against the planning and implementation of specific preventive and remedial interventions in high-risk groups and different age groups. The argument indicates that the resource investment in system-level and structural changes at the top is expected to also reduce the number of beneficiaries in need of intervention at the lower levels of the inverted pyramid as the population average prevalence rates of addictions decrease, with the subsequent cost savings in addictions-related social, economic, and health harm.

Ecological models target behaviour change at all levels. For instance, a multilevel smoking cessation programme at the workplace includes delivering behavioural change training for the individuals at the intrapersonal level, addressing immediately available social support at the interpersonal level, and implementing smoke-free workplace policies at the organizational level (Pantaewan and Kengganpanich, 2014).

5.6 Digital health

Digital health is defined as the 'use of information and communications technologies to improve human health, healthcare services, and wellness for individuals and across populations' (Kostkova, 2015). It has a high potential to implement preventive interventions in addictive substance use and behaviours. With an estimated number of 1.75 billion smartphone users worldwide in 2014, the use of mobile devices to access health-related information sources increased from 17 per cent in 2010 to 31 per cent in 2013 (http://www.emarketer.com/Article/Smartphone-Users-Worldwide-Will-Total-175-Billion-2014/1010536).

The 'digital divide' (i.e. haves and have-nots) has traditionally been related to differential affordability and geographical coverage of Internet and mobile services in populations. However, the focus of the digital divide has been widened from the need to provide affordable and universal access to assessing ways to also increase the interest in the uptake of the use of readily available inexpensive services which is of crucial interest in the design and implementation of population-level mobile health (mHealth)-based preventive interventions (Internet Society Global Internet Report, 2015). Even those users deeply immersed in social media and mobile apps may not spontaneously engage in extending their use to specific health topics, behaviours, and monitoring (Ralph et al., 2011). These two aspects, lack of access to digital services due to socioeconomic status or absence of interest, and uneasiness towards stigmatized health issues are of specific relevance when it comes to addressing addictive substance use and behaviours.

By 2013, over 31,000 health and medical apps were downloadable in the speedily growing software apps market; acceptance and demand for health apps has been part of larger societal trends to improve health and well-being through health literacy and behavioural change (Essany, 2013). The potential of apps has been shown to improve user retention in health behaviour interventions: in a number

Box 5.9 The potential of digital health throughout the prevention continuum

eHealth (computer-based) and mHealth (smartphone-based) solutions are expected to allow implementing large-scale population-level preventive interventions that can actually be tailored according to the physiological and motivational profiles and behavioural patterns of the individual users, and therefore to be used throughout the entire prevention continuum. Standardization, validation, and regulation of such health-promotion tools is still ongoing, hence the safe and widespread community use of *ICT-based prevention solutions* targeting addictive substance use and behaviours is still to be seen.

of selected studies on health apps targeting behavioural change, the mean retention rate for use of the app during the intervention was 79.6 per cent (Payne et al., 2015) (see Box 5.9).

Computer-tailored interventions providing personalized information and feedback to the individual user have been found to be effective in smoking prevention and cessation and decreasing alcohol intake (Riper et al., 2011). From a resource optimization perspective, the implementation of Internet-based (eHealth) tailored interventions targeting health-related behaviours, including alcohol use and smoking (Rooke et al., 2010; Smit et al., 2011, 2013), have been shown to improve cost-effectiveness in comparison with care as usual. Smartphone-based tools targeting health behaviour change can be expected to be similarly effective and cost-effective, and are seen as a promising way towards mixed prevention approaches, with a potential to focus simultaneously on the population as a whole, stratified population groups, and individuals using single intervention packages.

Adherence, that is, the extent to which a person follows an intervention as recommended, impacts on the likeliness and effectiveness of behaviour change. A number of factors including age, gender, health status, family status, employment status, and risk level of unhealthy lifestyle behaviours, have been found to interact with adherence to eHealth interventions (Reinwand et al., 2015). Therefore, both eHealth and mHealth interventions should carefully consider differential design needs and solutions depending on socioeconomic variables and personal characteristics of the targeted user groups, in addition to individual physiological and motivational profiles. Moreover, a number of contextual and behavioural elements have been found to facilitate the engagement and efficient use of health apps. These elements have a high relevance and potential when used in apps specifically targeting addictive substance use and behaviours, and include the identification of mood triggers and contextual cues, mood predictions, awareness of distressed behaviours and thoughts, real-time display of feedback and record of progress, easy and fast use, discreteness when used in public, and information on long-term health outcomes (Payne et al., 2015).

The market sector has produced an endless number of apps focusing on health-related behaviours, including mostly diet, smoking, and alcohol consumption. Some alcohol apps have been found to be actually intended to promote drinking (Weaver et al., 2013), while others unintentionally produce paradoxical effects. The findings of a large-scale, randomized, controlled study on brief intervention-based alcohol apps in university students show that a lot more research is still needed in order to prevent paradoxical effects such as increased frequency of drinking occasions, and also regarding intervention components, design-specific confounders, and gender specificities (Gajecki et al., 2014). As for cannabis apps, the most common content areas included cannabis strain classification, facts about cannabis, and cannabis food recipes, thus facilitating supply and use, whereas only one app provided information or resources on harm and treatment (Ramo et al., 2015).

Mobile health apps are not currently subject to formal validation and regulation, unless conceived as an accessory to a regulated medical device, or a mobile platform operating as a regulated medical device (FDA, 2015), thus in most cases it cannot be guaranteed that health apps offer evidence-based effective interventions, let alone validation in the general population. The safe and widespread community use of apps targeting addictive substance use and behaviours is yet to materialize.

Social networks modulate social norms which, in turn, are essential to promote sustainable behaviour changes, as individuals are expected to change their actions in view of the attitudes and behaviours of others around them (DeJong et al., 2006). The Framingham Heart Study is a longitudinal population-based cardiovascular study that started in 1948 and enrolled the third generation of participants in 2002 (Mahmood et al., 2014). The study has shown that health-related behaviours, including tobacco use (Christakis and Fowler, 2008) and alcohol intake (Rosenquist et al., 2010) are determined by social networks. Health-related lifestyle choices seem to reflect collective choices and pressures of the individual's connected groups of people, regardless of the geographical distance. Therefore, the widely spread online social network phenomenon seems to have a great potential in generalizing health-promoting behaviours through the spread of social norms.

The Web 2.0 context, which emphasizes user-generated content, usability, and interoperability, undoubtedly impacts on large-scale health beliefs and attitudes. The proliferation of Web 2.0 virtual health communities mostly based on user-generated content and multidirectional interaction and communication that go far beyond the traditional unidirectional read-only communication in terms of user participation, has become a challenge for existing health promotion and intervention models, resulting in an urgent need for innovative and more dynamic approaches in the design, deployment, and evaluation of ongoing health-related social media use and future social media-based health interventions (Chou et al., 2013).

Social media-based interventions also seem to have a potential to reach population segments who are medically or otherwise under-served or in socially and/or economically unfavourable situations and thus help alleviate health disparities. However, no social media interventions can be designed without first understanding a number of relevant factors, including differences in level and demand of health literacy,

Box 5.10 Social web modulate health attitudes and behaviours

Social networks modulate social norms which, in turn, are essential to promote sustainable behaviour changes, as individuals are expected to change their actions in view of the attitudes and behaviours of others around them. *Social media-based interventions* have a potential to impact on large-scale health beliefs and attitudes, as well as to reach population segments who are medically or otherwise underserved or in socially and/or economically unfavourable situations.

perceived content relevance and understanding, and reliability of the information source, and without innovative methods to assess effectiveness, based on descriptive and pilot studies. For instance, social network analysis was used to assess user and platform interactions in a large smoking cessation virtual community (Cobb et al., 2010). A combination of machine learning, natural language processing, network analysis, and statistics is increasingly being used to study population structures, human behaviour, and content patterns in social media based interactions around health topics (Ruths and Pfeffer, 2014).

Although the influence of social media on health behaviours needs further assessment, its capacity to modulate the social norm should be borne in mind, in particular when considering the strategies used by economic actors, such as the presence of alcohol marketing in social media specifically targeting brand loyalty and promoting routine daily alcohol consumption (Nicholls, 2012). The permeability and openness of social media allow monitoring and mapping the presence and diffusion of misinformation in large population groups, and an abusive use of peer-to-peer information exchange and personal advice sharing over evidence-based knowledge and guidance, as detected, for example, in Twitter quit smoking social networks (Prochaska et al., 2012) (see Box 5.10).

A decision and policy-making frame supported by information and communications technologies (ICT) and the use of the so-called 'big data' (i.e. massive or rapidly moving datasets usually collected through information sensing technologies, that are too large or complex to process using traditional database applications) are expected to exert great influence on public decision-making processes through capturing and representing the needs and interests of all stakeholders, in particular the public, in multidimensional policy domains exposed to high levels of uncertainty and change.

Effective policies targeting addictive substance use and behaviours need to be embedded and supported by the broad social, economic and environmental policy frame (World Health Organization, 2003). The availability of readily accessible ICT-based citizen participation platforms may encourage and extend public participation in both scientific research and politics and allow for multidirectional and multilayer communications, leading to enhanced perception of control, inclusiveness, and thus strengthened social cohesion (see Box 5.11).

> ## Box 5.11 What needs to be sorted out in order to safely use the potential of ICT and big data in prevention
>
> The potential of ICT-based and big data-supported policy making cannot be fully exploited without first further addressing some essential aspects related, for instance, to data mining from online social networks, imperfect or uncertain data, psychological and behavioural elements of decision-making, security, privacy, and ethical issues.

5.7 Towards a 'Culture of Health'

The premise of initiatives like 'Culture of Health' focuses on establishing health as a cultural norm and an integral part of all human actions, and aims at enabling everyone in society, regardless of their circumstances, to lead a healthy life throughout generations (Mockenhaupt and Woodrum, 2015). The concept advocates for population-centred structural changes as a means to reach massive and sustainable improvement in health and well-being.

Critical strategies include: (1) cross-sector collaboration in order to place health as a high priority and harmonize a socially responsible and meaningful 'resource investment in health determinants across sectors', and implement collaborative governance; (2) improvements of the physical, social, and economic environments in order to provide equitable opportunities for healthcare and healthy living for all and minimize the impact of living, employment, and leisure conditions on people's health outcomes; and (3) remodelling healthcare structures and systems in order to embed the appreciation and promotion of health in an integrated care model (see Box 5.12)

A population-level cultural change requires a sustained effort over generations, and identifying and addressing also behavioural, interpersonal, intergroup, and community factors able to reinforce and catalyse structural changes. Further research

> ## Box 5.12 Approaches based on a broad perspective of population health and well-being are needed
>
> Addressing the harm due to addictive substance use and behaviours in a socially equitable manner requires raising awareness of *addictive substance use and behaviours as whole-society problems*, which need to be addressed with the participation of the whole population. Inclusive and broad-minded initiatives like 'Culture of Health' optimally complement and positively shift high-risk-focused prevention and health promotion approaches, in line with the well-being frame and the drivers of harm described in Chapter 4.

using a transdisciplinary perspective is needed to integrate the existing knowledge on health topics from a variety of fields such as behavioural sciences, user-centred design, organizational studies, economics, implementation science, corporate ethics, game theory, and so on. It is crucial that the evidence from other fields is translated into a language accessible to all stakeholders and concrete uptake opportunities are identified for all sectors, paying special attention to the frame of reference of the health systems and structures.

5.8 Conclusions

Population-level strategies are based on the seemingly paradoxical situation, where the majority of cases of a disease come from a population at low or moderate risk of that disease, and only a minority of cases come from the high-risk population of the same disease. This situation applies when the population distribution of exposure is such that the majority of the people are not at high risk; and when the relative risk function between level of exposure and outcomes is linear, or otherwise in a function, that the risk differences between people with low to moderate risk, and with high risk levels, are not too large. In this case, the improvement of the norm, that is, the population mean, is indispensable for the improvement of the prevalence of the condition. Targeted interventions in high-risk groups are based on the situation where there is an exponential relationship between exposure and outcomes, for which greater health gain is achieved by reductions in high-risk groups. For outcomes due to exposure to addictive susbstances, risk curves vary between linear and exponential, depending on the outcome. Thus, a combination of a population strategy with a high-risk strategy is the most efficient approach in most situations. Segmenting the population into different strata according to the level of exposure to predictive risk factors is increasingly being considered as a 'third way' in between the high-risk and whole-population approaches.

Genetic mapping is essential to find novel treatment approaches for the group of high-risk individuals whose substance use and behaviour problems persist, despite the environmental and structural changes, and even specialized treatment. Genetic variations across population groups can be used in stratified prevention approaches focusing on overall risk resulting from the interaction of multiple determinants.

Interventions addressing addictive substance use and behaviours seem to work at their best when an ecological model is used, so that intrapersonal, interpersonal, organizational, and policy levels are simultaneously targeted. The levels of intervention may be represented in an inverted pyramid showing that, from top to bottom, each intervention level reaches a decreasing number of potential beneficiaries with decreasing potential of impacting on the population prevalence of a condition.

The potential of digital health, in particular multidirectional mHealth- and social media-based interventions calls for innovative and dynamic forms of research in order to support evidence-based design, implementation, and assessment guidelines for the rapidly growing health apps market. This need is even more pressing as economic actors are purposefully using both mobile apps and social media to influence systematically the social norms of alcohol use by promoting drinking as a central element of leisure and entertainment, and pushing for generalized routine daily consumption.

Addressing the harm due to addictive substance use and behaviours in a socially equitable manner requires raising awareness of addictive substance use and behaviours as whole-society problems, which need to be addressed with the participation of the whole population.

References

Agrawal A, Verweij KJH, Gillespie NA, Heath AC, Lessov-Schlaggar CN, Martin NG, and Lynskey MT (2012) The genetics of addiction—a translational perspective. *Transl Psychiatry* 2: e140.

Anderson P, Casswell S, Parry C, and Rehm J (2013) Alcohol. In: Leppo K, Ollila S, Peña S, Wismar M, and Cook S (eds) *Health in All Policies*. Helsinki: Ministry of Social Affairs and Health, pp. 224–53.

Bruun K, Pan L, and Rexed I (1975) *The Gentlemen's Club: International Control of Drugs and Alcohol* (Vol. 9). Chicago, IL: University of Chicago Press.

Burton H, Sagoo GS, Pharoah P, and Zimmern RL (2012) Time to revisit Geoffrey Rose: strategies for prevention in the genomic era? *Ital J Public Health* 9: e8865.

Carroll ML and Ciaffa J (2003) The Human Genome Project: a scientific and ethical overview. DNA from the Beginning. Available at: http://www.actionbioscience.org/genomics/carroll_ciaffa.html (accessed 6 June 2015).

Chou W, Prestin A, Lyons C, and Wen K (2013) Web 2.0 for health promotion: reviewing the current evidence. *Am J Public Health* 103: E9–18.

Christakis NA and Fowler JH (2008) The collective dynamics of smoking in a large social network. *N Engl J Med* 358: 2249–58.

Chuang YC, Chuang KY, and Yang TH (2013) Social cohesion matters in health. *Int J Equity Public Health* 12: 87.

Cobb N, Graham A, and Abrams D (2010) Social network structure of a large online community for smoking cessation. *Am J Public Health* 100: 1282–9.

DeJong W, Schneider SK, Towvim LG, Murphy MJ, Doerr EE, Simonsen N R, and Scribner RA (2006) A multisite randomized trial of social norms marketing campaigns to reduce college student drinking. *J Stud Alcohol* 67: 868–79.

Dick DM, Bernard M, Aliev F, Viken R, Pulkkinen L, Kaprio J, and Rose RJ (2009) The role of socioregional factors in moderating genetic influences on early adolescent behavior problems and alcohol use. *Alcohol Clin Exp Res* 33: 1739–48.

Essany M (2013) Mobile health care apps growing fast in number. Available at: http://mhealthwatch.com/mobile-health-care-apps-growing-fast-in-number-20052/ (accessed 11 October 2015).

FDA (2015) Mobile medical applications. Available at: http://www.fda.gov/downloads/MedicalDevices/DeviceRegulationandGuidance/GuidanceDocuments/UCM263366.pdf (accessed 11 October 2015).

Frieden TR (2010) A framework for public health action: the health impact pyramid. *Am J Public Health* 100: 590–5.

Gajecki M, Berman AH, Sinadinovic K, Rosendahl I, and Andersson C (2014) Mobile phone brief intervention applications for risky alcohol use among university students: a randomized controlled study. *Addict Sci Clin Pract* 9: 11.

Garcia-Closas M, Gunsoy NB, and Chatterjee N (2014) Combined associations of genetic and environmental risk factors: implications for prevention of breast cancer. *J Natl Cancer Inst* 106: djv127.

Gelernter J, Kranzler HR, Sherva R, Almasy L, Koesterer R, Smith AH, and Farrer LA (2014a) Genome-wide association study of alcohol dependence: significant findings in African-and European-Americans including novel risk loci. *Mol Psychiatry* **19**: 41–9.

Gelernter J, Sherva R, Koesterer R, Almasy L, Zhao H, Kranzler HR, and Farrer L (2014b) Genome-wide association study of cocaine dependence and related traits: FAM53B identified as a risk gene. *Mol Psychiatry* **19**: 717–23.

Gelernter J, Kranzler HR, Sherva R, Koesterer R, Almasy L, Zhao H, and Farrer LA (2014c) Genome-wide association study of opioid dependence: multiple associations mapped to calcium and potassium pathways. *Biol Psychiatry* **76**: 66–74.

Gell L, Bühringer G, McLeod J, Forberger S, Holmes J, Lingford-Hughes A, and Meier P (eds) (2016) *What Determines Harm from Addictive Substances and Behaviours?* Oxford: Oxford University Press.

Gornall J (2014) Europe under the influence. *BMJ* **348**: g1166.

Green LW and Allegrante JP (2011) /Healthy people 1980–2020: raising the ante decennially or just the name from public health education to health promotion to social determinants? *Health Educ Behav* **38**: 558–62.

Internet Society Global Internet Report (2015) The digital devide is not binary. Available at: http://www.wired.com/2015/01/the-digital-divide-is-not-binary/ (accessed 11 October 2015).

Kendler KS, Jacobson KC, Prescott CA, and Neale MC (2003) Specificity of genetic and environmental risk factors for use and abuse/dependence of cannabis, cocaine, hallucinogens, sedatives, stimulants, and opiates in male twins. *Am J Psychiatry* **160**: 687–95.

Khoury MJ, Gwinn M, Glasgow RE, and Kramer BS (2012) A population perspective on how personalized medicine can improve health. *Am J Prevent Med* **42**: 639–45.

Koob GF and Volkow ND (2010) Neurocircuitry of addiction. *Neuropsychopharmacology* **35**: 217–38.

Kostkova P (2015) Grand challenges in digital health. *Front Public Health* **3**: 134.

Kreitman N (1986) Alcohol consumption and the preventive paradox. *Br J Addict* **81**: 353–63.

Kumar S, Kingsley C, and DiStefano JK (2015) The Human Genome Project: where are we now and where are we going?. In: Duggirala R, Almasy L, Williams-Blangero S, Paul SFD, and Kole C (eds) *Genome Mapping and Genomics in Human and Non-Human Primates Genome Mapping and Genomics in Animals*. Berlin Heidelberg: Springer, pp. 7–31.

Kuntsche S, Gmel G, Knibbe RA, Kuendig H, Bloomfield K, Kramer S, and Grittner U (2006) Gender and cultural differences in the association between family roles, social stratification, and alcohol use: a European cross-cultural analysis. *Alcohol Alcohol* **41**: i37.

Lawton J (2002) Colonising the future: temporal perceptions and health-relevant behaviours across the adult lifecourse. *Sociol Health Illness* **24**: 714–33.

Li MD and Burmeister M (2009) New insights into the genetics of addiction. *Nat Rev Genet* **10**: 225–31.

Mahmood SS, Levy D, Vasan RS, and Wang TJ (2014) The Framingham Heart Study and the epidemiology of cardiovascular disease: a historical perspective. *Lancet* **383**: 999–1008.

Mäkelä P and Paljärvi T (2008) Do consequences of a given pattern of drinking vary by socioeconomic status? A mortality and hospitalisation follow-up for alcohol-related causes of the Finnish Drinking Habits Surveys. *J Epidemiol Commun Health* **62**: 728–33.

Marian AJ (2012) Challenges in medical applications of whole exome/genome sequencing discoveries. *Trends Cardiovasc Med* **22**: 219223.

Mechanic D (1997) The social context of health and disease and choices among health interventions. In: Brandt A and Rozin P (eds) *Morality and Health*. New York: Routledge, pp. 79–98.

Miller PG, de Groot F, McKenzie S, and Droste N (2011) Vested interests in addiction research and policy. Alcohol industry use of social aspect public relations organizations against preventative health measures. *Addiction* 106: 1560–7.

Ministry of Health Services and Ministry of Children and Family Development of British Columbia (2010) Healthy minds, healthy people: a 10-year plan to address mental health and substance use in British Columbia. Available at: http://www.health.gov.bc.ca/library/publications/year/2010/healthy_minds_healthy_people.pdf (accessed 4 June 2015)

Mockenhaupt R and Woodrum A (2015) Developing evidence for structural approaches to build a Culture of Health: a perspective from the Robert Wood Johnson Foundation. *Health Educ Behav* 42(1S): 15S–19S.

Nicholls J (2012) Everyday, everywhere: alcohol marketing and social media—current trends. *Alcohol Alcohol* 47: 486–93.

Pantaewan P and Kengganpanich M (2014) Factors predicting smoking behavior through multilevel interventions in the Royal Thai Army conscripts. *J Med Assoc Thai* 97(Suppl. 2): S123–30.

Payne HE, Lister C, West JH, and Bernhardt JM (2015) Behavioral functionality of mobile apps in health interventions: a systematic review of the literature. *JMIR mHealth uHealth* 3: e20.

Perka EJJr (2011) Culture change in addictions treatment: a targeted training and technical assistance initiative affects tobacco-related attitudes and beliefs in addiction treatment settings. *Health Promot Pract* 12(6 Suppl. 2): 159S–65S.

Prochaska JJ, Pechmann C, Kim R, and Leonhardt JM (2012) Twitter=quitter? An analysis of Twitter quit smoking social networks. *Tob Control* 21: pp. 447–9.

Ralph L, Berglas N, Schwartz S, and Brindis C (2011) Finding teens in TheirSpace: using social networking sites to connect youth to sexual health services. *Sex Res Soc Policy* 8: 38–49.

Ramo DE, Popova L, Grana R, Zhao S, and Chavez K (2015) Cannabis mobile apps: a content analysis. *JMIR Mhealth Uhealth* 3: e81.

Rehm J, Taylor B, Mohapatra S, Irving H, Baliunas D, Patra J, and Roerecke M (2010) Alcohol as a risk factor for liver cirrhosis—a systematic review and meta-analysis. *Drug Alcohol Review* 29: 437–45.

Rehm J, Zatonski W, Taylor B, and Anderson P (2011) Epidemiology and alcohol policy in Europe. *Addiction* 106(S1): 11–19.

Rehm J, Shield KD, Gmel G, Rehm MX, and Frick U (2013) Modeling the impact of alcohol dependence on mortality burden and the effect of available treatment interventions in the European Union. *Eur Neuropsychopharmacol* 23: 89–97.

Rehm J, Rehm MX, Shield KD, Gmel G, Frick U, and Mann K (2014) Reduzierung alkoholbedingter Mortalität durch Behandlung der Alkoholabhängigkeit [Decrease in alcohol-attributable mortality by treatment of alcohol dependence]. *Sucht* 60: 93–105.

Reinwand DA, Schulz DN, Crutzen R, Kremers SP, and de Vries H (2015) Who follows eHealth interventions as recommended? A study of participants' personal characteristics from the experimental arm of a randomized controlled trial. *J Med Internet Res* 17: e115.

Riper H, Spek V, Boon B, Conijn B, Kramer J, Martin-Abello K, and Smit F (2011) Effectiveness of E-self-help interventions for curbing adult problem drinking: a meta-analysis. *J Med Internet Res* 13: e42.

Rockhill B (2005) Theorizing about causes at the individual level while estimating effects at the population level. *Epidemiology* 16:124–9.

Rooke S, Thorsteinsson E, Karpin A, Copeland J, and Allsop D (2010) Computer-delivered interventions for alcohol and tobacco use: a meta-analysis. *Addiction* 105: 1381–90.

Rose G (1985) Sick individuals and sick populations. *Int J Epidemiol* 30: 427–32.

Rosenquist JN, Murabito J, Fowler JH, and Christakis NA (2010) The spread of alcohol consumption behavior in a large social network. *Ann Inter Med* 152: 426–33.

Ruths D and Pfeffer J (2014) Social sciences. Social media for large studies of behavior. *Science* 46: 1063–4.

Shield KD, Rylett MJ, Gmel G, and Rehm J (2013) Part 1. Trends in alcohol consumption and alcohol-attributable mortality in the EU in 2010. In: World Health Organization Regional Office for Europe (eds), *Status Report on Alcohol and Health in 35 European Countries 2013*. Copenhagen: WHO Regional Office for Europe, pp. 3–14.

Skog OJ (1999). The prevention paradox revisited. *Addiction* 94: 751–7.

Smit F, Lokkerbol J, Riper H, Majo MC, Boon B, and Blankers M (2011) Modeling the cost-effectiveness of health care systems for alcohol use disorders: how implementation of eHealth interventions improves cost-effectiveness. *J Med Intern Res* 13: e56

Smit ES, Evers SM, de Vries H, and Hoving C (2013) Cost-effectiveness and cost-utility of Internet-based computer tailoring for smoking cessation. *J Med Intern Res* 15: e57.

Solar O and Irwin A (2007) A Conceptual Framework for Action on the Social Determinants of Health: A Discussion Paper for the Commission on Social Determinants of Health. Geneva: World Health Organization.

Thorgeirsson TE, Geller F, Sulem P, Rafnar T, Wiste A, Magnusson KP, and Oskarsson H (2008) A variant associated with nicotine dependence, lung cancer and peripheral arterial disease. *Nature* 452: 638–42.

van El CG, Cornel MC, Borry P, Hastings RJ, Fellmann F, Hodgson SV, and de Wert GM (2013) Whole-genome sequencing in health care. *Eur J Hum Genet* 21: S1–5.

Weaver ER, Horyniak DR, Jenkinson R, Dietze P, and Lim MSC (2013) Let's get wasted! and other apps: characteristics, acceptability, and use of alcohol-related smartphone applications. *JMIR mHealth uHealth* 1: E9.

World Health Organization (2003) Addiction. In: Wilkinson R and Marmot M (eds) *Social Determinants of Health: The Solid Facts*. Geneva: World Health Organization, pp. 24–5.

World Health Organization (2014) *Global Status Report on Alcohol and Health 2014*. Geneva: World Health Organization.

Chapter 6

Policies and measures that impact on the harm done by addictive substances

6.1 **Introduction**

The harms that drugs can produce to both individuals and society have been known since ancient times. Because of this, societies have developed a range of initiatives and controls to minimize or reduce these harms, sometimes very efficiently, sometimes with no effect, or even with counterproductive effects. In historical societies, controls were enforced through tradition and peer pressure, while in modern societies action is taken through legislative initiatives and the development of health and social policies to address drug-related problems and try to minimize them (Hellman et al., 2016).

One of the cornerstones of democracy is that laws and policies are launched for the benefit of citizens, but quite often relevant pressure groups are able to lobby in order to promote laws and policies that favour their interests, despite having a negative impact on the population. Unfortunately, this happens in all economical sectors, and addictive products are no exception (Miller et al., 2016).

The need for evidence-based policies is an increasing demand from societies, and the public health field has been a pioneer in this request. Nevertheless, it is quite common to see useless policies remaining unchanged, while other policies with a good evidence base may take a long time to implement. In this chapter we make a critical review of drug policies, focusing on those that have proven effective, and exploring ways in which this effectiveness can be increased.

We take the view that humans have always lived and will continue to live with drugs, and this is why a rational approach to the problem needs to take into account the four areas addressed in this chapter: (1) how legal drugs can be modulated in a free market economy as they are not an ordinary commodity; (2) what the different strategies are that empower citizens to resist or moderate the use of addictive products; (3) what the harm-reduction strategies are that effectively reduce the negative impact of addictive products; and (4) how other policies (outside of direct drug control) may have an impact on the use of drugs and health. Finally, we review the impact global treaties on drugs have had until now and the implications for the future governance of addictions (see Box 6.1).

Box 6.1 Key elements of a rational drug policy

Humans have always lived with drugs, and this is why a rational drug policy needs to take into account four key aspects: (1) effective regulation of legal drugs in a free market; (2) strategies that empower citizens to resist or moderate the use of addictive products; (3) harm-reduction strategies that reduce the negative effect of addictive products; and (4) policies (outside of direct drug control) that have an impact on the use of drugs and well-being.

6.2 Counterbalancing market forces

In this section, the analysis will be restricted to the legal drugs, namely alcohol and tobacco. This does not imply that market forces are irrelevant in relation to illegal drugs, but it is with legal drugs that the phenomena we aim to describe can be seen most clearly. The first question is pretty obvious and fundamental: is there any need to modulate and counterbalance market forces?

The European Union (EU) economy is based on the free movement of persons, goods, and capital. Does it make sense to go against those principles? From a public health perspective there is no doubt that addictive products are not ordinary commodities (Babor, 2010), and hence deserve specific regulation.

There are at least three reasons to state that addictive products are not ordinary commodities and deserve specific regulation: (1) they produce direct and indirect harmful effects in consumers; (2) their use impacts on the health and well-being of third persons who are not consumers (passive users); and (3) these products stimulate brain systems, leading to an overestimation of their positive effects and underestimation of their negative effects, and even automatic use, all of which promote self-administration of these products.

The World Health Organization (WHO) and the World Economic Forum (WEF), identified in 2011 (Bloom et al., 2012; Wismar el al., 2013) the 'best buys' to prevent non-communicable diseases. Concerning alcohol and tobacco the best buys focus on controlling price, reducing accessibility, and forbidding advertisements.

6.2.1 Price

Governments have traditionally used taxes (custom taxes and excise duties) as a way to influence the final price of alcohol and tobacco. In the EU, these measures are used with a large heterogeneity concerning alcohol (European Comission, 2015b), and in a more harmonized way for tobacco (European Commission, 2015c): in 2015, excise taxes for wine ranged from €0 to €616.5 per hectolitre (mean 95.4; standard deviation (SD) 155.6), while excise taxes for tobacco ranged between €17.3 and €255.7 per 1000 cigarettes (mean 78.9; SD 63.7). Price has an inverse significant relationship with both alcohol and tobacco consumption and related problems.

Several studies have consistently shown that increases in real price lead to a decrease in alcohol-related problems (see OECD, 2015), including road fatalities

(Wagenaar, 2009a; Elder et al., 2010), crime, and alcohol-related morbidity (Mäkelä and Österberg, 2009).

Some authors, mainly those supporting the alcohol industry views, put into question the elasticity of alcoholic beverages (Grant and Leverton, 2009), but the impact of price on demand has been demonstrated extensively. Price elasticity represents the percentage of change in consumption that occurs when price increases by one per cent, holding other factors constant. So, a price elasticity of –0.7 indicates that a one per cent increase in price results in a 0.7 per cent decrease in alcohol consumption. Multiple reviews and meta-analyses have shown the impact of price on alcohol consumption. A meta-analysis (Wagenaar et al., 2009b) of 112 studies found an elasticity of –0.46 for beer, –0.69 for wine, and –0.80 for spirits. Their results show a highly significant relationship between alcohol tax or price measures and indices of sales or consumption of alcohol (aggregate-level correlation r = –0.44 for total alcohol).

Interestingly, because of the addictive properties of alcohol, actual consumption predicts future consumption and vice versa. This means that the price elasticity of alcohol is larger in the long term than in the short term (Xu et al., 2011). Grossman (1993) determined short- and long-term elasticities of alcohol on –0.41 and –0.65, respectively, while Gallet (2007) found elasticities of –0.52 for the short term and –0.82 for the long term. The fact that reducing actual consumption prevents future consumption adds to the preventive value of price (and taxes) for alcohol policies and becomes a key issue when targeting young people. Several studies have shown that moderate and heavy college drinkers are equally sensitive to price increases (Williams et al., 2005; Bloomfield et al., 2009), and reducing heavy drinking in this particular age group prevents future alcohol problems.

Price increases reduce alcohol consumption in the general population and, with slightly lower elasticities, also in heavy drinkers. A recent meta-analysis (Wagenaar et al., 2009b) identified ten studies on the impact of alcohol price or taxes in heavy drinkers. Eight of the ten studies found statistically significant effects and the simple mean of the ten elasticities reported was –0.28, a bit smaller than what was found for the general population (see Box 6.2).

The Sheffield Alcohol Policy Model (Brennan et al., 2014a) has modelled the impact of various policies on alcohol consumption, morbidity, and mortality, and has been extensively used to model different price policies. The minimum unit pricing (MUP) strategy has the advantage of targeting heavy drinkers, as they tend to drink cheaper

Box 6.2 In real terms, taxes on alcohol keep on decreasing

Increases in real price lead to a decrease in alcohol-related problems, including road fatalities, crime, and alcohol-related morbidity. Surprisingly, in real terms, taxes on alcohol have decreased consistently in most of Western countries since the 1970s.

alcohols and with the MUP policy these alcohols are better targeted. For example, according to the Sheffield model, the ban on below-cost selling (implemented in the UK in 2010) impacts on just one per cent of all the drinks consumed by harmful drinkers, while a MUP of 45 pence (0.5€) would affect 30.5 per cent of their drinks (Brennan et al., 2014b). At a population unit, the minimum pricing concept has successfully been tested in British Columbia, Canada, where an increase of ten per cent in the minimum price of alcohol led to a decrease of 1.5 per cent for beer, 8.9 per cent for wine, and 6.8 per cent for spirits (Stockwell et al., 2012).

Despite the consistent evidence accumulated, MUP is experiencing tremendous difficulties to be implemented owing to opposition from the alcohol industry. It is in itself an excellent case study to analyse the ability of the alcohol industry to lobby and actively try to block (often with success) the most promising policy initiatives. Scotland pioneered the adoption of the MUP. The Alcohol (Minimum pricing) Act (Scottish Parliament, 2012) was approved by Parliament in 2012 but the Scotch Whisky Association led a legal challenge, initially in Scotland and later at the EU Luxembourg Court, which has blocked the law until now.

The MUP was also to be implemented in the UK as a response to the rise in alcohol-related problems experienced in the last decade; in fact, the UK Prime Minister announced that the initiative would go ahead because 'the responsibility of being in government isn't always about doing the popular thing. It's about doing the right thing'. One year later the initiative was withdrawn, and the intense lobbying activity of the alcohol industry (discussed in more detail later) was the main driver of this U-turn (Gornall, 2014).

Price is one of the best tools to drive alcohol policy. Surprisingly, in real terms, taxes on alcohol have decreased consistently in most of Western countries since the 1970s. In the USA, for example (Xu et al., 2011), the real price (inflation adjusted) of the federal excise tax on beer had fallen from almost $31 per barrel in 1951, to around $6 per barrel in 2009. For the same period, the figures for distilled spirits fell from $35 to $6. Similar figures can be found in most of the EU countries (Österberg, 2011).

In the tobacco field, more than 100 studies, including from low-to-high-income countries, have shown that tobacco excise taxes can consistently reduce tobacco use. Significant increases in tobacco product prices help current smokers to stop and reduce consumption in those that keep on smoking (Chaloupka et al., 2011, 2012). Interestingly, the impact is higher in low-income populations and in youth. It is estimated that a ten per cent increase in price results in a four per cent decline in consumption in high-income population and eight per cent reduction in low-income groups, including youth (Jha et al., 2002). The impact of price in the onset age of smoking is also predicted but not so well documented owing to methodological limitations of the studies (Wilson et al., 2012; Guindon, 2014; Van Walbeek et al., 2013).

6.2.2 Availability

There are different ways to affect the availability of alcohol and tobacco products. Strategies can be directed to limit the number of outlets where those products are available and to limit the days and hours those outlets can be open. Other options include limiting access to certain high-risk populations, usually by setting age limits to purchase those products.

The relationship between alcohol outlet density and alcohol-related problems was established in the early 1990s in relation to injury and crime (Scribner et al., 1994, 1995; Speer et al., 1998) and has been confirmed in more recent studies (Liang and Chikritzhs, 2011), including longitudinal studies (Livingston, 2011).

Other studies have also shown a relationship between outlet density and alcohol-related morbidity and mortality (Richardson et al., 2015). Control of alcohol outlet density has been proposed as an effective system to reduce alcohol-related morbidity and mortality (Campbell et al., 2009).

Research on days and hours of opening the outlets and how this impacts alcohol-related problems is more scarce and subject to methodological limitations (Holmes et al., 2014). In any case, the available evidence is coherent with data on outlet density, and points in the direction that those are effective measures to reduce alcohol-related harm (Middleton et al., 2010).

In the tobacco field, the Framework Convention on Tobacco Control (FCTC) has allowed substantial progress, not only in the reduction of sales to minors (DiFranza, 2012), but also in the creation of smoke-free spaces. In recent years, most of the EU countries have implemented much more strict smoking bans in most public spaces (Martínez et al., 2014), and compliance with the bans is quite successful (European Commission, 2015a).

Availability is also an issue with illegal drugs. For example, Spain is one of the highest cannabis consumers in Europe, with up to 26.6 per cent of young people (aged 14–18 years) having smoked cannabis derivatives during the previous 12 months (Delegación del Gobierno para el Plan Nacional Sobre Drogas, 2014–2015). When asked about availability of cannabis products, two-thirds of teenagers considered it was easy or very easy to buy them. A clear consequence is that legal status and real status of drugs is not always coincident, and that whenever the use of drugs reaches a relevant percentage of population, availability tends to be correlated to the level of use.

In fact, cannabis provides a good example of the complexity linked to the regulation of availability. Moving away from strict prohibition, some jurisdictions have tried different options, like the coffee shops in Amsterdam (Monshouwer et al., 2011), the cannabis clubs in Catalonia (Diari Oficial de la Generalitat, 2015), the experiences of the states of Colorado and Washington in the USA, and the new approach promoted in Uruguay (Room, 2014). What all those experiences share is the interest in avoiding the criminalization of users, while impeding the unrestricted marketing and sales of cannabis products. Detractors of these innovative approaches claim that they may lead to an increase in drug use and drug-related problems. There is a need for research in order to assess the differential impact of each of those new strategies at a societal level.

6.2.3 **Marketing**

Marketing strategies have changed dramatically in recent years. The concept of a 'Global Marketing Strategy' has replaced the old idea of simply producing good advertisements. Companies are no longer interested in just successful advertisements; their aim is to reach a good placement of themselves and their products in front of consumers. Within this frame, sponsorship of activities or entities appealing to the consumer (i.e. music and sports events) has become a priority.

Also, sales strategies have become more sophisticated. Instead of providing clear explanations of the qualities of the products, the aim is now to create needs in the consumer. In the case of addictive products, creating needs that will later on be consolidated by the consumer becomes the ideal situation from a marketing perspective, even although this should be ethically (and legally) challenged.

These practices have led to the development of the neuromarketing concept. Neuromarketing studies consumers' sensorimotor, cognitive, and affective response to marketing stimuli, using technologies such as functional magnetic resonance imaging (fMRI) to measure activity in the reward areas of the brain. In other words, marketing experts are using the same technologies used by addiction neuroimaging experts but for obviously different reasons. It is clear this poses an ethical challenge that is even bigger when we talk about addictive substances like alcohol or tobacco.

In the tobacco field, marketing of tobacco products has been steadily controlled. Advertisement bans on tobacco products are already in place in most Western countries (World Health Organization, 2013), and this includes sponsorship of sports events (with the exception of Formula 1 races). At present, the major controversy is the plain packaging of cigarettes, an option that is fiercely opposed by the tobacco industry (McKee, 2013; Peeters et al., 2016).

Unfortunately, the positive experiences with tobacco have not set the scene to promote improvements in the alcohol field. It appears that the alcohol industry learnt from the lessons on what went wrong for the tobacco industry much faster than the policy-makers learnt how to translate the tobacco improvements into the alcohol arena. The alcohol industry argues that their marketing strategies do not affect global alcohol consumption and that it just produces branding effects. Nevertheless, evidence shows that adolescents exposed to alcohol advertisements, even on the Internet (Anderson et al., 2009), tend to increase their alcohol consumption. A clear correlation has also been shown between the number of alcohol-sponsored sports events an adolescent has seen and their drinking later on (De Bruijn, 2013) (see Box 6.3).

An area that is especially sensitive relates to the impact of alcohol advertisements on patients who are recovering from an alcohol use disorder. Neuroimaging studies show that alcohol advertisements produce an attentional bias (Myrick et al., 2004) and an overstimulation of brain reward circuitry (Volkow et al., 2011) in

Box 6.3 Effective regulation of alcohol advertising is lacking in most countries

Alcohol advertisements favour adolescent drinking and may jeopardize the recovery of patients suffering an alcohol use disorder. This raises important ethical issues, but regulation of alcohol advertising is lacking in Europe. Most of the EU governments have given up their regulatory role and accept the self-regulation codes proposed by the alcohol industry.

patients suffering from a substance use disorder. So, in short, apart from the impact on the general population, the evidence shows that alcohol advertisements favour adolescent drinking and may jeopardize the recovery of patients suffering an alcohol use disorder. Beyond the situations that raise important ethical issues, the regulation of alcohol advertising is still very unsatisfactory in Europe. In fact, most of the EU governments have given up their regulatory role and accept the self-regulation codes proposed by the alcohol industry. Unfortunately, these codes are often broken, and self-regulatory measures have proven ineffective in these cases.

6.3 **Managing corporate influence**

At the time this book is written, non-governmental organizations and scientists have just resigned from the EU Alcohol and Health Forum, another excellent case study in itself. The EU Alcohol and Health Forum was created, in theory, to provide support to the EU alcohol strategy, but, in fact, became a mechanism for the alcohol industry to block the development and full implementation of the strategy. Unexpectedly, the European Commission decided to postpone 'sine die' the development of a new alcohol strategy, despite the evidence that alcohol consumption in Europe is the highest in the world, and despite requests of the European Parliament and several member countries.

A similar example can be found with MUP in the UK, a proposal publicly announced by the UK's prime minister that suddenly faded away from the political agenda (Gornall, 2014). It is interesting to see how corporate influence has been managed in two different jurisdictions: Scotland and England.

In Scotland, the industry tried but failed to block the MUP and the Alcohol (Minimum Pricing) Act (Scottish Parliament, 2012), which was passed by the Scottish Parliament in May 2012. However, a legal challenge was brought by the Scotch Whisky Association and two other trade bodies, Spirits Europe and the Comité Européen des Entreprises Vins, which argued it breached European law. The legal bid was rejected by the Court of Session in Edinburgh in 2013, but, not surprisingly, it was appealed and the case was referred to the European Court of Justice. Three years later, the case is still open and the Scottish Health Authorities have not been able to implement the MUP policy.

In England, the alcohol industry reacted faster, and used their lobbying influence to block the MUP initiative, even although the UK's prime minister had publicly stated it would be implemented. An impact assessment lead by the Home Office was published in November 2012 (GB Home Office, 2012), with strong arguments in favour of setting a MUP of 45 pence per unit of alcohol.

The case of MUP has been studied as an example of how public health issues can be put high on the agenda of the general public (Patterson et al., 2015). It also serves as proof that even when there's general concern, the industry is still able to manage to defend its interests and block public health initiatives that would be saving lives and costs to society.

Industry has direct access to politicians and it has been well documented how they approached both politicians and policy-makers during and after the public hearings period of the MUP in the UK (Gornall, 2014). A similar strategy was used with the launch of the EU alcohol strategy and the creation of the Alcohol and Health Forum (De Bruijn, 2008), where the alcohol industry lobbied in order to have a dominant position in the Forum, and has managed later on to block the initiatives for a new EU alcohol strategy. Interestingly, both at UK and EU level, the forums where industry and public health actors have gathered have had the same end: the industry obtaining their goals and scientists finally pulling out of the Forums.

These tactics are not new, and, in fact, they have already been described in detail a few years ago in the tobacco area (Neuman et al., 2002). One of the best documented strategies used by the alcohol industry is the so called 'revolving door'. It is defined as 'a movement of personnel between roles as legislators and regulators and the industries affected by the legislation and regulation. In some cases the roles are performed in sequence but in certain circumstances may be performed at the same time. Political analysts claim that an unhealthy relationship can develop between the private sector and government, based on the granting of reciprocated privileges to the detriment of the nation and can lead to regulatory capture' (Miller and Harkins, 2013; Wikipedia, 2015). Clear examples of senior civil servants being hired by the alcohol industry have been documented; one of the cases is extremely relevant as the person had previously been involved in the development of the MUP in Scotland.

In summary, the evidence shows that partnering with the addictive industries does not pay off. The lobbying activities of those industries are profit oriented, and their claims of being 'public health' oriented are just part of their communication strategies. Lessons learnt should include that economical actors with vested interests should be kept outside when public health policy decisions are taken.

6.4 **Empowering citizens**

Modern societies are expected to put citizens first when deciding on policies and priorities. From this perspective, empowerment of citizens becomes a key element of all policies that focus on public health and well-being. When it comes to addictive products, empowerment can be promoted at different levels. In order to give a coherent overview of the various forms that can be used to empower citizens, we will group them in five different areas: creating awareness, dealing with stigma, decriminalizing drug use, providing advice and treatment services, and making the best use of eHealth and mHealth technologies.

6.4.1 **Creating awareness**

Governments try to provide their citizens with information that is meant to have relevant societal value, but, apart from governments, there are many other actors trying to influence citizens. In the case of addictive products, all industries involved use sophisticated global marketing strategies to defend their positions. While general mass media campaigns on alcohol and tobacco have failed to prove any effect on citizen's behaviour (Edwards, 1997), targeted actions, and especially when reinforced legally (i.e. drink and driving (Elder et al., 2004), smoke-free designated areas (Hyland et al., 2012), etc.), have proven to be successful. In a way, it could be said that enforcement is part of the global marketing strategies of governments, as the creation of popular awareness on the dangers of addictive products is a necessary step towards the adoption of less popular measures to control these products and vice versa.

6.4.2 Dealing with stigma

In its Greek origins, stigma was a mark that was burnt on the skin of criminals or slaves in order to identify them easily. Psychiatric diseases are highly stigmatized all over the world (Fabrega, 1991; Byrne, 2001). Alcohol use disorders have a higher stigma than other mental disorders (Schomerus et al., 2011). Disorders related to illegal drugs are even more stigmatized, and nowadays smokers start to face a transition from being 'trendy' to being stigmatized (Stuber et al., 2008). Even although it is well established in our societies, there are a lot of reasons to combat stigma.

At the users' level, stigma worsens their condition by increasing feelings of denial and guilt, deteriorating sense of self-efficacy, delaying help seeking behaviours, and creating social isolation that, in turn, makes things worse. At a societal level, stigma leads to inappropriate responses to the problems. Treatments are offered too late and often in inadequate settings, which, in turn, tend to reinforce the stigma. Thanks to stigma, patients are held responsible for their condition, and this a priori vision obscures clinicians' and health and social systems' vision in seeing what the real needs are of those affected (Schomerus et al., 2011). This, in turn, leads to partial and inefficient treatments with poor outcomes, closing a self-fulfilling prophecy loop.

Even although quite a lot is known about stigma (Link and Phelan, 2001), the reasons underlying it, and how it delays treatment-seeking behaviour (Vogel et al., 2007; Glass et al., 2014), we are still lacking evidence on effective ways to overcome it at personal, clinical, and societal levels. Recent experience inspired by another stigmatized condition (HIV) show that sympathetic portrayal of successfully treated individuals may lead to a decrease in stigmatization (McGinty et al., 2015). This fact points to the relevance of providing effective treatments to those in need.

According to the Social Identity Theory (Tajfel and Turner, 1986), just creating the group 'addicts' (vs the rest who are 'non-addicts') contributes to the creation of stigma. Hence, if addictions were considered as a continuum, instead of an 'on-off' phenomenon, people would find it easier to identify themselves along this continuum without feeling different from the rest (see Chapter 2).

6.4.3 De-criminalizing drug use

Since the Opium Wars of the nineteenth century, there are quite a few examples of how vested interests influence the way drugs are approached (Costa Storti and De Grauwe, 2009). Western societies can no longer ignore the fact that they have promoted and exported their own drugs (alcohol and tobacco), while criminalizing the use of drugs from foreign cultures (i.e. cocaine, heroin, cannabis, khat, etc.). This has been done under the umbrella of international treaties and still, today, we are worried about the dangers posed by illegal drugs to Western adolescents, while ignoring the harm alcohol is already creating in African societies. The War on Drugs was declared by Richard Nixon in 1972 and almost half a century later it is not only obvious that it failed to reach its goals, but it also produced serious 'collateral' damages. In the context of a 'war on drugs', drug users are easily seen as enemies who need to be prosecuted, not citizens that need support. Criminalization of drug users leads to high rates of incarceration. In the USA, from a total of 2.3 million adults incarcerated, 64.5 per cent (1.5 million) met DSM-IV criteria for a substance use disorder (Bollinger et al., 2010). On top of that, it is well established that deprived social groups are at more risk of being incarcerated than wealthier groups, even if their prevalence of drug use is lower. Criminalization usually creates more problems than it solves, and, paradoxically, drug problems are an important unsolved problem in most of the prisons (Fazel et al., 2006).

Despite the overwhelming evidence, movements towards de-criminalization are slow. At a global level, one of the most relevant initiatives is the Global Commission on Drug Policy (GCDP). The aim of the GCDP is 'to bring to the international level an informed, science-based discussion about humane and effective ways to reduce the harm caused by drugs to people and societies' (Global Commission on Drug Policy, 2014). Their position is quite strong, as they claim the War on Drugs failed in its aim to banish drugs, and they advocate for the decriminalization of drug use by those who do not produce harm to others.

Along these lines and at a country level, one of the most interesting experiences is the Portuguese initiative to decriminalize drug use. The Portuguese National Strategy for the Fight Against Drugs (Lei n.º 30/2000, de 29 de Novembro REGIME JURÍDICO DO CONSUMO DE ESTUPEFACIENTES; http://www.pgdlisboa.pt/leis/lei_mostra_articulado.php?nid=186&tabela=leis&so_miolo= (acccesed 25 September 2015)) was set in place in 2000. Its evaluation shows that social costs associated with drug use decreased by 12 per cent at the end of the first five years, and the reduction reached 18 per cent 11 years after the implementation of the strategy (Gonçalves et al., 2015). Interestingly, even although the reduction in the legal system costs is the main driver of the reduction of costs, in the longer term reductions in the health-system costs have also played a relevant part.

Although different, the regulation of legal cannabis use in Uruguay, Colorado, and Washington State may also have an impact in the same direction, even although those changes are too recent to be evaluated.

6.4.4 Advice and treatment services

Health is one of the most essential components of well-being, and modern societies recognize the right of their citizens to live in healthy environments and to receive medical care when needed. Europe is the most advanced region of the world in this aspect, but in the area of addictive behaviours the unmet needs are highly significant, especially when the high prevalence of some addictive behaviours is taken into account.

In the case of tobacco, the most common addiction, only seven per cent of smokers who tried to quit sought support from a health professional (European Commission, 2015a). It may be argued that some of them did not want any support, but given the low success rates and the scarcity of treatments provided at a primary healthcare level, a simpler explanation is that treatment and advice are not offered to those in need. On top of this, even pharmacological options like nicotine replacement therapy are offered at very expensive prices (especially when compared with the price of nicotine in the cigarettes (Bertram et al., 2007)).

In the case of alcohol, data show that alcohol use disorder is the least-treated mental disorder in Europe, with 92 per cent of those in need not receiving any treatment (Alonso et al., 2004). In the USA the treatment gap is also high: three out of four USA citizens with alcohol-related problems will not receive any formal treatment (Dawson et al., 2005) (see Box 6.4).

Identification of alcohol dependence is sometimes difficult, but even when correctly identified, this may not lead to action. In a recent European study (Rehm et al., 2015) three out of four patients identified by their general practitioner as meeting criteria for alcohol dependence did not receive any treatment nor advice to reduce their drinking. For a complete picture, we must add the fact that there is a time gap of around 10 years between the establishment of dependence and attendance for treatment (Gual et al., 2013).

According to the European Monitoring Centre for Drugs and Drug Addiction (EMCDDA), over one million EU citizens receive treatment for addiction to illegal drugs in a given year (EMCDDA, 2011a). Estimates of the population in need are difficult to make as reliable data on the prevalence of addictive disorders across the EU are not available. An EU diabetic citizen should probably expect similar treatments and standards of care in most of the EU countries, but this would not be the case if this citizen suffers a substance use disorder. Diversity here also means inequality. In some countries (or regions) specialized treatment is offered within mental health facilities, while in other countries they are completely independent. Funding bodies are also diverse, and when they are different from the health department this tends to create difficulties to promote a seamless treatment and to facilitate coordination among professionals.

Diversity is also reflected in the available clinical guidelines. Data collected by the EMCDDA (2011b) show that 17 EU countries do not have harm reduction guidelines and, further, 50 per cent of the guidelines are not evidence based, and often not in concordance with the evidence based 2009 WHO guidelines on the treatment of opioid dependence (which include opioid substitution treatment among other options).

A major problem is that services are not integrated, and the average primary care practitioner, for example family doctors, psychologist, nurse, or teacher, are not required as part of their core training to develop skills in detecting or intervening

Box 6.4 Access to treatment and standards of care are very heterogeneous

Over one million EU citizens receive treatment for addiction to illegal drugs in a given year. Access to treatment and standards of care are very heterogeneous in the EU, leading to important inequalities.

with substance use disorders, keeping treatment in this field as highly specialized, unregulated, and limited to those with the most severe need.

6.4.5 **Information and communications technologies and mHealth**

As discussed in Chapter 5, there is no doubt that new technologies can play a key role in the empowerment of citizens. The Internet is a huge and valuable source of information for both, patients and professionals. Web-based programs have shown their efficacy to screen and provide advice to some groups at risk (Bhochhibhoya et al., 2015), and the wide dissemination of smartphones has led to the development of multiple apps devoted to help people with substance use disorders, specially alcohol and tobacco (Crane et al., 2015).

But this is probably the beginning of a revolution. The next generation of apps will be much more interactive, will gather data from sensors (movement, heart rate, blood alcohol level, anxiety level, etc.), and provide a more personalized and interactive advice in real time (Boulos et al., 2014). Those changes will transform the relationship with health professionals and can offer opportunities to the patients to deal with the stigma in a more efficient way.

6.5 **Shifting use to safer delivery systems or safer drugs**

Opioid substitution treatments (OST) can be considered the paradigm of a shift to safer delivery systems. Quite often they have been considered a harm reduction strategy, while it may be more appropriate to consider them simply as one of the treatments for opiate use disorders (Fareed et al., 2001, 2011). OST was first introduced in the USA in the early 1960s, and, despite the evidence of their impact in the treated population, its wide dissemination took very long in some countries (and is still not available in some countries, e.g., Russia), mostly for ideological reasons. Professionals and policy-makers were quite often against the idea of patients recovering without being abstinent from any drug. Unfortunately, the late adoption of OST led to much higher mortality rates when the AIDS epidemic started, from cross-infection in intravenous heroin users (Torrens et al., 2013). Even today, when OST is supported by extensive evidence and included in numerous treatment guidelines (including those of the WHO), those programmes are not yet implemented in a few EU countries. Syringe exchange programmes and supervised injecting facilities are another good example of harm reduction approaches that have faced more ideological than scientific opposition (Small and Drucker, 2007).

As mentioned in Chapter 4, the tobacco field has witnessed during the last few years the rise of e-cigarettes. From a public health perspective there is still an ongoing debate on whether the e-cigarettes may be useful tools to reduce the harm produced by tobacco or, on the contrary, they will lead to an increase in the number of smokers. While the debate is ongoing (Odum et al., 2012; Bullen et al., 2013), one of the most surprising things is how fast e-cigarettes have spread across Europe without relevant legal constraints. It may also be presented as a good example of how the industry moves much faster than policy-makers. As pointed out by Hall et al. (2015), some health authorities have been very permissive, allowing a free market, while others have taken a prohibitionist approach that precludes the use of a tool that may serve to decrease harm and even to stop smoking. From a public health perspective it would be much better if a coherent regulatory approach was taken, so that access to this option was guaranteed to those who may benefit from it, while simultaneously avoiding its massive diffusion through commercial circuits. However, the exceptionally varied regulations in different countries may, in the end, yield clear epidemiological evidence of each approach.

In the alcohol field, shifts from one type of drink to another have been studied, and even unsuccessfully promoted through taxation (Herttua et al., 2008) in some countries. In some cases changes in a healthy direction have happened as a natural result of the market evolution. For example, in Southern Europe (France, Greece, Italy, Portugal, and Spain) alcohol consumption declined from 14 litres per person per year in 1974 to 10.4 litres in 1992. This relevant reduction was associated with a shift in drinking patterns, with beer increasing its consumption by 36.6 per cent and wine reducing in the same period by 43 per cent (Gual and Colom, 1997). Lowering the strength as a means to reduce the global number of grams of alcohol put in the market is a strategy that has been proposed (see Chapter 4) but has not been implemented except in Sweden, even although it is feasible from both a legal and a practical view. On the one hand, from a legal perspective, the EU has already set a strength limit for the spirits traded in the EU (European Parliament, 2008), while on the other hand, from a practical view, drinks like non-alcoholic and low-alcohol beers are already in the market are also appealing to drinkers (Segal and Stockwell, 2009) and may also be contributing to decreased alcohol consumption, even although data here are lacking. Substitution may also occur within different drugs. Some authors suggest that the rise of cannabis use is reducing the use of alcohol (Subbaraman, 2014) and could have a positive effet at a public health level, but data are not yet available to confirm this possibility (see Weissenborn and Nutt, 2012).

There are several other measures that have successfully been implemented to reduce the negative impact of alcohol, like the enforcement of drink driving laws which has taken place in most EU countries (Bernhoft et al., 2008). Also in the USA the gradual increase in legal age for drinking from 18 to 21 years has had a huge impact on road deaths (Wagenaar, 1983). Another area where action has taken place is in the analysis of drinking environments in order to make them safer. These are complex situations, and it has been shown in different European cities that young people tend to preload (drink before they go to the entertainment areas) and they can show significant levels of intoxication when arriving at venues (Hughes et al., 2011a).

Nevertheless, some of the characteristics of the venues—like crowding, permissive environments, loud music, cheap alcohol availability, poor cleanliness, a focus on dancing, and poor staff practice—are clearly associated with increased risks of alcohol-related problems and offer room for improvement through policy measures, even although measures need to be customized to the local drinking patterns that still may present relevant variations across Europe (Hughes et al., 2011b).

6.6 **Non-health policies**

The WHO has made a relevant investment in the development of the Health in All Policies (HiAP) strategy. Quite often tobacco and alcohol are used as relevant examples of the need to take health into account when developing policies that are not directly related to health (Anderson et al., 2013). The WHO director general, Margaret Chan, stated it clearly: 'The health and medical professions can plead for lifestyle changes and tough tobacco legislation, can treat patients and issue the medical bills, but they cannot re-engineer social environments in ways that encourage healthy behaviours'. And when it comes to alcohol, tobacco, and other addictive products, quite often decisions are taken in sectors that are far from health but have an important impact on health, well-being, and sustainability. The rise of non-commmunicable diseases, most of them linked to lifestyle (obesity, diabetes, hypertension, etc.), puts a tremendous stress on social/healthcare care systems of all societies, but, paradoxically, the policies that have an impact on these lifestyles are designed in other sectors, and often give priority to the profits of multinational corporations, even if this is detrimental for the whole country in the long run.

The detrimental effects of drugs on individuals and society are, to a large extent, related to the immediate drivers of harm, and those drivers are often dependent on policies issued by non-health sectors (see Chapter 4). One specific aspect that needs to be mentioned is the additive relationship between addictive products and health and social inequalities (see Chapter 3). On one hand, the evidence shows that addictive products create more harm in deprived populations; on the other hand, addictions lead to social exclusion processes that, in turn, make it more difficult to recover.

6.7 **The impact of global treaties in the drug problem**

There is no doubt that a large and sustained effort has been put into place by most of the states in the world in order to agree and maintain the United Nations' treaties on drugs (United Nations Office on Drugs and Crime, 2013a), namely the Single Convention on Narcotics from 1968 amended in 1972, the Convention on Psychotropic Substances from 1971, and the United Nations Convention Against Traffic in Narcotic Drugs and Psychotropic Substances approved in 1988. More than 40 years of Conventions allow for an in-depth analysis of its successes and failures, and, unfortunately, the latter are very predominant, especially in developing or transitional countries (Reuter et al., 2009). According to the United Nations Office on Drugs and Crime the number of drug users worldwide rose from 203 millions in 2008 to 243 million in 2012 (United Nations Office on Drugs and Crime, 2014). Interestingly, the number of novel psychoactive substances identified in 2013 was higher than the number of drugs controlled by the treaties (United Nations Office on Drugs and Crime, 2013b)(see Box 6.5).

The situation is no better when dealing with the most classical drugs. Opium production has steadily increased since the 1980s (Global Commission on Drug Policy, 2014), as has the potency of heroin, cocaine, and cannabis in the markets, while its

> ## Box 6.5 Drugs do not have to be promoted (legal) or criminalized (illegal); they need to be regulated
>
> Legal drugs are not an ordinary commodity and that is why there is a need to regulate their price and availability, and to ban their promotion. Those key measures are known as the *three best buys* and are endorsed by the WEF and the WHO. However, criminalization of illegal drugs creates more problems than it solves, and decriminalization does not lead to increased use but helps to decrease social and health costs.

price has decreased substantially (Werb et al., 2013). Even although these figures in themselves should raise criticisms with regard to the efficacy of the conventions (Strang et al., 2012), most of the contest comes from the 'side effects' attributable to the international drug conventions: violence, crime, corruption, illicit markets, and social exclusion, among others (Room and Reuter, 2012; LSE Expert Group on the Economics of Drug Policy, 2014; Kleiman et al., 2015).

Interestingly, some advocates for change (Global Commission on Drug Policy, 2014) present the WHO's FCTC (World Health Organization, 2003) as an example of how to move forward. Even although tobacco prevalence has decreased in Western countries, the total number of smokers is expected to increase from 967 million in 2012 to 1100 million in 2015, mainly owing to the population growth (Ng et al., 2014). Even although the FCTC is clearly a move forward in the control of the impact of tobacco in societies, it also must be acknowledged that an outcome evaluation is lacking, as most of the evaluations performed focus on process rather than on outcomes. In any case, compared with alcohol it is clear that tobacco is a few steps ahead, and, in fact, several voices have claimed for the need of a framework convention on alcohol (Casswell and Thamarangsi, 2009).

In summary, global treaties have not had a real positive impact on the field of illegal drugs, have allowed a few steps forward in the tobacco arena, and are still very much needed in the alcohol field, where the alcohol industry is playing an active role in undermining international initiatives (i.e. the European Alcohol Plan (World Health Organization, 2012)).

6.8 Conclusions

Addictive products pose a challenge to modern societies. The factors that influence how addictive products impact on societies are multiple and interactions between those factors are usually complex. Yet, societal responses tend to be simple (labelling products as legal or illegal) and poorly evidence based. Legal products tend to be extensively marketed, while illegal products tend to be criminalized. In both cases, these approaches are proving ineffective in terms of harm reduction.

Drugs are not an ordinary commodity and that is why there is a need to regulate their price and availability, and to ban their promotion through marketing strategies in their various forms. Those key measures are known as the *three best buys* and are endorsed by the WEF and the WHO.

However, criminalization of illegal drugs creates more problems than it solves, and there are experiences that show that decriminalization does not lead to increased use, but helps to decrease social and health costs.

Decriminalization is one of the strategies proposed to empower citizens, but there are a few more that need to be brought altogether. A very relevant one is access to treatment in appropriate settings, which needs to be improved in most countries. Normalization of treatment settings also leads to a decrease in the stigma associated with addictive behaviours.

Addictive behaviours are not a problem that can be made to disappear from Earth through a 'war on drugs'. Instead, we have to face the reality that the global treaties have proven unsuccessful. Addictive products will continue to be used. There are, however, effective ways to minimize their impact on individuals and society through a variety of strategies.

Finally, the way addictive products impact on society depends not only on the products, but also on the living conditions of citizens, as happens with most health conditions. This is why policies that deal with addictive products should also be considered in global policy making, as promoted by the 'Health in all policies' approach of the WHO.

References

Alonso J, Angermeyer MC, Bernert S, Bruffaerts R, Brugha TS, Bryson H, et al. (2004) Use of mental health services in Europe: results from the European Study of the Epidemiology of Mental Disorders (ESEMeD) project. *Acta Psychiatr Scand Suppl* **109**: 47–54.

Anderson P, de Bruijn A, Angus K, Gordon R, and Hastings G (2009) Impact of alcohol advertising and media exposure on adolescent alcohol use: a systematic review of longitudinal studies. *Alcohol Alcohol* **44**: 229–43.

Anderson P, Casswell S, Parry C, and Rehm J (2013) Health in all policies.Seizing opportunities, implementing policies. Available at: http://www.euro.who.int/__data/assets/pdf_file/0007/188809/Health-in-All-Policies-final.pdf (accessed 26 October 2016).

Babor TF (2010) Alcohol: no ordinary commodity—a summary of the second edition. *Addiction* **105**: 769–79.

Bernhoft IM, Hels T, and Hansen AS (2008) Trends in drink driving accidents and convictions in Denmark. *Traffic Inj Prev* **9**: 395–403.

Bertram MY, Lim SS, Wallace AL, and Vos T (2007) Costs and benefits of smoking cessation aids: making a case for public reimbursement of nicotine replacement therapy in Australia. *Tob Control* **16**: 255–60.

Bhochhibhoya A, Hayes L, Branscum P, and Taylor L (2015) The use of the internet for prevention of binge drinking among the college population: a systematic review of evidence. *Alcohol Alcohol* **50**: 526–35.

Bloom DE, Cafiero E, Jané-Llopis E, Abrahams-Gessel S, Reddy Bloom L, Fathima S, et al. (2012) The global economic burden of noncommunicable diseases. Available at: https://www.hsph.harvard.edu/program-on-the-global-demography-of-aging/WorkingPapers/2012/PGDA_WP_87.pdf (accessed 26 October 2016).

Bloomfield K, Rossow I, and Norström T (2009) Changes in alcohol-related harm after alcohol policy changes in Denmark. *Eur Addict Res* 15: 224–31.

Bollinger LC, Chenault KI, Dolan PR, Ganzi VF, Tuggle CC, and Roth MI (2010). Behind bars II: substance abuse and america's prison population. Available at: http://www.centeronaddiction.org/addiction-research/reports/substance-abuse-prison-system-2010 (accessed 26 October 2016).

Boulos MNK, Brewer AC, Karimkhani C, Buller DB, and Dellavalle RP (2014) Mobile medical and health apps: state of the art, concerns, regulatory control and certification. *Online J Public Health Inform* 5: 229.

Brennan A, Meier P, Purshouse R, Rafia R, Meng Y, Hill-Macmanus D, et al. (2014a) The Sheffield alcohol policy model—a mathematical description. *Health Economics* 24: 1368–88.

Brennan A, Meng Y, Holmes J, Hill-McManus D, and Meier PS (2014b) Potential benefits of minimum unit pricing for alcohol versus a ban on below cost selling in England 2014: modelling study. *BMJ* 349: g5452.

Bullen C, Howe C, Laugesen M, McRobbie H, Parag V, Williman J, and Walker N (2013) Electronic cigarettes for smoking cessation: a randomised controlled trial. *Lancet* 382: 1629–37.

Byrne P (2001) Psychiatric stigma. *Br J Psychiatry* 178: 281–4.

Campbell CA, Hahn RA, Elder R, Brewer R, Chattopadhyay S, Fielding J, et al. (2009) The effectiveness of limiting alcohol outlet density as a means of reducing excessive alcohol consumption and alcohol-related harms. *Am J Prev Med* 37: 556–69.

Casswell S and Thamarangsi T (2009) Reducing harm from alcohol: call to action. *Lancet* 373: 2247–57.

Chaloupka FJ, Straif K, and Leon ME (2011) Effectiveness of tax and price policies in tobacco control. *Tob Control* 20: 235–8.

Chaloupka FJ, Yurekli A, and Fong GT (2012) Tobacco taxes as a tobacco control strategy. *Tob Control* 21: 172–80.

Costa Storti C and De Grauwe P (2009) The cocaine and heroin markets in the era of globalisation and drug reduction policies. *Int J Drug Policy* 20: 488–96.

Crane D, Garnett C, Brown J, West R, and Michie S (2015) Behavior change techniques in popular alcohol reduction apps. *J Med Internet Res* 17: e118.

Dawson DA, Grant BF, Stinson FS, Chou PS, Huang B, and Ruan WJ (2005) Recovery from DSM-IV alcohol dependence: United States, 2001–2002. *Addiction* 100: 281–92.

De Bruijn A (2008) No reason for optimism: the expected impact of commitments in the European commission's alcohol and health forum. *Addiction* 103: 1588–92.

De Bruijn A (2013) Exposure to online alcohol marketing and adolescents' binge drinking: a cross-sectional study in four European countries. In: Anderson P, Braddick F, Reynolds J, and Gual A (eds) *Alcohol Policy in Europe: Evidence from AMPHORA*. Available at: http://www.amphoraproject.net/w2box/data/e-book/AMPHORA%20ebook.pdf (accessed 26 October 16).

Delegación del Gobierno para el Plan Nacional Sobre Drogas (2014–2015) Encuesta Estatal sobre uso de Drogas En Enseñanzas Secundarias (Estudes). Available at: http://www.pnsd.msssi.gob.es/profesionales/sistemasInformacion/sistemaInformacion/pdf/2016_ESTUDES_2014-2015.pdf (accessed ??).

Diari Oficial de la Generalitat (2015) *RESOLUCIÓN SLT/32/2015, de 15 de enero, por la que se aprueban criterios en materia de salud pública para orientar a las asociaciones cannábicas y sus clubes sociales y las condiciones del ejercicio de su actividad para los ayuntamientos de Cataluña.* Barcelona: Catalan Parliament.

DiFranza JR (2012) Which interventions against the sale of tobacco to minors can be expected to reduce smoking? *Tob Control* 21: 436–42.

Edwards G (1997) Alcohol policy and the public good. *Addiction* 92: S73–9.

Elder RW, Shults RA, Sleet DA, Nichols JL, Thompson RS, and Rajab W (2004) Effectiveness of mass media campaigns for reducing drinking and driving and alcohol-involved crashes: a systematic review. *Am J Prev Med* 27: 57–65.

Elder RW, Lawrence B, Ferguson A, Naimi TS, Brewer RD, Chattopadhyay SK, et al. (2010) The effectiveness of tax policy interventions for reducing excessive alcohol consumption and related harms. *Am J Prev Med* 38: 217–29.

European Commission (2015a) Attitudes of Europeans towards tobacco and electronic cigarettes. Available at: http://ec.europa.eu/public_opinion/archives/ebs/ebs_429_en.pdf (accessed on 26 October 2016).

European Commission (2015b) Excise duty tables. Part I alcoholic beverages (2015). Available at: http://ec.europa.eu/taxation_customs/index_en.htm# (accessed 24 May 2016).

European Commission (2015c) Excise duty tables. Part III manufactured tobacco. Available at: http://ec.europa.eu/taxation_customs/taxation/excise_duties/index_en.htm (accessed 24 May 2016).

European Monitoring Centre for Drugs and Drug Addiction (2011a) Cost and financing of drug treatment services in Europe: an exploratory study. Available at: http://www.emcdda.europa.eu/attachements.cfm/att_143682_EN_TDSI11001ENC.pdf (accessed 30 May 2016).

European Monitoring Centre for Drugs and Drug Addiction (2011b) Guidelines for the treatment of drug dependence: a European perspective. Available at: http://www.emcdda.europa.eu/attachements.cfm/att_144638_EN_SI_treatment-guidelines-p3.pdf (accessed 30 May 2016).

European Parliament (2008) Regulation (EC) No 110/2008 of the European Parliament and of the Council, L 269. *Off J Eur Commun* ??: 1–15 (accessed 24 May 2016).

Fabrega H (1991). Psychiatric stigma in non-Western societies. *Compr Psychiatry* 32: 534–51.

Fareed A, Casarella J, Amar R, Vayalapalli S, and Drexler K (2010) Methadone maintenance dosing guideline for opioid dependence, a literature review. *J Addict Dis* 29: 1–14.

Fareed A, Vayalapalli S, Stout S, Casarella J, Drexler K, and Bailey SP (2011) Effect of methadone maintenance treatment on heroin craving, a literature review. *J Addict Dis* 30: 27–38.

Fazel S, Bains P, and Doll H (2006) Substance abuse and dependence in prisoners: a systematic review. *Addiction* 101: 181–91.

Gallet CA (2007) The demand for alcohol: a meta-analysis of elasticities. *Aust J Agr Resour Econ* 51: 121–35.

GB Home Office (2012) A Minimum unit price for alcohol. Available at: https://www.gov.uk/government/uploads/system/uploads/attachment_data/file/157763/ia-minimum-unit-pricing.pdf (accessed30 May 2016).

Glass JE, Williams EC, and Bucholz KK (2014) Psychiatric comorbidity and perceived alcohol stigma in a nationally representative sample of individuals with DSM-5 alcohol use disorder. *Alcohol Clin Exp Res* 38: 1697–1705.

Global Comission on Drug Policy (2014) Taking control. Pathways to drug policies that work. Available at: http://static1.squarespace.com/static/53ecb452e4b02047c0779e59/t/540da6ebe4b068678cd46df9/1410180843424/global_commission_EN.pdf (accessed 31 May 2016).

Gonçalves R, Lourenço A, and Da Silva SN (2015) A social cost perspective in the wake of the Portuguese strategy for the fight against drugs. *Int J Drug Policy* **26**: 199–209.

Gornall J (2014) Alcohol and Public Health. Under the influence. *BMJ* **348**: f7646.

Grant M and Leverton M (2009) *Working Together to Reduce Harmful Drinking.* Hove: Routledge.

Grossman M (1993) The economic analysis of addictive behavior. In Hilton ME ad Bloss G (eds) *Economics and the Prevention of Alcohol Related Problems. National Institute on Alcohol Abuse and Alcoholism Research Monograph No. 25, NIH Pub. No. 93–513.* Bethesda, MD: National Institute on Alcohol Abuse and Alcoholism, pp. 91–123.

Gual A and Colom J (1997) Why has alcohol consumption declined in countries of southern Europe? *Addiction* **92**(Suppl.): S21–31.

Gual A, He Y, Torup L, van den Brink W, and Mann K (2013) A randomised, double-blind, placebo-controlled, efficacy study of nalmefene, as-needed use, in patients with alcohol dependence. *Eur Neuropsychopharmacol* **23**: 1432–42.

Guindon GE (2014) The impact of tobacco prices on smoking onset in Vietnam: duration analyses of retrospective data. *Eur J Health Econ* **15**: 19–39.

Hall W, Gartner C, and Forlini C (2015) Ethical issues raised by a ban on the sale of electronic nicotine devices. *Addiction* **110**: 1061–7.

Hellman M, Berridge V, Duke K, and Mold A (eds) (2016) *Concepts of Addictive Substances and Behaviours Across Time and Place.* Oxford: Oxford University Press.

Herttua K, Mäkelä P, and Martikainen P (2008) Changes in alcohol-related mortality and its socioeconomic differences after a large reduction in alcohol prices: A natural experiment based on register data. *Am J Epidemiol* **168**: 1110–18.

Holmes J, Guo Y, Maheswaran R, Nicholls J, Meier PS, and Brennan A (2014) The impact of spatial and temporal availability of alcohol on its consumption and related harms: a critical review in the context of UK licensing policies. *Drug Alcohol Rev* **33**: 515–25.

Hughes K, Quigg Z, Bellis MA, van Hasselt N, Calafat A, Kosir M, et al. (2011a) Drinking behaviours and blood alcohol concentration in four European drinking environments: a cross-sectional study. *BMC Public Health* **11**: 918.

Hughes K, Quigg Z, Eckley L, Bellis M, Jones L, Calafat A, et al. (2011b) Environmental factors in drinking venues and alcohol-related harm: The evidence base for European intervention. *Addiction* **106**(Suppl. 1): 37–46.

Hyland A, Barnoya J, and Corral JE (2012) Smoke-free air policies: past, present and future. *Tob Cont* **21**: 154–61.

Jha P, Chaloupka FJ, Chaloupka FJ, Moore J, et al. (2002) Tobacco addiction. Chapter 46 in *Disease Control in Developing Countries.* Available at: http://dcp-3.org/sites/default/files/dcp2/DCP46.pdf (last accessed 26 October 2016).

Kleiman MAR, Caulkins JP, Jacobson T, and Rowe B (2015) Violence and drug control policy. In: Donnelly PD and Ward CL (eds) *Oxford Textbook of Violence Prevention.* Oxford: Oxford University Press.

LSE Expert Group on the Economics of Drug Policy (2014) *Ending the Drug Wars.* London: London School of Economics.

Liang W and Chikritzhs T (2011) Revealing the link between licensed outlets and violence: Counting venues versus measuring alcohol availability. *Drug Alcohol Rev* **30**: 524–35.

Link BG and Phelan JC (2001) Conceptualizing stigma. *Annu Rev Sociol* **27**: 363–85.

Livingston M (2011) A longitudinal analysis of alcohol outlet density and domestic violence. *Addiction* **106**: 919–25.

McGinty EE, Goldman HH, Pescosolido B, and Barry CL (2015) Portraying mental illness and drug addiction as treatable health conditions: effects of a randomized experiment on stigma and discrimination. *Soc Sci Med* **126**: 73–85.

McKee M (2013) European Union's tobacco products directive. *BMJ* **347**: f6196.

Mäkelä P and Österberg E (2009) Weakening of one more alcohol control pillar: a review of the effects of the alcohol tax cuts in Finland in 2004. *Addiction* **104**: 554–63.

Martínez C, Martínez-Sánchez JM, Robinson G, Bethke C, and Fernández E (2014) Protection from secondhand smoke in countries belonging to the WHO European Region: an assessment of legislation. *Tob Control* **23**: 403–11.

Middleton JC, Hahn RA, Kuzara JL, Elder R, Brewer R, Chattopadhyay S, et al. (2010) Effectiveness of policies maintaining or restricting days of alcohol sales on excessive alcohol consumption and related harms. *Am J Prev Med* **39**: 575–89.

Miller D, Harkins C, and Schlögl M (2016) *Impact of Market Forces on Addictive Substances and Behaviours.* Oxford: Oxford University Press.

Miller D and Harkins C (2013) Revolving doors and alcohol policy: a cautionary tale - ALICE RAP. Available at: http://www.alicerap.eu/blog/120-revolving-doors-and-alcohol-policy-a-cautionary-tale.html (accessed 01 June 2016).

Monshouwer K, Van Laar M, and Vollebergh WA (2011) Buying cannabis in 'coffee shops.' *Drug Alcohol Rev* **30**: 148–56.

Myrick H, Anton RF, Li X, Henderson S, Drobes D, Voronin K, and George MS (2004) Differential brain activity in alcoholics and social drinkers to alcohol cues: relationship to craving. *Neuropsychopharmacol* **29**: 393–402.

Neuman M, Bitton A, and Glantz S (2002) Tobacco industry strategies for influencing European Community tobacco advertising legislation. *Lancet* **359**: 1323–30.

Ng M, Freeman MK, Fleming TD, Robinson M, Dwyer-Lindgren L, Thomson B, et al. (2014) Smoking prevalence and cigarette consumption in 187 countries, 1980-2012. *JAMA***311**: 183–92.

Odum LE, O'Dell KA, and Schepers JS (2012) Electronic cigarettes: do they have a role in smoking cessation? *J Pharm Pract* **25**: 611–14.

OECD (2015) *Tackling Harmful Alcohol Use : Economics and Public Health Policy.* Paris: OECD Publishing.

Österberg EL (2011) Alcohol tax changes and the use of alcohol in Europe. *Drug Alcohol Rev* **30**: 124–9.

Patterson C, Katikireddi SV, Wood K, and Hilton S (2015) Representations of minimum unit pricing for alcohol in UK newspapers: a case study of a public health policy debate. *J Public Health* **37**: 40–9.

Peeters S, Costa H, Stuckler D, McKee M, and Gilmore AB (2016) The revision of the 2014 European tobacco products directive: an analysis of the tobacco industry's attempts to 'break the health silo'. *Tob Control* **25**: 108–17.

Rehm J, Allamani A, Vedova R Della, Elekes Z, Landsmane I, Manthey J, et al. (2015) General practitioners recognizing alcohol dependence: a large cross-sectional study in 6 European countries. *Ann Fam Med* **13**(1): 28–32.

Reuter P, Trautmann F, Pacula RL, Kilmer B, Gageldonk A, and van der Gouwe D (2009) Assessing Changes in Global Drug Problems, 1998–2007. RAND Technical Report. Available at: http://www.rand.org/pubs/technical_reports/TR704.html (accessed 26 October 2016).

Richardson EA, Hill SE, Mitchell R, Pearce J, and Shortt NK (2015) Is local alcohol outlet density related to alcohol-related morbidity and mortality in Scottish cities ? *Health Place* **33**: 172–80.

Room, R. (2014). Legalizing a market for cannabis for pleasure: Colorado, Washington, Uruguay and beyond. *Addiction*, *109*(3), 345–351. http://doi.org/10.1111/add.12355

Room R and Reuter P (2012) How well do international drug conventions protect public health? *Lancet* **379**: 84–91.

Schomerus G, Lucht M, Holzinger A, Matschinger H, Carta MG, and Angermeyer MC (2011) The stigma of alcohol dependence compared with other mental disorders: a review of population studies. *Alcohol Alcohol* **46**: 105–12.

Scottish Parliament (2012) Alcohol (Minimum Pricing) (Scotland) Act (2012). Scottish Parliament. Available at: http://www.legislation.gov.uk/asp/2012/4/pdfs/asp_20120004_en.pdf (accessed 31 May 2016).

Scribner RA, MacKinnon DP, and Dwyer JH (1994) Alcohol outlet density and motor vehicle crashes in Los Angeles County cities. *J Stud Alcohol* **55**: 447–53.

Scribner RA, MacKinnon DP, and Dwyer JH (1995) The risk of assaultive violence and alcohol availability in Los Angeles county. *Am J Public Health* **85**: 335–40.

Segal DS and Stockwell T (2009) Low alcohol alternatives: a promising strategy for reducing alcohol related harm. *Int J Drug Policy* **20**: 183–7.

Small D and Drucker E (2007) Closed to reason: time for accountability for the International Narcotic Control Board. *Harm Reduct J* **4**: 13.

Speer PW, Gorman DM, Labouvie EW, and Ontkush MJ (1998) Violent crime and alcohol availability: relationships in an urban community. *J Public Health Policy* **19**: 303–18.

Stockwell T, Auld MC, Zhao J, and Martin G (2012) Does minimum pricing reduce alcohol consumption? The experience of a Canadian province. *Addiction* **107**: 912–20.

Strang J, Babor TF, Caulkins J, Fischer B, Foxcroft DR, and Humphreys K (2012) Drug policy and the public good: Evidence for effective interventions. *Lancet* **379**: 71–83.

Stuber J, Galea S, and Link BG (2008) Smoking and the emergence of a stigmatized social status. *Soc Sci Med* **67**: 420–30.

Subbaraman MS (2014) Can cannabis be considered a substitute medication for alcohol? *Alcohol Alcohol* **49**: 292–8.

Tajfel H and Turner JC (1986) The social identity theory of intergroup behavior. In Worchel ?? and Austin ?? (eds) *Psychology of Intergroup Relations*, 2nd edition,. Chicago, IL: Burnham, pp. 7–24.

Torrens M, Fonseca F, Castillo C, and Domingo-Salvany A (2013) Methadone maintenance treatment in Spain: the success of a harm reduction approach. *Bull World Health Organ* **91**: 136–41.

United Nations Office on Drugs and Crime (2013a) The international drug control conventions. Available at: https://www.unodc.org/documents/commissions/CND/Int_Drug_Control_Conventions/Ebook/The_International_Drug_Control_Conventions_E.pdf (accessed 31 May 2016).

United Nations Office on Drugs and Crime (2013b) World Drug Report 2013. Available at: https://www.unodc.org/unodc/secured/wdr/wdr2013/World_Drug_Report_2013.pdf (accessed 26 October 2016).

United Nations Office on Drugs and Crime (2014) *World Drug Report 2014.* New York: Oxford University Press.

Van Walbeek C, Blecher E, Gilmore A, and Ross H (2013) Price and tax measures and illicit trade in the framework convention on tobacco control: what we know and what research is required. *Nicotine Tob Res* 15: 767–76.

Vogel DL, Wade NG, and Hackler AH (2007) Perceived public stigma and the willingness to seek counseling: the mediating roles of self-stigma and attitudes toward counseling. *J Counsel Psychol* 54: 40–50.

Volkow ND, Wang GJ, Fowler JS, Tomasi D, and Telang F (2011) Addiction: beyond dopamine reward circuitry. *Proc Natl Acad Sci U S A* 108: 15037–42.

Wagenaar AC (1983) Raising the legal drinking age in Maine: impact on traffic accidents among young drivers. *Int J Addict* 18: 365–77.

Wagenaar AC, Maldonado-Molina MM, and Wagenaar BH (2009a) Effects of alcohol tax increases on alcohol-related disease mortality in Alaska: time-series analyses from 1976 to 2004. *Am J Public Health* 99: 1464–70.

Wagenaar AC, Salois MJ, and Komro KA (2009b) Effects of beverage alcohol price and tax levels on drinking: a meta-analysis of 1003 estimates from 112 studies. *Addiction* 104: 179–90.

Weissenborn R and Nutt DJ (2012) Popular intoxicants: what lessons can be learned from the last 40 years of alcohol and cannabis regulation? *J Psychopharmacol* 26: 213–20.

Werb D, Kerr T, Nosyk B, Strathdee S, Montaner J, and Wood E (2013) The temporal relationship between drug supply indicators: an audit of international government surveillance systems. *BMJ Open* 3: e003077.

Wikipedia. (2015). Revolving door (politics). Available at: https://en.wikipedia.org/wiki/Revolving_door_%28politics%29 (accessed 2 September 2016).

Williams J, Chaloupka FJ, and Wechsler H (2005) Are there differential effects of price and policy on college students' drinking intensity? *Contemp Econ Policy* 23: 78–90.

Wilson LM, Avila Tang E, Chander G, Hutton HE, Odelola OA, Elf JL, et al. (2012) Impact of tobacco control interventions on smoking initiation, cessation, and prevalence: a systematic review. *J Environ Public Health* 2012: 961724. Available at: https://www.ncbi.nlm.nih.gov/pmc/articles/PMC3376479/pdf/JEPH2012-961724.pdf(accessed on 26 October 2016).

Wismar M, McKee M, Ernst K, Srivastava D, and Busse R (2013) *Measurement of and Target-setting for Well-being: An Initiative by the WHO Regional Office for Europe.* World Health Organization, Copenhagen.

World Health Organization (2003) The Framework Convention on Tobacco Control. *Glob Health Promot* 17(1 Suppl.): 76–80.

World Health Organization (2012) *European Alcohol Action Plan 2012–2020 Implementing Regional and Global Alcohol Strategies.* World Health Organization, Copenhagen.

World Health Organization (2013) *WHO Report on the Global Tobacco Epidemic.* World Health Organization, Geneva.

Xu X, Ph D, and Chaloupka FJ (2011) Trends in alcoholic beverage taxes and prices. *Alcohol Res Health* 34: 236–46.

Chapter 7

Empowering young people to manage drug-related risk

7.1 **Introduction**

The transition from childhood to young adulthood involves maturational changes in all domains of life, including important biological and neural maturation, changes to one's social context requiring autonomy and personal responsibility, and environmental changes, including exposure to new opportunities for enrichment and risk for harm. This developmental period is also marked by high rates of risk-taking behaviours, including drug use, and is a period during which symptoms of chronic mental health disorders begin to manifest.

There is much known about risk factors for drug-related harm, which include environmental, psychosocial and genetic factors. Yet public health and prevention strategies have traditionally been universal and generic in nature. The current chapter will review risk factors for drug-related harm in the population and the intervention strategies that most target these risk factors in youth. An effort will also be made to review evidence, when available, on targeted intervention strategies, which have received far less attention in systematic reviews on preventing drug-related harm. Finally, we review resilience factors unique to this developmental period which could be harnessed in new interventions to promote risk management among young people as a form of prevention.

7.2 **Drug use in young people**

While the burden of disease, social costs, and disability associated with drug use is considerable (Begg et al., 2007; Collins and Lapsley, 2008; Degenhardt et al., 2008) across the lifespan, the peak of this disability occurs in those aged 15–24 years (Andrews et al., 2001). Despite alcohol having a minimum legal purchase age in most Western countries, young people continue to consume alcohol, and the majority of adolescents report trying alcohol in their lives (National Health and Medical Research Council, 2001; Hibell et al., 2007; National Institute on Drug Abuse, 2008). In Europe, an average of around 90 per cent of young people (defined in the corresponding study as 15–16 year olds) reported having ever tried alcohol in their lives, 80 per cent reported consuming alcohol in the past 12 months, and 60 per cent in the past month (Hibell et al., 2007). Approximately 60 per cent of young people report having ever tried a cigarette in their life; half of these young people had a cigarette in the past month and only two per cent had smoked a packet within the last month (Hibell et al., 2007). These statistics clearly highlight the need to rethink policies simply focused on legal age limits for access to drugs in Europe. This point is further emphasized when we look at rates of illegal drug use in young people. In Europe, 20 per cent of young people reported lifetime cannabis use, and seven per cent reported having ever used an illegal drug other than cannabis in their life (Hibell et al., 2007).

In North America, despite having made great strides in reducing adolescent drinking rates, illicit substance use remains significantly above national targets for health promotion and disease prevention (Substance Abuse and Mental Health Services Administration (SAMHSA), 2015; Health Canada, 2014). In 2014, cannabis use and non-medical use of psychotherapeutics were the most common types of illicit drug use by North American adolescents and there is little evidence that rates of cannabis use have changed over the last 10 years. More concerning is that rates of adolescent substance abuse and dependence remain high and unchanged over this period (SAMHSA, 2015).

Acute effects of excessive use of alcohol by adolescents can lead to memory loss, blackouts, injuries, violence, risky sexual behavior, suicide, overdose, or death (National Health and Medical Research Council, 2001; Loxley et al., 2004). Longer-term or chronic harms resulting from alcohol use in young people are less well studied and complicated by the role of premorbid vulnerability factors and chaotic drug use patterns that are often recurrent and relapsing. In the long term, excessive use of alcohol among adolescents can lead to cognitive impairment, neural abnormalities, damage to the pancreas and liver (cirrhosis), stomach ulcers, increased risk of some cancers, poorer mental health, including increased anxiety and depression, and even suicide (Windle et al., 1992; Degenhardt et al., 2001; National Health and Medical Research Council, 2001; Loxley et al., 2004; Alanti et al., 2005; Tapert et al., 2005; Baker and Velleman, 2007; Back and Brady, 2008; Back et al., 2009; Hall et al., in press).

The acute effects of cannabis use on adolescents are also well studied and include anxiety, panic, depressive feelings, short-term memory impairments, psychotic-like experiences, and slowing of reaction time (Scheier and Botvin, 1995; Degenhardt et al., 2001; Hall et al., 2001; Hall, 2006; Wittchen et al., 2007; Yucle et al., 2008; Fergusson et al., 2009; Mackie et al., 2013). Early onset (before the age of 17 years) and frequent use of cannabis can also increase the risk of developing later sustained heavy use of cannabis, using other illegal drugs, and experiencing related harms (Coffey et al., 2002; Patton et al., 2007). One particular concern is the increased risk for psychosis, particularly among those with genetic and/or familial predisposition to psychosis (e.g. Arseneault et al., 2004; Caspi et al., 2005; Mackie et al., 2013). The longer-term effects associated with chronic or heavy use of cannabis are robust and include increased risk of developing chronic bronchitis and cancers of the digestive tract and lungs, poor attention and memory, reduced academic performance, and school dropout (Tien and Anthony, 1990; Thomas, 1996; Hall, 1998, 2006; Degenhardt and Hall, 2001; Hall et al., 2001, 2004; Van Os et al., 2002; Zammit et al., 2002; Semple et al., 2005; Wittchen et al., 2007; Chabrol et al., 2008) (see Box 7.1).

Box 7.1 Prevention requires substantially more investment

Investment in prevention research and delivery typically represents less than one per cent of all costs of drug use to society in a given year (see Rehm, 2006), despite demonstrated substantial cost savings resulting from each delayed or prevented case of drug-related harm (e.g. Hurley, et al., 2004).

7.3 Age of initiation and when to intervene

Early initiation to substance use has been recognized as a strong risk factor for the later development of substance use disorder, comorbid mental health problems, and more severe course of substance use disorder (Gruber et al., 1996; Anthony and Petronis, 1995; Teesson et al., 2005; Grant et al., 2006; Behrendt et al., 2009). The earlier the age of initiation of regular drinking, the greater the risk of developing alcohol-related disorder, as well as related harms such as violence and injuries (Gruber et al., 1996; Grant et al., 2006). Similarly, earlier age of initial use and onset of regular use of cannabis is associated with greater risk of developing sustained heavy use and related harms such as psychosis (Patton et al., 2007; Behrendt et al., 2009; Mackie et al., 2013).

It is therefore extremely important to consider the timing of programme delivery and policies that impact youth drug use before regular and excessive drug use has begun. The onset of drug use in adolescence coincides with the occurrence of critical developmental periods in terms of social and emotional well-being (Spooner et al., 1996; Simmons and Blyth, 2008) and critical brain development (Sowell et al., 2004; Tapert et al., 2005). It is a time when young people are highly motivated to become more independent, autonomous, and develop the skills they need to decrease dependence on families and traditional structures (e.g. schools), in order to experience new things, be accepted by peers, and forge new opportunities for themselves. This is a time when the prefrontal cortex (involved in judgement, decision-making, and control of emotional responses) is maturing, which involves pruning of grey matter and refining of connections across the brain (Gogtay et al., 2004). Decision-making (Luna and Sweeney, 2004) and susceptibility to immediate rewards (Galvan et al., 2006) are brain functions that have been shown to evolve during the adolescent period as a result of these brain changes. It has been hypothesized that early exposure to drugs interferes with important neuromaturation. Evidence from animal studies is mounting suggesting that early exposure to drugs, particularly alcohol and at high doses, has neurotoxic effects on the adolescent brain (e.g. Vetreno and Crews, 2015). Equally, biological processes implicated in addiction such as sensitization and tolerance to certain psychoactive substances can be observed following single drug-using events (Kameda et al., 2011). Additionally, adolescence and prior stress exposure appear to render individuals more sensitive to the sensitization process (Kameda et al., 2011; Matuszewich et al., 2014). This might explain why early-onset drug use is so robustly linked to future regular heavy use and, more broadly, to many other mental health and psychosocial outcomes.

Box 7.2 Youth-relevant policies must be based on findings from cognitive and developmental neuroscience

Current drug policies must align themselves with these findings and focus on developing effective strategies for delaying onset of drug-use behaviours that have the most severe consequences for young people both from a neurotoxicity and a social perspective. According to the growing literature suggesting impact of drug use on cognitive development, not only will these emergent policies and programmes reduce future drug-related harmful behaviour, but they will also have the potential to increase intellectual and functional capacity in young people in the general population more broadly.

Evidence for humans is limited by the lack of longitudinal data and experimental designs, but what there is also suggests an association between early-onset drug misuse and neurocognitive impairment (e.g. Cservenka and Nagel, 2012; Squeglia et al., 2014) (see Box 7.2).

Drawing on the literature emerging from the traumatic brain injury field, once we have a clear picture of the neurodevelopmentally toxic effects of early-onset drug use, neuropsychologically informed interventions can be developed to support families and youth in their recovery from early-onset drug use during treatment (e.g. Kurowski et al., 2014), which currently do not exist.

7.4 Risk and protective factors for substance use

While many youth illegally experiment with legal and illegal drugs as they transition to adulthood, not all initiate at very early ages or make the transition to excessive use, or experience harm from their drug use. Thirty decades of longitudinal research have identified a number of robust risk factors for heavy drug use, many of which are observable or manifest as problems in adolescence (e.g. Castellanos-Ryan et al., 2012; Whelan et al., 2014). It has been suggested that the most promising solutions to effective prevention of substance use disorders is to target risk factors and enhance protective factors in interventions before drug use has its onset (Hawkins et al., 1992; Conrod and Nikolaou, 2016). We first briefly review the evidence for risk and protective factors, and then discuss new and emerging intervention approaches that more directly address these targets.

The numerous risk and protective factors strongly implicated in the development of drug use can be divided into three main categories: (1) Genetic factors (biological predispositions to drug use); (2) individual factors, which include personality, attitudes, beliefs, and early childhood characteristics (Hawkins et al., 1992; Spooner et al., 1996; Scheier et al., 1997; Loxley et al., 2004; Stockwell et al., 2004); and (3) environmental/contextual factors, which include peer (Oetting and Lynch, 2003; Kuntsche et al., 2006), family, and societal factors affecting pressure to use, drug availability, and acceptability of drug use behaviours; see Newton et al. (2010) for a review.

7.5 **Youth-informed drug and alcohol policy for the twenty-first century**

Policies relevant to youth drug use have traditionally been developed by adults and often validated using adult data. There is a recognition that for public health policies and health services to be more effective for youth, researchers and policy-makers must strive to engage youth when developing effective and sustainable solutions to public health problems. In the following sections we review the traditional policies aimed at reducing youth drug-related harm, with a particular focus on how they could be modified while taking into account youth-relevant data and perspectives.

7.5.1 **Limiting youth access to substances through age limits**

Statistics on the multiple harms experienced by young people who use drugs have renewed interest in evidence-based intervention programmes and policies that can be initiated early, before problems begin to cause disability, and educational and social harms (Spooner and Hall, 2002). Policies that simply focus on accessibility have been widely studied, but rarely within an experimental design, making it difficult to infer causal relationships to youth drug use and related harms. The other difficulty in this area is that such policies are often implemented within a specific sociopolitical context, making it very difficult to associate a specific policy with a particular outcome. Nevertheless, there are a number of important studies that do shed some light on this issue.

The Health Behaviour in School-aged Children (HBSC) study provides an opportunity to examine cross-sectionally the relationship between a country's legal drinking age and average age of onset, binge drinking rates, and problem-drinking symptoms among 11, 13, and 15 year olds across 37 countries. This study reported relationships between minimum purchasing age and weekly alcohol consumption by adolescents, but did not show such policies to be related to frequency of drunkenness in adolescents, which was predicted by adult consumption patterns (Bendtsen et al., 2014). By contrast, using a quasi-experimental design, a USA study was able to capitalize on the implementation of major policy changes around legal drinking age and was able to show that drinking rates, alcohol-related problems, and automobile accidents among young people were significantly reduced following adoption of policies that increased legal drinking age limits (e.g. Ferguson et al., 2007; Ponicki et al., 2007).

How to reconcile these two sets of findings? It is possible that age limits are important in cultures where young people have early and regular access to automobiles, such as in rural and suburban contexts in the USA. Accordingly, it has been suggested that it might be important to separate the age at which young people learn to drive and begin to experiment with alcohol and that policies that force young people to stage the age at which they go through these two developmental milestones will help them to transition into these two adult behaviours responsibly and with less risk.

Following the recognition of the role of alcohol in a significant portion of motor vehicle accidents, France has adopted a number of driving regulations, including one directed at young drivers, holding them to different driving standards than older, more seasoned drivers. The blood alcohol limit for novice drivers (less than three years of driving experience) has been reduced to 0.02 per cent, which is the same level as that applied to bus drivers in France. North American evaluations of graduated licensing laws have demonstrated a significant reduction in drinking behavior and alcohol-related vehicle fatalities (Fell et al., 2011).

With respect to cannabis-relevant policies, laws that allow for similar regulation of cannabis use while driving have proven difficult to implement owing to the difficulties associated with testing for acute cannabis intoxication and have not been widely studied in terms of their effects on drug-related harms in young people. Nevertheless, as European governments begin to adopt new drug policies, including decriminalizing policies, they must begin to explore more creative policies for young people that go beyond legal access limits. Like France's recent regulations, policies should be based on an understanding of the contexts in which young people are most at risk of experiencing harm from drugs and the drugs that have the most potential to interfere with normal (neuro)maturation and development. Taking France's example, is it possible to develop youth-relevant policies that will help young people to adopt gradually harm-free drug-use patterns, for example allowing them to have legal access to low-potency nicotine or cannabis in smokeless forms, so that they can experiment with substances without having to interact with the illegal drug market, expose themselves to carcinogens, and unregulated high-potency tobacco or tetrahydrocannabinol agents that have been linked to sustained heavy use and psychosis risk in young people.

7.5.2 Enforcing age limits without causing harm

Within this realm of drug-related policies, there are also considerations for how we manage young people who violate such laws. While it is true that the more strictly legal drinking and smoking laws are enforced, the greater the benefits on youth drug use (see Chapter 6), it is important that such policies do not inadvertently lead to consequences for drug-using young people that are as or even more harmful than the drug use itself. Consequences for violating such laws can often lead to sentences that interfere with travel to or access to mainstream education and other personally valued activities, social isolation or embarrassment, and incarceration. This is one reason why the American Academy of Pediatrics did not recommend the use of drug testing in schools (Levy et al., 2015), and why school inclusion is advocated in many school drug strategies.

Similarly, youth drug courts have been evaluated with respect to their potential to help divert drug-using young people away from incarceration by forcing them to attend treatment. Youth drug courts have been shown to be effective when they implement evidence-based treatment programmes (e.g. Henggeler et al., 2012). However, many more policies should be considered earlier in the pathway to harmful drug use as young people begin to experiment with drug use. While policies such as mandated treatment might be cost-effective considering the alternative (e.g. incarceration), they remain expensive and invasive relative to solutions that can be implemented earlier in the developmental course of a drug use trajectory. Finally, recognizing that there are significant inequalities in criminal justice and health systems with respect to how young minority men are provided with services (see Chapter 3), there is even more reason to try to avoid using such systemic interventions as the only deterrent for harmful drug use in young people.

7.5.3 Pricing policies and youth substance use

Some policies are not relevant in specific contexts or populations and it is important that policies are also targeted to the needs of specific youth subcultures. For example, underage drinking and binge drinking are prevalent among young people living in cultures where alcohol is highly accessible and inexpensive, and in urban centres where sanctions against impaired driving are less of a deterrent for young people. In such contexts, young people still suffer from alcohol and drug-related injuries, which can account for as much as 20 per cent of all accident and emergency room visits (Hoskins and Benger, 2012).

Pricing laws clearly impact adult consumption behaviour and consequences, and recent reviews also suggest that such benefits also extend to adolescents (Xu and Chaloupka, 2011), including benefits to academic performance and risky sexual behaviours. It has also been suggested that minimum pricing laws have the potential to be specifically relevant to the prevention of alcohol-related harm among young people, owing to their limited financial independence.

Nevertheless, in many Western countries, alcohol is marketed so cheaply that a person can purchase enough alcohol to become legally intoxicated for less than the cost of lunch. Limiting accessibility to single-serving containers or extra-large container sizes and minimum pricing will no doubt reduce excessive drinking among young people. These principles should also be explored in contexts where drug policies involve decriminalization. It will be very important to adopt concurrently policies that will allow governments to control drug prices in ways that are relevant to young people. Otherwise, young people will continue to access cheaper, unregulated, and often unsafe alternatives to the more expensive, safer option.

It should also be noted that young people do not necessarily choose to consume the cheapest brands, and price does not appear to dictate their behaviour in the same way as it might for adults (e.g. Albers et al., 2014). The relationship between socio-economic status and drug use in adolescence can in some cases be the inverse of that observed in adults (Patrick et al., 2012). Policies deemed evidenced-based from research on adults should not be directly applied to young people without proper evaluation, and there is a need for more youth-focused research in this area. Another advantage to regulated drug markets is that marketing strategies can be developed to set prices according to behavioural economics research which will tell us at what point certain attributes of a drug (e.g. price, brand, availability, potency) will tip a young person over into an illegal drug market. Simply focusing on legal age limits and enforcement can detrimentally interfere with our ability to understand and shape youth drug use towards safer alternatives.

7.6 **Youth and the digital world**

Pricing policies cannot fully protect young people against the use and harmful use of illegal drugs, which, despite their illegal nature, remain highly accessible in places where young people tend to aggregate, such as school playgrounds, parks, public transit stations, shopping malls, and, more recently, over the Internet. For these reasons, policies and programmes that allow for better supervision of such environments, particularly those which involve well-supervised and scheduled after-school activities, have been shown to have highly protective effects on adolescent drug use and antisocial behaviours (Gottfredson, 2012). With the emergence of new retail operations focusing on spaces for children to play and interact, similar teen-focused products have the potential to provide young people with these protective benefits. Yet, very few businesses other than digital products have developed around this potential market.

The Australian Headspace brand is an example of youth-focused, community-based services that have the potential to provide at-risk youth with safe environments for gathering, seeking social support, and youth-friendly health services. While the evidence has yet to demonstrate that such a system provides any protective effect on youth drug use, particularly at the population level, this model is certainly being considered as a possible solution to youth mental health and drug-related problems and one which provides alternatives to restrictive regulatory policies.

Equally, social media products must begin to address their role in promoting opportunities for accessing drugs and for promoting drug-related attitudes and behaviours in young people. Policies that allow for new emerging drugs to be temporarily banned for up to 12 months have been used to help governments stay on top of the rapidly evolving nature of the synthetic drug market that is now available online. Such policies allow toxicologists a period of time to conduct necessary research on the toxicity and in some cases addictive potential of a drug in order to inform longer-term policies. However, it remains difficult to limit access to information on how to set up chemical laboratories at home and where to legally access compounds to produce certain banned drugs. This is the case for drugs such as gamma-hydroxybutyric acid (GHB), gamma-butyrolactone (GBL), and 1,4-butanediol (1,4-BD), which are almost exclusively used by young people, and which have very severe toxicity profiles.

Considering that such drugs are mostly used in specified contexts that are not well supervised (e.g. unsupervised parties and raves), it is possible to implement interventions that encourage young people to adopt more evidence-based harm reduction behaviours in high-risk contexts. For example, young people are naturally inclined to engage in harm-reduction strategies (Fernández-Calderón et al., 2014). Public health programmes must expand the extent to which young people are engaged in developing harm-reduction solutions so that programmes facilitate youth resilience behaviours, particularly among the most hard to reach. These programmes should be implemented regardless of whether the target behaviours are deemed legal or illegal. Digital tools and hotlines to report drug-related incidences, pop-up or mobile emergency services (such as has been done in London, UK, around the GHB and GBL epidemic), and the use of crowdsourcing and social media as a way to develop and spread effective peer-to-peer messages (e.g. Coley et al., 2013) are all examples of how young people can be engaged in their digital world to impact dramatically the efficacy of public health interventions to promote safer drug-taking environments.

7.6.1 Digital marketing and young people

The majority of the Western world has adopted advertising bans on alcohol and nicotine products, particularly targeted at young people, in reaction to the established relationship between advertising exposure and risk for onset and escalation of drinking and smoking (see Anderson et al., 2009). However, a number of other forms of marketing continue to influence adolescent drug use that requires attention in current policies. Alcohol and tobacco cues continue to be highly prevalent in media relevant to young people, but it has been difficult to document the role of industry in other marketing actions, such as portraying heavy drinking or smoking as normative, rather than specific product and brand placements. Social media platforms now provide digital marketers with opportunities to use interactive techniques, giving them access to information on relationships between individuals and communities and allowing them to monitor and track who influences whom and the sources of greatest influence on youth (see review by Montgomery et al., 2012) and most national policies focusing on advertising to children have not been sufficiently updated to address these new practices. Furthermore, many of these policies treat adolescents like adults, despite clear evidence that reward and self-control behaviours are under-developed in adolescents relative to adults (Sowel and Thompson, 2004; Casey et al., 2011). Finally, the interactive nature of current marketing strategies is intentionally used to further compromise decision making ability (e.g. distraction or tapping into reward-seeking behaviours through gaming and contests).

Despite being held to the same regulatory standards as offline advertising and marketing strategies (e.g. Federal Trade Commission guidelines for governing endorsements/testimonials in advertisement), social media websites are dominated by advertisements and references to excessive drinking, smoking, and drug use at all times of the day and with very little restriction. For example, many drinks companies sponsor and/or advertise on youth-popular sites on Instagram, Facebook, and Twitter, in addition to hosting their own websites, which often contain youth-relevant content such as games, videos, competitions, and prizes. Many advertising codes restrict alcohol marketing to children by preventing advertisements being shown on television until after 20.30, yet these rules do not appear to be enforced when it comes to Internet-based advertising. Instagram and YouTube have no age restrictions on viewers, but they do allow alcohol companies to link their television advertisements on youth-relevant sites. Furthermore, in order to protect the important contribution of social media sites to the dissemination of free speech, under many federal laws, Acts such as the Communications Decency Act (CDA) in the USA immunize social media websites from responsibility of harm caused by the content published by a third party. Public health policy and research communities have failed to keep up with the rapid and evolving pace of social media, particularly

> ## Box 7.3 While policies designed to limit youth access to addictive substances should be implemented, they must have a harm-reduction approach and should not lead to more harm than the substance use itself
>
> Traditional regulatory approaches targeting age limits, price, advertising, and access are effective, and should be implemented for newly regulated substances. However, new drug policies must go beyond these policies to develop youth-relevant strategies that will help youth to:
>
> avoid punitive consequences of some regulatory policies (e.g., exclusion or incarceration);
>
> delay onset of use until late adolescence;
>
> naturally adopt harm-reduction strategies in drug-using contexts;
>
> moderate drug use in high-risk situations, for example while driving or in the first few years of learning to drive;
>
> access resources and interventions to address important individual risk factors such as unemployment, mental health problems, academic underachievement, and family history of heavy substance use.

youth-relevant products, limiting our ability to make recommendations for how to manage and regulate such influences on young people, but acts such as the CDA make it very difficult to protect youth on the internet (*Doe v. MySpace*, 528 F.3d 413 (5th Cir. 2008)). Until such policies are in place, the burden is on young people and their parents to monitor online activity and the type of content that young people are being exposed to through social media (see Box 7.3).

7.7 Interventions promoting well-being

7.7.1 Parental supervision and training

Family-based prevention approaches typically aim at supporting the development of parenting skills, including parental support, nurturing behaviours, clear communication, establishing and enforcing clear boundaries or rules, and parental monitoring. At least two systematic reviews have assessed the efficacy of various family-based programmes on adolescent drug-use outcomes (Petrie et al., 2007; Foxcroft and Tsertsvadze et al., 2011) and concluded that some parent-based programmes can be mildly effective in the short and long term, particularly approaches that emphasize active parental involvement, as well as developing skills in social competence, self-regulation, and parenting (Petrie et al., 2007). All but two of the numerous studies reviewed were conducted in the USA and neither of these two was shown to be effective in reducing children's alcohol use (Koning et al., 2009). There is a need to continue to understand how interventions that enhance parental supervision and involvement in their children's lives impact on youth drug use, particularly outside the context of the USA. Furthermore, there is a need to modernize these family-based interventions to help guide parents in managing the impact of social media on their childrens' drug use. To date, not a single parent intervention has focused specifically on Internet behaviours (and supervision thereof) as a form of youth drug and alcohol prevention.

7.7.2 **Economic and social conditions promoting well-being**

There are a number of risk factors for drug use that are relevant to the current socio-economic situation in Europe, including unemployment, social isolation, homeless-ness, low academic achievement or drop-out, and hopelessness (see Chapter 3). With as many as 50 per cent of young people now unemployed in some parts of Europe, there is a very pressing need to identify ways to counteract these socioeconomic pressures on young people and their risk for drug use. Furthermore, there is evidence that during this economic crisis, the most vulnerable (e.g. those with mental health needs) are most likely to suffer in terms of losing employment and income (e.g. Evans-Lacko et al., 2013). While it has been suggested that young people are more at risk for drug use during economic crises, the empirical research is limited but does suggest that young people are more likely to use and sell drugs during eco-nomic downturns (Arkes, 2011). There is evidence that the financial crisis in Greece is causally related to the observed increase in suicide rates and major depression in the general population, and to the increase in communicable diseases, namely tuber-culosis, among sex workers and drug users (Kentikelenis et al., 2014) related to a cut in funding for harm-reduction practices. With unemployment comes lack of health-care coverage, particularly among the long-term unemployed. According to a recent report, what really stands out as a consequence of the dramatic economic change in Europe is the increase in death by 'alcohol abuse' and suicide, relative to all other possible causes of mortality (Stuckler et al., 2009). By contrast, young people are less likely to die from car accidents with increases in unemployment, likely owing to the fact that fewer young people can afford to drive during economic crises (Stuckler et al., 2009). According to these data, it is essential that governments direct their lim-ited resources during economic crises to measures that keep young people employed and that help to sustain harm-reduction practices among vulnerable populations.

7.7.3 **Universal school-based programmes**

Schools offer the ideal location to implement policies and interventions to large audi-ences while keeping costs low (Botvin and Griffin, 2003), and access to prevention programmes are increasing for young people in the Western world. However, the majority of school-based programmes and policies are not evidence-based, have not been evaluated, or show minimal effects in reducing drug use and related harms (White and Pitts, 1998; Tobler et al., 2000; Botvin and Griffin, 2007; Faggiano et al., 2008). Some have even reported iatrogenic effects of evidence-based programmes when implemented under unsupported implementation models (Sloboda et al., 2009). Many programmes are based on the premise that simply educating young peo-ple about the harms associated with drugs will lead to reduced drug use, and fail to recognize the important role of individual differences in risk for drug-related harm.

It is now clear that while programmes that focus on drug education can increase knowledge of drug-related harms, they do not necessarily lead to changes in behaviours (see and Foxcroft (2006) and Faggiano et al. (2010) for review). A number of systematic reviews have concluded that of the universal programmes that have been well evaluated, those that show efficacy on drug-related behaviours are those that (at least theoretically) promote development of skills and resilience.

More recently, the use of Internet technology has been shown to facilitate implementation of universal drug-prevention programmes, yielding larger effects on adolescent behaviour (see Newton et al., 2009a), but there has yet to be a study that directly compares these different implementation models. Importantly, effective programmes, to date, have always involved an adult facilitator, face-to-face interactions (rather than web-only contact), and peer interactions (rather than didactic teaching or testimonials) (see Newton et al., 2010 for review). In particular, we highlight the demonstrated efficacy of the Life Skills Programme (Botvin et al., 1995, 2001), UnPlugged (Faggiano et al., 2007), Strengthening Families Programme (Spoth et al., 2001, 2002), and the Climate Programme (Newton et al., 2009b). However, none of these programmes attempts to address additional well-established risk factors for drug use, including genetic factors, personality, and psychopathology, which might explain their small effects on drug-use outcomes generally (Foxcroft, 2006; Faggiano et al., 2008; but see Newton et al., 2009b). Moreover, these programmes remain unavailable to the majority of the population due to a number of implementation barriers, including lack of national regulation of school-based prevention, lack of national registries of evidence-based programmes (see Faggiano et al., 2014), and, most importantly, lack of governmental agencies taking on the responsibility of disseminating evidence-based programmes in ways that assure intervention fidelity and sustainability.

7.7.4 Targeted interventions strategies

Findings from twin and adoption studies have robustly shown heritable influences on alcohol-, cannabis-, opiate-, cocaine-, and tobacco-related behaviours and problems, suggesting a genetic predisposition to sustained heavy drug use (Hawkins et al., 1992; Spooner, et al., 1996; Lynskey et al., 2002; Loxley et al., 2004; Volkow and Li, 2007). These studies suggest that multiple genetic factors are implicated in drug use and related harm, and that there are likely multiple genetically mediated pathways, including an impulsive/disinhibited behaviours pathway, a negative affect/psychopathology pathway, and a reward-sensitivity pathway (see Sher et al., 2000; Castellanos-Ryan and Conrod, 2012; Conrod and Nikolaou, 2016). Not only do these risk pathways have the potential to interact to further increase risk, but they have also been shown to interact with key environmental factors to further increase risk (e.g. childhood maltreatment (Byrd and Manuck, 2014)). Finally, high-risk family studies, twin studies, and prospective molecular genetic studies have all demonstrated that part of what is inherited in the predisposition to drug use is the genetic influence on personality and psychopathology (Stewart et al., 1998; Laucht et al., 2006; Hicks et al., 2013). Castellanos-Ryan and Conrod (2013) and Conrod and Nikolaou (2016) have outlined the role of different genetically mediated psychological traits in the risk for adolescent drug use, which include impulsivity, thrill seeking, anxiety sensitivity, and hopelessness. These traits are also implicated in risk for other forms of psychopathology and can explain why substance use disorders are so highly comorbid with other mental health disorders.

Drug policies must do more to translate current knowledge on risk for substance use disorders to prevention as there are very few evidence-based programmes available to children of drug-using parents. Most policies will first focus on safety of the child, and then the influence of the parent's behaviour on child development, but very few programmes directly target risk factors that are understood as being *inherent to the genetic predisposition*. Consequently, a recent systematic review of prevention programmes targeting children of substance-using parents identified only one programme as having effects on the substance use behaviour of adolescents. One approach that has been shown to be highly effective in preventing drug use and drug-related harm in high-risk young people is the Preventure Programme, which targets four personlity risk factors in school-based cognitive–behavioural interventions delivered to groups of adolescents who report high levels of these traits in a school-wide screening. This programme has been shown to help adolescents delay onset of drinking, binge drinking, illegal drug use, other mental health problems, and reduces risk for problematic drug use among those at risk (Conrod et al., 2006, 2008, 2010, 2013, Mahu et al., 2015; and see Conrod, 2016 for review). Furthermore, as the genetic predisposition to drug-related harm also appears to express itself through age of onset of use (likely through the influence of genetically mediated personality risk factors), there is evidence that this targeted approach to prevention can have broader population-level effects on youth drug use by delaying use among those most likely to be the first to use in a given peer network (Conrod et al., 2013).

Another example of school-based interventions targeting genetically mediated risk factors for drug use includes a classroom-based programme for children with disruptive and aggressive temperaments, which have also been shown to be genetically mediated and longitudinally linked to vulnerability of sustained heavy use (e.g. Kim-Cohen et al., 1999, 2006). Interesting mediational analysis showed that when one such targeted programme was delivered to 5–7-year-old children, it was effective in reducing adolescent drug use 11 years later through its influence on other impulsive behaviours and the promotion of positive peer relationships (Castellanos-Ryan et al., 2013).

Review of the available evidence on targeted interventions suggests that they are impactful and, through the interaction between genetic and non-genetically determined risk factors, such interventions can broadly impact high- and low-risk individuals (e.g. Conrod et al., 2013; Newton et al., 2016) on a variety of outcomes (e.g. psychopathology; see O'Leary-Barrett et al., 2013). While national drug and alcohol policies often recognize the need to target vulnerable populations, very little effort has been dedicated to the study and broader implementation of targeted intervention programmes, despite a much larger investment in research on biological risk for drug-related harm or more universal approaches to drug prevention. Decision-makers might be concerned about the potential stigmatizing effects of targeted prevention strategies, but there is little evidence that students receiving targeted mental health interventions in schools report feeling stigmatized (e.g. Rapee et al., 2006; O'Leary-Barrett et al., submitted). Again, supporting resources that facilitate evidence-to-practice activities are desperately needed (see Faggiano et al., 2014). These resources can be used to help decision-makers in the community synthesize prevention science research, which has the tendency to be complex from a quantitative methods perspective, access training on evidence-based programmes (e.g. through train-the-trainer models), make decisions about the need to adapt programmes for particular socioenvironmental contexts, and, most importantly, continue to evaluate implementation efforts.

7.7.5 Indicated interventions for young people

Considering our proposal to reframe addictive behaviours as regular, heavy use over time (see Chapter 2) and the negative effects of such use on young people, a number of early intervention/indicated prevention approaches have been developed to help young people reduce their excessive drug use before it becomes a problem. Personal feedback interventions (PFIs) provide normative feedback on drinking patterns, peak blood alcohol level, alcohol-related problems, and personal risk factors (e.g. dependence symptoms, family history) (Linehan et al., 1999; Cronce and Larimer, 2011). PFIs can be stand-alone interventions or provided within the context of a brief motivational intervention (BMI). BMIs are usually delivered in one or two sessions and aim to increase the individual's motivation and readiness to change their drug-use behavior and help guide them through the change process (Dimeff et al., 1999). Facilitators of both types of interventions use a motivational interviewing style, which presents feedback in an empathetic, non-judgemental manner (Miller and Rollnick, 2002).

Cronce and Larimer (2011) reviewed individual-based alcohol prevention programmes for college students and found a lack of support for didactic education and awareness programmes but found consistent support for the efficacy of brief, personalized, individual motivational feedback interventions, alcohol expectancy challenge interventions and other types of brief alcohol interventions, and stand-alone personal feedback interventions. More recently, Tanner-Smith et al. (2015) conducted a number of meta-analyses summarizing the effectiveness of PFIs for adolescent drinkers on drinking, smoking, and illegal drug use outcomes. While they found consistent effects of PFIs on drinking outcomes, smoking behaviour was not shown to reduce following such interventions, regardless of whether they directly targeted smoking behaviour or not. Similarly, PFIs and BMIs more generally have only been shown to be inconsistently effective in reducing illegal drug use among drug-using adolescents and young adults. More recently, there has been a trend towards screening and providing brief interventions in primary care practices to help heavy drinkers and drug users reduce their use. Again, while screening and BMIs in primary care appear to be effective in reducing drinking outcomes in patients, studies do not support the use of screening and brief interventions in primary care for illegal drug use (e.g. Saitz et al., 2014). More recently, the use of mHealth strategies have been successfully applied to PFIs to allow for more economical ways to deliver effective brief interventions to young heavy drinkers. These studies show promising results with respect to the use of Internet-based and text messaging-based PFIs for alcohol (e.g. Suffoletto et al., 2014).

7.8 **Multicomponent programmes**

Greater number and greater persistence of risk factors within an individual over time are associated with greater risk for substance use disorders (Hawkins et al., 1992; Loxley et al., 2004). Therefore, it would seem logical to incorporate a multicomponent approach to prevention aimed at reducing risks and enhancing protective factors across a number of risk dimensions (Hawkins et al., 1992; Spooner et al., 1996). In some cases, multicomponent programmes are shown to be more effective (e.g. combining age limits and minimum pricing; see Chapter 6). However, many other reviews have demonstrated that multicomponent programmes do not show any benefits over and above well-implemented single component intervention programmes (see Stewart et al., 2013 for review). Possible explanations for these findings are that communities might be under-resourced and therefore overwhelmed when administering multicomponent programmes, potentially compromising the quality of the multiple components. Alternatively, well-implemented single-component programmes have the potential to impact indirectly on other secondary processes, outcomes or populations such that no additional benefit can be detected, as suggested above for indirect 'herd' effect of targeted programmes (Conrod et al., 2013).

7.9 **Conclusions**

Considering that there are multiple pathways to drug use and drug-related harm, and a number of interacting biological, psychological, and environmental influences along these trajectories, drug-prevention policies need to be comprehensive, will require long-term investment, and organizational structures to support them appropriately. Unfortunately, this is not the case at the moment. Investment in prevention research and delivery typically represents less than one per cent of all costs of drug use to society in a given year (see Rehm et al., 2006). This lack of investment is surprising considering that a number of economic models have demonstrated substantial cost savings resulting from each delayed or prevented case of drug-related harm (e.g. Hurley et al., 2004).

Drug and alcohol prevention requires strong governance and coordinated investment by multiple public sectors and ministries with long-term views of human health and well-being. This is an area that remains detrimentally under-invested in and will require strong advocacy from the public for improved conditions. As governments begin to contemplate new drug policies, which include legalization and regulation, it is essential that public health advocates seize an opportunity to insist that incomes from sumptuary taxes are meaningfully re-invested into drug prevention research and programme delivery. Traditionally, such 'sin' taxes have been seen as being used to pay for the costs of harmful behaviours to society and have been criticized as not necessarily having the desired impact on drug use. Governments must change the way such taxes are used as they adopt new drug policies, where substantially more investment should be directed upstream in the course of this potentially lifelong problem, rather than toward acute and costly services downstream.

Box 7.4 Measures must be taken to increase access to evidence-based interventions to prevent and reduce harm to young people and to assure quality implementation of such programmes

Evidence-based programmes remain unavailable to the majority of the population owing to a number of implementation barriers. Therefore, governments should support resources that facilitate evidence-to-practice activities (see Faggiano et al., 2014). These resources can be used to help decision-makers in the community:

♦ synthesize prevention science research, which has the tendency to be complex from a quantitative methods perspective;

♦ access evidence-based programmes and training on such programmes;

♦ make decisions about the need to adapt programmes for particular socioenvironmental contexts;

♦ continue to evaluate implementation efforts.

There are a number of examples where state and provincial governments in North America and Scandinavia have been required to invest a certain percentage of income from alcohol or gaming taxes to research and treatment services (e.g. alcohol sales in State of Washington and gaming sales in Canada and Sweden). Such policies have the potential to direct more evidence-based programmes towards young people in society. They deserve much more public attention and debate than they are currently given (see Box 7.4).

References

Alanti R, Lawlor DA, Najman JM, Williams GM, Bor W, and O'Callaghan M (2005) Is there really a 'J-shaped' curve in the association between alcohol consumption and symptoms of depression and anxiety? Findings from the Mater-University Study of Pregnancy and its outcomes. *Addiction* **100**: 643–51.

Albers AB, DeJong W, Naimi TS, Siegel M, and Jernigan DH (2014) The relationship between alcohol price and brand choice among underage drinkers: are the most popular alcoholic brands consumed by youth the cheapest? *Subst Use Misuse* **49**: 1833–43.

Anderson P, Chisholm D, and Fuhr DC (2009) Effectiveness and cost-effectiveness of policies and programmes to reduce the harm caused by alcohol. *Lancet* **373**: 2234–46.

Andrews G, Henderson S, and Hall W (2001) Prevalence, comorbidity, disability and service utilisation: overview of the Australian National Mental Health Survey. *Br J Psychiatry* **178**: 145–53.

Anthony JC and Petronis KR (1995) Early-onset drug use and risk of later drug problems. *Drug Alcohol Depend* **40**: 9–15.

Arkes J (2011) Recessions and the participation of youth in the selling and use of illicit drugs. *Int J Drug Policy* **22**: 335–40.

Arseneault L, Cannon M, Witton J, and Murray RM (2004) Causal association between cannabis and psychosis: examination of the evidence. *Br J Psychiatry* **184**: 110–17.

Back SE and Brady KT (2008) Anxiety and substance use disorders: Diagnostic and treatment considerations. *Psychiatr Ann* **38**: 724–9.

Back SE, Waldrop AE, and Brady KT (2009) *Anxiety in the Context of Substance Abuse.* Arlington, VA: American Psychiatric Publishing.

Baker A and Velleman R (2007) *Clinical Handbook of Co-existing Mental Health and Drug and Alcohol Problems.* London: Routledge.

Begg S, Vos T, Barker B, Stevenson C, Stanley L, and Lopez AD (2007) *The Burden of Disease and Injury in Australia 2003.* Canberra: AIHW.

Behrendt S, Wittchen H, Hofler M, Lieb R, and Beesdo K (2009) Transitions from first substance use to substance use disorders in adolescence: is early onset associated with a rapid escalation? *Drug Alcohol Depend* **99**: 68–78.

Bendtsen P, Damsgaard MT, Huckle T, Casswell S, Kuntsche E, Arnold P, et al. (2014) Adolescent alcohol use: a reflection of national drinking patterns and policy? *Addiction* **109**: 1857–68.

Botvin GJ and Griffin KW (2003) Drug abuse prevention curricula in schools. In: Sloboda Z and Bukoski WJ (eds) *Handbook of Drug Abuse Prevention: Theory, Science and Practice.* New York: Kluwer Academic/ Plenum Publishers, pp. 45–74.

Botvin GJ and Griffin KW (2007) School-based programmes to prevent alcohol, tobacco and other drug use. *Int Rev Psychiatry* **19**: 607–15.

Botvin GJ, Baker E, Dusenbury L, Botvin EM, and Diaz T (1995) Long-term follow-up results of a randomized drug abuse prevention trial in a White middle-class population. *JAMA* **273**: 1106–12.

Botvin GJ, Griffin KW, Diaz T, and Ifill-Williams M (2001) Preventing binge drinking during early adolescence: one- and two-year follow-up of a school-based preventive intervention. *Psychol Addict Behav* **15**: 360–5.

Byrd AL and Manuck SB (2014) *MAOA*, childhood maltreatment and antisocial behavior: meta-analysis of a gene–environment interaction. *Biol Psychiatry* **75**: 9–17.

Casey B, Jones RM, and Somerville LH (2011) Braking and accelerating of the adolescent brain. *J Res Adolesc* **21**: 21–33.

Caspi A, Moffitt TE, Cannon M, McClay J, Murray R, Harrington H, et al (2005) Moderation of the effect of adolescent-onset cannabis use on adult psychosis by a functional polymorphism in the catechol-O-methyltransferase gene: longitudinal evidence of a gene X environment interaction. *Biol Psychiatry* **57**: 1117–27.

Castellanos-Ryan N, Conrod PJ, Vester JBK, Strain E, and Galanter M (2012) Personality and substance misuse: evidence for a four-factor model of vulnerability. In: Vester JBK, Strain E, Galanter M, and Conrod PJ(eds) *Drug Abuse and Addiction in Medical Illness*, Vols 1 and 2. New York: Humana/Spring Press, pp. 47–62.

Castellanos-Ryan N, Séguin JR, Vitaro F, Parent S, and Tremblay RE (2013) Impact of a 2-year multimodal intervention for disruptive 6-year-olds on substance use in adolescence: randomised controlled trial. *Br J Psychiatry* **203**: 188–95.

Chabrol H, Chauchard E, and Girabet J (2008) Cannabis use and suicidal behaviours in high-school students. *Addict Behav* **33**: 152–5.

Coffey C, Carlin JB, Degenhardt L, Lynskey M, and Sanci L (2002) Cannabis dependence in young adults: an Australian population study. *Addiction* 97: 187–94.

Coley HL, Sadasivam RS, Williams JH, Volkman JE, Schoenberger YM, Kohler CL, et al. (2013) Crowdsourced peer- versus expert-written smoking-cessation messages. *Am J Prev Med* 45: 543–50.

Collins DJ and Lapsley HM (2008) *The Costs of Tobacco, Alcohol and Illicit Drug Abuse to Australian Society in 2004/05*. Canberra: Commonwealth of Australia.

Conrod P (2016) Personality-targeted interventions for substance misuse. *Curr Addict Rep* (in press).

Conrod P, Stewart SH, Comeau N, and Maclean AM (2006) Preventative efficacy of cognitive behavioural strategies matched to the motivational bases of alcohol misuse in at-risk youth. *J Clin Child Adolesc Psychol* 35: 55–63.

Conrod PJ, Castellanos N, and Mackie C (2008) Personality-targeted interventions delay the growth of adolescent drinking and binge drinking. *J Child Psychol Psychiatry* 49: 181–90.

Conrod PJ, Castellanos N, and Strang J (2010) Brief, personality-targeted coping skills interventions prolong survival as a non-drug user over a two-year period during adolescence. *Arch Gen Psychiatry* 67: 85–93.

Conrod PJ, O'Leary-Barrett M, Newton N, Topper L, Castellanos-Ryan N, Mackie C, and Girard A (2013) Effectiveness of a selective, personality-targeted prevention program for adolescent alcohol use and misuse: a cluster randomized controlled trial. *JAMA Psychiatry* 70: 334–42.

Cronce JM and Larimer ME (2011) Individual-focused approaches to the prevention of college student drinking. *Alcohol Res Health* 34: 210–21.

Cservenka A and Nagel BJ (2012) Risky decision-making: An fMRI study of youth at high risk for alcoholism. *Alcohol Clin Exp Res* 36: 604–15.

Degenhardt L and Hall WD (2001) The association between psychosis and problematic drug use among Australian adults: findings from the National Survey of Mental Health and Wellbeing. *Psychol Med* 31: 659–68.

Degenhardt L, Hall W, and Lynskey M (2001) Alcohol, cannabis and tobacco use among Australians: a comparison of their associations with other drug use and use disorders, affective and anxiety disorders, and psychosis. *Addiction* 96: 1603–14.

Degenhardt L, Chiu W, Sampson N, Kessler RC, Anthony JC, Angermeyer M, et al. (2008) Toward a global view of alcohol, tobacco, cannabis, and cocaine use: findings from the WHO World Mental Health Surveys. *PLOS Med* 5: 1053–67.

Dimeff LA, Baer JS, Kivlahan DR, and Marlatt GA (1999) *Brief Alcohol Screening and Intervention for College Students*. New York: Guilford Press.

Evans-Lacko S, Knapp M, McCrone P, Thornicroft G, and Mojtabai R (2013) The mental health consequences of the recession: economic hardship and employment of people with mental health problems in 27 European countries. *PLOS ONE* 20138: e69792.

Faggiano F, Richardson C, Bohrn K, Galanti MR, and EU-Dap Study Group (2007) A cluster randomized controlled trial of school-based prevention of tobacco, alcohol and drug use: the EU-Dap design and study population. *Prev Med* 44: 170–3.

Faggiano F, Vigna-Taglianti FD, Versino E, Zambon A, Borraccino A, and Lemma P (2008) School-based prevention for illicit drugs use: a systematic review. *Prev Med* 46: 385–96.

Faggiano F, Vigna-Taglianti F, Burkhart G, Bohrn K, Cuomo L, Gregori D, et al. (2010). The effectiveness of a school-based substance abuse prevention program: 18-month follow-up of the EU-Dap cluster randomized controlled trial. *Drug Alcohol Depend* 108: 56–64.

Faggiano F, Minozzi S, Versino E, and Buscemi D (2014) Universal school-based prevention for illicit drug use. *Cochrane Database Syst Rev* 12: CD003020

Fell JC, Jones K, Romano E and Voas R (2011) An evaluation of graduated driver licensing effects on fatal crash involvements of young drivers in the United States. *Traffic Inj Prev* 12: 423–31.

Ferguson SA, Teoh ER, and McCartt AT (2007) Progress in teenage crash risk during the last decade. *J Safety Res* 38: 137–45.

Fergusson DM, Boden JM, and Horwood LJ (2009) Tests of causal links between alcohol abuse or dependence and major depression. *Arch Gen Psychiatry* 66: 260–6.

Fernández-Calderón F, Lozano-Rojas Ó, Rojas-Tejada A, Bilbao-Acedos I, Vidal-Giné C, Vergara-Moragues E, and González-Saiz F. (2014) Harm reduction behaviors among young polysubstance users at raves. *Subst Abus* 2014; 35:45–50.

Foxcroft D (2006) Alcohol education: absence of evidence or evidence of absence. *Addiction* 101: 1057–9.

Foxcroft DR and Tsertsvadze A (2011) Universal family-based prevention programs for alcohol misuse in young people. *Cochrane Database Syst Rev* 9: CD009308

Galvan A, Hare TA, Parra CE, Penn J, Voss H, Glover G, et al. (2006) Earlier development of the accumbens relative to orbitofrontal cortex might underlie risk-taking behaviour in adolescents. *J Neurosci* 26: 6885–92.

Gogtay N, Giedd JN, Lusk L, Hayashi KM, Greenstein D, Vaituzis AC, et al. (2004) Dynamic mapping of human cortical development during childhood through early adulthood. *Proc Natl Acad Sci U S A* 101: 8174–9.

Gottfredson DC (2012) *Schools and Delinquency.* Cambridge: Cambridge University Press.

Grant J, Scherrer J, Lynskey M, Lyons MJ, Eisen S, Tsuang MY, et al. (2006) Adolescent alcohol use is a risk factor for adult alcohol and drug dependence: evidence from a twin design. *Psychol Med* 36: 109–18.

Gruber E, DiClements R, Anderson M, and Lodico M (1996) Early drinking onset and its association with alcohol use and problem behaviour in late adolescent. *Prev Med* 25: 293–300.

Hall WD (1998) Cannabis use and psychosis. *Drug Alcohol Rev* 17: 433–44.

Hall W (2006) The mental health risks of adolescent cannabis use. *PLOS Med* 3: 1–2.

Hall W, Degenhardt L, and Teesson M (in press). Understanding comorbidity: broadening the research base. *Addict Behav.*

Hall W, Degenhardt L, and Lynskey M (2001) *The Health and Psycholgical Effects of Cannabis Use.* Canberra: National Drug Strategy.

Hall W, Degenhardt L, and Teesson M (2004) Cannabis use and psychotic disorders: an update. *Drug Alcohol Rev* 23: 433–43.

Hawkins JD, Catalano RF, and Miller J (1992) Risk and protective factors for alcohol and other drug problems in adolescence and early adulthood: implications for substance abuse prevention. *Psychol Bull* 112: 64–105.

Health Canada (2011) Major findings from the Canadian Alcohol and Drug Use Monitoring Survey (CADUMS). Available at: http://www.hc-sc.gc.ca/hc-ps/drugs-drogues/stat/index-eng.php (accessed 15 September 2016).

Henggeler SW, McCart MR, Cunningham PB, and Chapman JE (2012) Enhancing the effectiveness of juvenile drug courts by integrating evidence-based practices. *J Consult Clin Psychol* **80**: 264–75.

Hibell B, Guttormsson U, Ahlström S, Balakireva O, Bjarnason T, Kokkevi A, et al. (2007) *The 2007 ESPAD Report: Substance Use Among Students in 35 European Countries*. Stockholm: The European School Survey Project on Alcohol and Other Drugs.

Hicks BM, Foster KT, Iacono WG, and McGue M (2013) Genetic and environmental influences on the familial transmission of externalizing disorders in adoptive and twin offspring. *JAMA Psychiatry* **70**: 1076–83.

Hoskins R and Benger J (2012) What is the burden of alcohol-related injuries in an inner city emergency department? *Emerg Med J* **30**: e21.

Hurley SF, Scollo MM, Younie SJ, English DR, and Swanson MG (2004) The potential for tobacco control to reduce PBS costs for smoking-related cardiovascular disease. *Med J Aust* **181**: 252–5.

Kameda SR, Fukushiro DF, Trombin TF, Procopio-Souza R, Patti CL, Hollais AW, et al. (2011) Adolescent mice are more vulnerable than adults to single injection-induced behavioral sensitization to amphetamine. *Pharmacol Biochem Behav* **98**: 320–4.

Kentikelenis A, Karanikolos M, Reeves A, McKee M, and Stuckler D. (2014) Greece's health crisis: from austerity to denialism. *Lancet* **383**: 748–53.

Kim-Cohen J, Caspi A, Taylor A, Williams B, Newcombe R, Craig IW, and Moffitt TE (2006) MAOA, maltreatment, and gene-environment interaction predicting children's mental health: new evidence and a meta-analysis. *Mol Psychiatry* **11**: 903–13.

Koning IM, Vollebergh WAM, Smit F, Verdurmen JEE, van den Eijnden RJJM, et al. (2009) Preventing heavy alcohol use in adolescents (PAS): cluster randomized trial of a parent and student intervention offered separately and simultaneously. *Addiction* **104**: 1669–78.

Kuntsche E and Delgrande Jordon M (2006) Adolescent alcohol and cannabis use in relation to peer and school factors: results of multilevel analyses. *Drug Alcohol Depend* **84**: 167–74.

Kurowski BG, Wade SL, Kirkwood MW, Brown TM, Stancin T, and Taylor HG (2014) Long-term benefits of an early online problem-solving intervention for executive dysfunction after traumatic brain injury in children: a randomized clinical trial. *JAMA Pediatr* **168**: 523–31.

Laucht M, Esser G, and Schmidt MH (2006) Developmental outcome of infants born with biological and psychosocial risks. *J Child Psychol Psychiatry* **38**: 843–53.

Levy S, Schizer M; Committee on Substance Abuse, American Academy of Pediatrics. (2015) Adolescent drug testing policies in schools. *Pediatrics* **135**: e1107–12.

Linehan MM, Schmidt H, Dimeff LA, Craft JC, Kanter J, and Comtois KA (1999) Dialectical behavior therapy for patients with borderline personality disorder and drug-dependence. *Am J Addict* **8**: 279–92.

Loxley W, Toumbouruo JW, Stockwell T, Haines B, Scott K, Godfrey C, et al. (2004) *The Prevention of Substance Use, Risk and Harm in Australia: A review of the Evidence*. Canberra: Ministerial Council on Drug Strategy.

Luna B and Sweeney JA (2004) The emergence of collaborative brain function: fMRI studies of the development of response inhibition. *Ann N Y Acad Sci* **1021**: 296–309.

Lynskey M, Heath AC, and Nelson AC (2002) Genetic and environmental contributions to cannabis dependence in a national young adult twin sample. *Psychol Med* **32**: 195–207.

Mackie CJ, O'Leary-Barrett M, Al-Khudhairy N, Castellanos-Ryan N, Struve M, Topper L, and Conrod P (2013) Adolescent bullying, cannabis use and emerging psychotic experiences: a longitudinal general population study. *Psychol Med* **43**: 1033–44.

Mahu IT, Doucet C, O'Leary-Barrett M, and Conrod PJ (2015) Can cannabis use be prevented by targeting personality risk in schools? Twenty-four-month outcome of the adventure trial on cannabis use: a cluster-randomized controlled trial. *Addiction* **110**: 1625–33.

Matuszewich L, Carter S, Andersen E, Friedman RD, and McFadden LM (2014) Persistent behavioral and neurochemical sensitization to an acute injection of methamphetamine following unpredictable stress. *Behav Brain Res* **272**: 308–13.

Miller WR and Rollnick S (2002) *Motivational Interviewing, Second Edition: Preparing People for Change*. New York: Guilford Press.

Montgomery KC, Chester J, Grier SA, and Dorfman L (2012) The new threat of digital marketing. *Pediatr Clin North Am* **59**: 659–75.

National Health and Medical Research Council (2001) *Australian Alcohol Guidelines: Health Risks and Benefits*. Canberra: NHMRC.

National Institute on Drug Abuse (2008) *Monitoring the Future: National Results on Adolescent Drug Use*. Bethesda, MD: National Institutes of Health.

Newton NC, Andrews G, Teesson M, and Vogl LE (2009a) Delivering prevention for alcohol and cannabis using the internet: A cluster randomised controlled trial. *Prev Med* **48**: 579–84.

Newton NC, Vogl LE, Teesson M, and Andrews G (2009b). CLIMATE Schools Alcohol Module: cross-validation of a school-based prevention programme for alcohol misuse. *Aust N Z J Psychiatry* **43**: 201–7.

Newton N, Teesson M, Vogl L, and Andrews G (2010) Internet-based prevention for alcohol and cannabis use: final results of the Climate Schools course. *Addiction* **105**: 749–59.

Oetting ER and Lynch RS (2003) Peers and the prevention of adolescent drug use. In: Sloboda Z and Bukoski WJ (eds) *Handbook of Drug Prevention: Theory, Science and Practice*. New York: Kluwer Academic/Plenum Publishers, pp. 101–27.

O'Leary-Barrett ML, Pihl RO, and Conrod PJ (2016) Youth self-report responses to school-based personality-targeted interventions and their relationship to 12 months drinking outcomes. Presented at the 64th Annual Meeting of the American Academy of Child and Adolescent Psychiatry October 23–28, 2016, New York, New York.

O'Leary-Barrett M, Topper L, Al-Khudhairy N, Pihl RO, Castellanos-Ryan N, and Mackie C (2013) Two-year impact of personality-targeted, teacher-delivered interventions on youth internalizing and externalizing problems: a cluster-randomized trial. *J Am Acad Child Adolesc Psychiatry* **52**: 911–20.

Patrick ME, Wightman P, Schoeni RF, and Schulenberg JE (2012) Socioeconomic status and substance use among young adults: a comparison across constructs and drugs. *J Stud Alcohol Drugs* **73**: 772–82.

Patton G, Coffey C, Lynskey MT, Reid S, Hemphill S, Carlin JB, et al. (2007) *Trajectories of Adolescent Alcohol and Cannabis Use Into Young Adulthood*. Melbourne: Centre for Adolescent Health.

Petrie J, Bunn F, and Byrne G (2007) Parenting programmes for preventing tobacco, alcohol or drugs misuse in children < 18: a systematic review. *Health Educ Res* **22**: 177–91.

Ponicki WR, Gruenewald PJ, and LaScala EA. (2007) Joint impacts of minimum legal drinking age and beer taxes on US youth traffic fatalities, 1975 to 2001.*Alcohol Clin Exp Res* **31**: 804–13.

Rapee RM, Wignall A, Sheffield J, Kowalenko N, Davis A, McLoone J, and Spence SH (2006) Adolescents' reactions to universal and indicated prevention programs for depression: perceived stigma and consumer satisfaction. *Prev Sci* **7**: 167–77.

Rehm J, Gnam W, Popova S, Baliunas D, Brochu S, Fischer B, et al. (2007) The costs of alcohol, illegal drugs, and tobacco in Canada, 2002. *J Stud Alcohol Drugs* **68**: 886–95.

Saitz R, Palfai TP, Cheng DM, Alford DP, Bernstein JA, Lloyd-Travaglini CA, et al. (2014) Screening and brief intervention for drug use in primary care: the ASPIRE randomized clinical trial. *JAMA* **312**: 502–13.

Scheier LM and Botvin GJ (1995) Effects of early adolescent drug use on cognitive efficacy in early-late adolescence: a developmental structural model. *J Subst Abuse* **7**: 379–404.

Scheier LM, Botvin GJ, and Baker E (1997) Risk and protective factors as predictors of adolescent alcohol involvement and transitions in alcohol use: a prospective analysis. *J Stud Alcohol* **58**: 652–67.

Semple DM, McIntosh AM, and Lawrie SM (2005) Cannabis as a risk factor for psychosis: systematic review. *J Psychopharmacol* **19**: 187–94.

Sher KJ, Bartholow BD, and Wood MD (2000) Personality and substance use disorders: a prospective study. *J Consult Clin Psychol* **68**: 818–29.

Simmons RG and Blyth D (2008) *Moving Into Adolescence: The Impact of Pubertal Change and School Context*. New Brunswick: Transaction Publishers.

Sloboda Z, Stephens RC, Stephens PC, Grey SF, Teasdale B, Hawthorne RD, et al. (2009) The Adolescent Substance Abuse Prevention Study: a randomized field trial of a universal substance abuse prevention program. *Drug Alcohol Depend* **102**: 1–10.

Sowell ER, Thompson PM, and Toga AW (2004) Mapping changes in the human cortex through out the span life. *Neuroscientist* **10**: 372–92.

Spooner C and Hall W (2002) Public policy and the prevention of substance-use disorders. *Curr Opin Psychiatry* **15**: 235–9.

Spooner C, Mattick R, and Howard J (1996) *The Nature and Treatment of Adolescent Substance Abuse Monograph No. 26*. Sydney: National Drug and Alcohol Research Centre.

Spoth RL, Redmond C, and Shin C (2001) Randomized trial of brief family interventions for general populations: adolescent substance use outcomes 4 years following baseline. *J Consult Clin Psychol* **69**: 627–42.

Spoth RL, Guyll M, and Day SX (2002) Universal family-focused interventions in alcohol-use disorder prevention: cost-effectiveness and cost-benefit analyses of two interventions. *J Stud Alcohol* **63**: 219–28.

Squeglia LM, Jacobus J, Nguyen-Louie TT, and Tapert SF (2014) Inhibition during early adolescence predicts alcohol and marijuana use by late adolescence. *Neuropsychology* **28**: 782–90.

Stewart SH, Pihl RO, Conrod PJ, and Dongier M (1998) Functional associations among trauma, PTSD, and substance-related disorders. *Addict Behav* **23**: 797–812.

Stewart SH, Conrod PJ, Latvala A, Wiers RW, and White HR (2013) Prevention of alcohol use and misuse in youth: a comparison of north american and european approaches. In: De Witte P and Mitchell Jr MC. (eds) *Underage Drinking: A Report on Drinking in the Second Decade of Life in Europe and North America*. Leuven: Presses Universitaires de Louvain, pp. 147–209.

Stockwell T, Toumbouruo JW, Letcher P, Smart D, Sanson A, and Bond L (2004) Risk and protective factors for different intensities of adolescent substance use: when does the prevention paradox apply? *Drug Alcohol Rev* 23: 67–77.

Stuckler D, Basu S, Suhrcke M, Coutts A, and McKee M (2009) The public health effect of economic crises and alternative policy responses in Europe: an empirical analysis *Lancet* 374: 315–23.

Substance Abuse and Mental Health Services Administration (2015) *Results from the 2014 National Survey on Drug Use and Health: Summary of National Findings*, NSDUH Series H-46, HHS Publication No. (SMA) 13-4795. Rockville, MD: Substance Abuse and Mental Health Services Administration.

Suffoletto B, Kristan J, Callaway C, Kim KH, Chung T, Monti PM, and Clark DB. (2014) A text message alcohol intervention for young adult emergency department patients: a randomized clinical trial. *Ann Emerg Med* 64: 664–72.

Tanner-Smith EE, Steinka-Fry KT, Hennessy EA, Lipsey MW, and Winters KC (2015) Can brief alcohol interventions for youth also address concurrent illicit drug use? Results from a meta-analysis. *J Youth Adolesc* 44: 1011–23.

Tapert SF, Caldwell L, and Burke C (2005) Alcohol and the adolescent brain: Human studies. *Alcohol Res Health* 28: 205–12.

Teesson M, Degenhardt L, Hall W, Lynskey M, Toumbourou J, and Patton G (2005) Substance use and mental health in longitudinal perspective. In: Stockwall T, Grueneald P, Toumbourou J, and Loxley W (eds) *Preventing Harmful Substance Use: The Evidence Base for Policy and Practice*. Chichester: John Wiley and Sons, pp. 43–52.

Thomas H (1996) A community survey of adverse effects of cannabis use. *Drug Alcohol Depend* 42: 201–7.

Tien AY and Anthony JC (1990) Epidemiological analysis of alcohol and drug use as risk factors for psychotic experiences. *J Nerv Ment Dis* 178: 473–80.

Tobler NS, Roona MR, Ochshorn P, Marshall DG, Streke AV, and Stackpole KM (2000) School-based adolescent drug prevention programs: 1998 meta-analysis. *J Prim Prevent* 20: 275–336.

Van Os J, Bak M, Hanssen M, Bijl RV, De Graaf R, and Verdoux H (2002) Cannabis use and psychosis: a longitudinal population-based study. *Am J Epidemiol* 156: 319–27.

Vetreno RP and Crews FT (2015) Binge ethanol exposure during adolescence leads to a persistent loss of neurogenesis in the dorsal and ventral hippocampus that is associated with impaired adult cognitive functioning. *Front Neurosci* 9: 35.

Volkow ND and Li TK (2005) Drugs and alcohol: treating and preventing abuse, addiction and their medical consequences. *Pharmacol Ther* 108: 3–17.

Whelan R, Watts R, Orr CA, Althoff RR, Artiges E, Banaschewski T, et al. (2014) Neuropsychosocial profiles of current and future adolescent alcohol misusers. *Nature* 512: 185–9.

White D, and Pitts M (1998) Review: educating young people about drugs: a systematic review. *Addiction* 93: 1475–87.

Windle M, Miller-Tutzauer C, and Domenico D (1992) Alcohol use, suicidal behaviour, and risky activities among adolescents. *J Res Adolesc* 2: 137–330.

Wittchen H, Frohlich C, Behrendt S, Gunther A, Rehm J, Zimmermann P, et al. (2007) Cannabis use and cannabis use disorders and their relationship to mental disorders: a 10-year prospective-longitudinal community study in adolescents. *Drug Alcohol Depend* 88S: S60–70.

Xu X and Chaloupka FJ (2011) The effects of prices on alcohol use and its consequences. *Alcohol Res Health* 34: 236–45.

Yucle M, Solowij N, Respondek C, Whittle S, Fornito A, Pantelis C, et al. (2008) Regional brain abnormalities assocaited with long-term heavy cannabis use. *Arch Gen Psychiatry* 65: 694–701.

Zammit S, Allebeck P, Andreasson S, Lundberg I, and Lewis G (2002) Self-reported cannabis use as a risk factor for schizophrenia in Swedish conscripts in 1969: Historical cohort study. *BMJ* 325: 1199–201.

Chapter 8

Government leadership
for whole-of-society approaches

8.1 Introduction to the European public policies

According to Díaz (1998), there are different historical factors that have contributed to the current consumerist model of drugs (Arif, 1981; Comas, 1985), among which the development of the pharmaceutical industry, the emergence of synthetic addictive compounds, and the process of globalization are determinant. More concretely, three general trends on how addictions have been tackled by Western European governments can be identified: the moral paradigm, the assistentialist, and the public health approach.

The moral paradigm emerged at the beginning of the twentieth century as a reactive and puritan response to the popularization of drugs and promoted a moral crusade against drugs. This approach considers drug consumption as a weakness and a lack of self-control. Hence, the moral attitude towards consumers is both to stigmatize and 'save' drug consumers who are sinners and vicious. Treatment was mainly provided either by 'beneficiary houses' or by health professionals, who, as noted later, a few decades later embraced an assistentialist approach. The moral paradigm was especially promoted in the USA by the temperance movements, which were exported internationally through conferences, conventions, and international agreements (Shanghai 1909, The Hague 1912, 1913, and 1914, and Geneva 1925, 1931, and 1936) (Hellman et al., 2015).

In essence, the new economic model emerging after the Second World War, the development of the welfare state in Western Europe and a growing middle class are key factors in understanding the emergence of the assistentialist paradigm. Hence, treatments were based on prescription and abstinence, and relapse was considered a failure. This approach established a clear power relation between the doctor and the patient (Foucault, 1963), with the former representing the knowledge and the latter considered as an outsider that science has to heal.

Finally, the public health approach emerged hand in hand with the heroin and cocaine boom during the 1970s and the 1980s. At first, in order to respond to this, most countries opted for an assistance strategy, which had as a final aim total abstinence. Although the public health approach has the same long-term goal as the assistentialist one, that is, total abstinence, it also embeds intermediate goals focused on

Box 8.1 Western European historical trends in policies on addictions

Three historical trends on how addictions have been tackled by Western European governments can be identified: the moral paradigm, the assistentialist, and the public health approach. The public health approach embeds goals focused on preserving health and improving the quality of life of drug consumers.

preserving health (e.g. via methadone programmes) and improving the quality of life of drug consumers (e.g. via needle exchange) (see Box 8.1).

8.2 Normalization: the need of new models

Western societies have been forced to find new forms of governance and renewed policies to counteract and better adapt to these realities. Nowadays, consumption of drugs is a primary activity in itself for young people, so does not require any kind of justification, and is compatible with any recreational activity (Díaz et al., 2004). Currently, the pathways towards the European public policies on addiction are characterized by three trends, depending on the substance (Trautmann, 2013), that co-exist at both national and European levels and are often interrelated.

The first one, decriminalization of drug use, is especially relevant in the governance of illegal drugs like heroin and cannabis. Characterized as a health-oriented policy, decriminalization actions no longer regard drug consumers as criminals but as ill patients. Furthermore, consumption and/or possession of small quantities for personal use are generally treated as misdemeanour and not as a criminal offence (Reuter and Trautmann, 2009).

The second trend is the wider introduction of harm reduction for both illegal and legal substances. Since the beginning of the twenty-first century, harm-reduction acceptance has significantly increased among European countries. This has even been embraced and promoted by international organizations such as the European Union (EU), the World Health Organization (WHO), and the United Nations (UN), and is recognized as a key characteristic of public health-oriented policy.

The final trend is a shift from repression to regulation, the most relevant approach for licit substances like alcohol and tobacco, and also observed in cannabis with recent experiences in different countries where governments have opted for a regulatory approach (see Box 8.2).

Box 8.2 Current European trends in policies on addictions

Three current European trends in public policies on addictions: decriminalization of drug use; wider introduction of harm-reduction policies for both illegal and legal substances; and a shift from repression to regulation.

8.3 **Governance of addictions: a wicked issue**

In the last few decades, the complexity of dealing with public policies has increased mainly owing to what are known as 'wicked problems' (Rittel and Webber, 1973), which, by definition, are inherently resistant to clear and agreed solutions (Kickert et al., 1997; Stoker, 1998; Bovaird, 2004). As Mendoza and Vernis state (2008: 392): 'the need to respond to "wicked social problems" require public agencies to be prepared to work in partnership with other public, civil society and business organisations'.

Moreover, Lozano et al. (2008: 19) add that 'the governance of our complex and interdependent societies will not be possible unless we turn the sense of responsibility among their many social actors into one of co-responsibility'. Hence, public and private (profit and non-profit) sectors come together to address issues, solve problems, and provide services that are too complex and/or costly for any organization to handle on its own (O'Toole, 1997).

We rely on the most recent definition of governance understood from a relational point of view, which takes into consideration what governments, private companies, and third-sector organizations are doing in the governance of addiction field either in partnership with the government or by themselves. Hence, governance is understood as 'the processes and structures of public policy decision making and management that engage people across the boundaries of public agencies, levels of government, and/or the public, private and civic spheres in order to carry out a public purpose that could not otherwise be accomplished' (Emerson et al., 2012: 2).

The complexity of addictions and drug issues leaves no doubt that this is a wicked problem that must be tackled by different levels of governments in collaboration with non-governmental organizations (NGOs) and businesses. Addiction governance is recognized as a complex area that does not follow the traditional linear model (problem–options–solution–implementation) and that is influenced by various factors that intervene in this policy-making owing to its implications on society and the controversy that it generates (Ritter and Bammer, 2010).

By taking governance as the reference framework we assume that private companies and not-for-profit organizations do play a role when deciding and implementing drug and addiction policies. Addiction governance is influenced by many stakeholders, public, private, and non-profit coming from different fields: health, justice, public order, safety, economy, trade, and so on. This wide range of stakeholders, and also the international domain related to drug trafficking and the EU, makes the governance of addictions more complex.

All the EU countries plus Norway involve, at least to some extent, non-profit organizations in decision-making and especially in the implementation process. However, as with other health issues, businesses have been identified with the industry, either from tobacco or alcohol, and other stakeholders focused on lobbying the governments so they do not increase taxes and embrace evidence-based regulative approaches. Thus, as anybody would expect, the industry aims to protect its own interests, boosting earnings and minimizing business losses.

A further complexity to add to the drugs and addictions issue is the double standard and stigma traditionally applied to drug consumers. Traditions, cultures and

Box 8.3 What is 'governance'?

Governance: the processes and structures of public policy decision-making and management that engage people across the boundaries of public agencies, levels of government, and/or the public, private, and civic spheres in order to carry out a public purpose that could not otherwise be accomplished.

the fact that Europe is the principal producer of alcoholic beverages worldwide has meant, and continues to mean, that the consumption of alcohol is not seen as an addiction. This does not provoke the unified response and rejection that it would deserve, especially if we consider the high level of harm it causes in our societies. However, the consumption of other substances, and those who consume them, suffer discriminatory attitudes from many sectors of society, attitudes that are clearly affected by the collective imagery. Therefore, the distinction of legal and illegal drugs in the context of normalization we are living is no longer valid (see Box 8.3).

8.4 **Models of governance of addictions**

Ysa et al. (2014) identify 19 key policy characteristics that have been used to cluster 28 European countries into four different groups (see Table 8.1). Some of the grouped countries may seem strange to the reader, especially if they have traditional models

Table 8.1 Models of governance of addictions in Europe

Model	Characteristics	Countries
1 Trendsetters in illegal substances	These countries combine a well-being and relational management strategy with a comprehensive structure	Belgium, Czech Republic, Germany, Italy, Luxemburg, Netherlands, Portugal, and Spain
2 Regulation of legal substances	These countries have strict regulation on legal substances (tobacco and alcohol)	Finland, France, Ireland, Norway, Sweden, and the UK
3 Transitioning model	This group gathers the most divergent countries of the sample. They do not follow a clear trend	Austria, Bulgaria, Cyprus, Denmark, Poland, and Slovenia
4 Traditional approach	Countries within this cluster have still not embraced the three trends. They have a 'safety and disease' strategy combined with a 'substance-based structure'	Estonia, Greece, Hungary, Latvia, Lithuania, Malta, Romania, and Slovakia

Source: data from Ysa T, Colom J, Albareda A, Ramon A, Carrión M, and Segura L. *Governance of Addictions: European Public Policies*. Oxford: Oxford University Press, Copyright © 2014 Oxford University Press.

in mind, but the addiction field poses some challenges and complexities, and contextual factors (geopolitics), culture and traditions, among others, that have a high impact in their governance.

8.4.1 Model 1: trendsetters in illegal substances

The first model is determined by its strategy for illegal substances, which, apart from taking into account prevention and treatment, gives much importance to harm-reduction policies. A distinctive characteristic of this model is the fact that the clustered countries decriminalize possession of illegal substances (i.e. a shift from repression to regulation and from criminal to administrative law). Furthermore, they have realtively weaker policies for alcohol and tobacco (Österberg and Karlsson, 1998; Joossens and Raw, 2010). Model 1 includes Continental and Mediterranean welfare states (Esping-Andersen, 1990; Ferrera, 1996), and all these countries have developed well-being-oriented policies by placing the Ministry of Health as the responsible institution. This results in their giving much weight to harm-reduction policies, decriminalizing possession of illegal substances, proactively developing policies aimed at coping with drug-related problems, embracing a health-oriented rather than a security-oriented approach and protecting the public and society in general instead of the individual. However, when it comes to evidence-based regulation of legal substances, model 1 states have still not introduced measures related to production, distribution, age limits, taxes, and advertising and marketing, which still are not as developed as in other states.

8.4.2 Model 2: regulation of legal substances

Countries in this second model, regulation of legal substances, do not focus on decriminalization but implement evidence regulations aimed at reducing the levels of alcohol and tobacco consumption, and enhancing societal well-being. It is worth noting that all model 2 countries have developed evidence and research-based regulations aimed at reducing the levels of legal substance consumption, preventing heavy use over time, and improving the overall well-being of the population. These countries have complex structures for dealing with drugs, that is, they devolve implementation to decentralized structures, involve non-profit organizations in the decision-making, and have a sound trajectory dealing with drugs. In fact, this model gathers countries with different welfare state traditions: Nordic, Anglo-Saxon, and Continental countries (Esping-Anderson, 1990). It is worth noting here that the Nordic and the Anglo-Saxon countries are pioneers in evidence-based research.

8.4.3 Model 3: transitioning model

Here we find the most divergent and most peculiar group of countries: Austria, Bulgaria, Cyprus, Denmark, Poland, and Slovenia. Those are countries in transition regarding the governance of addictions, from this model to the other three. These countries are characterized by placing the Ministry of Health as the main responsible institution, and foster treatment, prevention, and harm reduction above supply-reduction measures. Moreover, these countries have been clustered together for not having a set of characteristics: decriminalization of possession, injection rooms, tobacco control, and public-health aims. Regarding structure, these countries do not tackle legal and illegal substances together; hence, they focus on the substances rather than on addictions. Furthermore, none of the countries involve non-profit and private organizations in the decision-making process.

8.4.4 Model 4: traditional approach

In model 4, we primarily find central and eastern European countries that became EU member states during the first decade of the twenty-first century; the only exceptions in this respect are Greece and Malta. These countries have been classified as having a 'safety and disease' strategy combined with a 'substance-based' structure. All these countries, except for Greece, give the responsibility to manage drug and addiction policies to the Prime Minister, the Ministry of Interior, the Ministry of Justice, or the Ministry of Social Affairs. These countries are entrance points for illegal substances and for smuggling alcohol and tobacco, which, to some extent, could justify the supply-reduction approach. There is little involvement of private and non-profit stakeholders in the decision-making process and regional administrations are involved neither in the policy-making nor in the implementation process. We must not forget that these countries have recently become members of the EU and still are incorporating most of the guidelines and the 'well-being and relational management' strategy promoted by this institution.

It is worth noting that none of the four European models embraces the three trends mentioned at the beginning of this chapter, simultaneously: decriminalization of use and possession of illegal substances, broader acceptance for harm reduction perspectives, and an increasing focus on regulative politics. This shows that policy-making is subject to contingency factors, such as path-dependency frames, as well as to different forces and traditions that cannot be ignored when reframing previous approaches. Those countries embracing a regulatory approach do not have many decriminalization and harm-reduction policies and vice versa.

At the same time, the governance of addictions has its own levers, coming from the contingent combination of context (state factors) and the logistics of policy (strategy and structure). Moreover, the results from research lead to the conclusion that strategy determines structure in the governance of addictions in Europe. Thus, when a

---

Box 8.4 Four models of governance of addictions in Europe

Four models of governance of addictions coexist in Europe: (1) trendsetters in illegal substances; (2) regulation of legal substances; (3) transitioning model; and (4) traditional approach. None of the models implemented in European countries has yet been able to maximize results both for legal and illegal substances, while pursuing a societal well-being.

country embraces a well-being and relational management strategy, it consequently develops a more comprehensive organizational structure. In other words, the more harm reduction, regulation, and decriminalization, the more involvement of multi-level governance and multi-stakeholder participation it needs. The finding that strategy determines structure is also justified by the fact that none of the 28 counties analysed has a well-being and relational management strategy combined with a substance-based structure (see Box 8.4).

8.5 Connecting government: the whole of government challenge

The harm done by addictive substances is contributed to by many sectors in the public and private spheres. Further, policies and approaches to reducing the harm lie largely outside the health sector. They include sectors such as trade, agriculture, criminal justice, finance, commercial communications, education, and employment (see Table 8.2 for the 2015 US costs of tobacco, alcohol, and illegal drugs, where there is more than $700 billion annually in costs related to crime, lost of work productivity, and healthcare).

Drug addiction treatment has been shown to reduce associated health and social costs by far more than the cost of the treatment itself. According to several conservative estimates (NIDA, 2012), every dollar invested in addiction treatment programs yields a return of between $4 and $7 in reduced drug-related crime, criminal justice costs, and theft. When savings related to healthcare are included, total savings can exceed costs by a ratio of 12:1. Major savings to the individual and to society also stem from fewer interpersonal conflicts; greater workplace productivity; and fewer drug-related accidents, including overdoses and deaths.

To tackle effectively the complex issues that addictions present, approaches that involve the whole of government and the whole of society are needed. The purpose of this framework is

- to align different stakeholder contributions to a set of high-level outcomes defined for the government as a whole (economic affairs, social affairs, international affairs, and government affairs);
- to shape the governance model of addictions in EU countries;
- to steer the global system so that it is more conducive to meeting overriding objectives.

Table 8.2 US 2015 cost of addictions

	Healthcare	Overall
Tobacco	$130 billion	$295 billion
Alcohol	$25 billion	$224 billion
Illegal drugs	$11 billion	$193 billion

Reproduced from National Institute on Drug Abuse (NIDA), *Trends & Statistics*, http://www.drugabuse.gov/related-topics/trends-statistics, accessed 02 Jul. 2015, Copyright © 2015 NIH/NIDA.

In recent years, there has been a change in emphasis away from structural disaggregation, and single-purpose organizations towards a more integrated approach to public service delivery. Variously termed 'one-stop government', 'joined-up government', and 'whole-of-government' (Christensen and Laegreid, 2007), the movement from isolated silos in public administration to formal and informal networks is a global trend. The whole of government denotes public service agencies working across portfolio boundaries to achieve a shared goal and an integrated government response to particular issues. Approaches can focus on policy development, programme management, and service delivery.

In the new governance of addictive substances, there are many imperatives that make being successful at 'whole-of-government' work increasingly important. In a context of putting policies to the service of inclusive and people-centred sustainable well-being, integrated policy approaches, enabled by cohesive institutional mechanisms, contribute to the overall objectives. The absence of a 'whole-of-government' approach, by contrast, can inhibit progress, where limited coordination can undermine societal outcomes, delivery of services, provision of (geopolitical) security, and inclusive processes.

The implementation of a 'whole-of-government' approach for addictions will nevertheless require changes in governance structures and practices. It requires governments to provide leadership for 'whole-of-society' approaches to reducing the harm done, and if well-being is the approach the EU would like to aim for, the role of the health sector in coordinating relevant approaches is key. To realize a national strategy, strong leadership is required. One necessary measure is the establishment of a coordinating authority with authority across departmental and ministerial boundaries to facilitate strategy and decision-making. Top government officials then have the authority to steer process redesign efforts, facilitating communication among departments, highlight best practices, and leverage shared solutions. In most countries adding to the complexity is the fact that an increasing number of these services are delivered on behalf of a government by a network of private and non-profit organizations. Government can also bring together those key stakeholders across ministries and agencies, define shared needs, identify potential gaps and redundancies in implementing strategic goals, and guide government innovation in service delivery for addictions.

To avoid the inefficiencies inherent in earlier efforts to reorganize government agencies into single large units, networked service delivery needs to focus on engaging existing agencies in joint problem solving without realignment of formal authorities. This involves defining the framework for the 'whole of government' for addictions, with defined roles of the public, as well as the private, sector. If effective 'whole of government' is to materialize, governments must have a long-term coherent vision that identifies, articulates, and advocates the benefits of a one-stop approach to addictions.

We find that 'whole-of-government' approaches remain 'works in progress'. Despite a few promising innovations and pilot projects, individual governments continue to struggle in their efforts to define the purposes of policy integration; to formulate a strategic vision to guide their efforts; to create robust structures of coordination; to

> ### Box 8.5 Whole-of-government approach to deal with complexity
>
> Governance is influenced by many stakeholders—public, private, and non-profit—coming from different fields: health, justice, public order, safety, economy, and trade, plus an international domain related to drug trafficking and the EU. To tackle addictions issues effectively, the whole-of-government approach is needed, from single-purpose organizations towards a more integrated approach.

build critical civilian capabilities to address priority addictions governance needs; and to evaluate the impact of new strategies and policies (see Box 8.5).

8.6 The 'whole-of-government' approach for addictive substances

A better governance for addictions, far different from the widely known 'war against drugs', is possible. As this chapter shows, there are already countries with outstanding achievements in building complex solutions to complex problems. But none of the four models in Europe has yet been able to maximize results both for legal and illegal substances, while pursuing societal well-being. There is still room for improvement in all of the four models. The challenge is now how to bring the best from the different models into one governance model when there are so many variables and stakeholders involved.

It will be difficult to have an EU-wide approach as historical paths, socioeconomic standards, values, and geostrategic locations affect the levels of consumption and the final governance of addictions. Nonetheless, as the EU has done in the last two decades, it proves useful to establish minimum requirements and recommendations in order to promote harmonization, especially that driven by evidence-based research. The EU is promoting policies towards a comprehensive policy structure for addictions and lifestyles, while embracing a co-production strategy for a well-being outcome.

Governments should provide leadership for whole-of-society approaches to be able to deliver global solutions to both individuals and society, and not just reactive partial programmes. What we propose henceforth in this chapter is to define the constructs that compose this model into which European governments seem to be moving, and where public leadership is key.

Two constructs follow: strategy and structure. Regarding strategy in policies, this means to move from 'safety and disease approach' to focus more on a 'well-being and relational management approach'. This asks for developments moving from placing efforts in supply-reduction policies to dealing with high levels of social acceptance for tackling drugs and addictions (thus individual actions will be respected as long as they do not risk the freedom of another individual). The main issue is taking into account the social consequences of substance consumption and substance addictions and dealing with them through harm-reduction policies. Countries in Europe moving towards this extreme of the continuum decriminalize drug use and tend to develop evidence-based policies, previously contrasted with research and aimed at protecting public and society in general through regulation.

The second construct, structure, is based on countries' organizational structures when dealing with substances and addictions. The 'whole-of-government' approach would require moving from 'substance-based policies', which split policies (and structures) regarding substances, towards a 'comprehensive policy'. The aim is to overcome a reactive policy-making approach to the issue (policies and

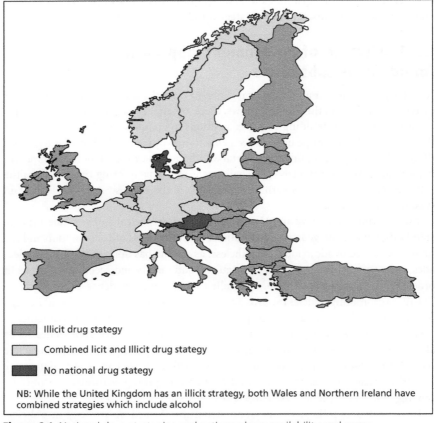

Figure 8.1 National drug strategies and actions plans: availability and scope.

Source: data from EMCDDA, *European Drug Report 2015: Trends and developments*. EMCDDA Office for Official Publications of the European Communities, Luxembourg, Copyright © 2015 European Monitoring Centre for Drugs and Drug Addiction, http://www.emcdda.europa.eu/attachements.cfm/att_239505_EN_TDAT15001ENN.pdf, accessed 01 Nov. 2015.

Box 8.6 Main drivers for a whole-of-government governance for addictions

Strategy

- Government's comprehensive strategies for addictions, combining legal and illegal substances, and behaviours.
- Treat the issue as a whole, focusing on well-being. The impact of harm done independently of substance or behaviour. Multi-causation.
- Anticipatory and innovative policies vs reactive ones.
- Regulative approach.
- International coordination.

Structure

- Coordinated networked governance.
- Break silos inside government: health and social, legal departments, justice, international treaties, well-being.
- Local and regional public policies to create policy communities and networks for responses, not losing sight of a common strategy.
- Avoid creation of new organizational structures with the introduction of new addictive products.

structures are only built when a problem appears, creating silos for any new addiction), towards embracing holistic political strategies, including substances, either legal or illegal, and behaviours (see Figure 8.1 for the current situation in Europe). Some countries are walking this path, which normally leads to more complex networked structures.

In this respect governments should provide leadership for embracing a regulative approach, decriminalization, and harm reduction policies. Box 8.6 proposes the main drivers for a whole-of-government governance for addictions, in the variables of strategy and structure (see Box 8.7).

Box 8.7 Regulation of stakeholders participation in policy making

For a whole-of-government approach, the relation with stakeholders should establish the rules of the game regarding which phase of the policy cycle and which typologies of stakeholders can provide a contribution for the public good, simultaneously to their own interests.

8.7 Two main challenges: economic crisis and the role of the private sector

To aim for this model of whole of government, proper use of the governance model and steering towards well-being strategies and governance structures to develop comprehensive policies, two main governance challenges currently have to be taken into account in Europe: the effects of the economic crisis, and the contested role of the private sector in addictions policies.

In 2008 and the years that followed, Europe experienced a severe economic crisis, which presents a challenge to public finances (for the different impact of the crisis on countries, see Olivera, 2013). The European Monitoring Centre for Drugs and Drug Addiction (EMCDDA) report on the crisis (EMCDDA, 2014) concluded, first, that austerity led to reductions in spending in those categories of government activity that encompass most drug-related initiatives: public order and safety, health, and social protection (see Table 8.3); second, that countries that experienced greater levels of austerity tended to show greater reductions in expenditure; and, third, that bigger cuts in public expenditure were registered in health than in public safety and social protection. The EMCDDA's 2015 data for the period 2009–12 shows a decline in public spending on health in most countries, compared with the pre-recession period

Table 8.3 Average growth (%) of public expenditure for health, social protection, and public order and safety in Europe after the recession

	Group 1	Group 2	Group 3	Group 4	EU27 and Norway
Health					
2000–07	4.0	4.8	4.5	8.0	**5.6**
2010	1.7	−0.9	1.1	−7.0	**−1.4**
2011	1.6	0.3	−0.3	−4.6	**−0.8**
Social protection					
2000–07	2.2	3.7	3.7	3.9	**3.9**
2010	17	0.3	2.1	−1.1	**0.7**
2011	0.7	−0.6	−0.2	−2.3	**−0.6**
Public order and safety					
2000–07	2.4	5.1	4.4	67	**4.7**
2010	1.8	24	0.5	0.4	**1.3**
2011	1.4	−25	−1.8	−3.3	**−1.5**

Note. Group 1: Germany, Luxembourg, Malta, the Netherlands, Austria, Sweden, and Norway; Group 2: Belgium, Czech Republic, Denmark, Estonia, Romania, Slovenia, and Finland; Group 3: Bulgaria, France, Italy, Cyprus, Hungary, Poland, and UK; Group 4: Ireland, Greece, Spain, Latvia, Lithuania, Portugal, and Slovakia.

Reproduced from European Monitoring Centre for Drugs and Drug Addiction, *Financing drug policy in Europe in the wake of the economic recession*, EMCDDA Papers, Publications Office of the European Union, Luxembourg, Copyright © 2014 European Monitoring Centre for Drugs and Drug Addiction.

2005–07, with reductions of more than ten percentage points in many European countries (EMCDDA, 2015).

Simultaneously, according to data from the WHO (World Health Organization, 2011), the economic contraction has led to a deterioration in some of the factors protective of mental health (e.g. social capital, welfare protection, and healthy workplaces), while increasing risk factors (poverty, poor education, deprivation, high debt, unemployment, job insecurity, and stress).

In the years to come, we will have to take into account how the effects of the economic crisis in Europe have affected countries in balancing austerity measures with high-quality addictions policies. In some countries the high levels of debt have led to a reduction of social services' budgets. Simultaneously, there is also the risk that substance use and related harm will increase as a consequence of high unemployment rates. However, some countries deeply affected by the crisis, such as Portugal, stand out as having innovative policies; thus, these factors are not mutually exclusive.

By taking governance as our reference framework we assume that, as with many other 'wicked' public issues, addictions can no longer be addressed by governments alone. There is a need to enhance better results from collaboration and to promote the involvement of organizations in order to maximize the outcomes to society and its well-being (European Commission, 2006; Council of the European Union, 2012; O'Gorman and Moore, 2012). Governance frameworks show that government bodies cannot do everything, and that interventions are far more effective when they are integrated with various institutions in civil society (United Nations, 2004; NIDA, 2005) (see Figure 8.2). Research institutions, not-for-profit organizations, individuals with problems, families, professionals, media, and even businesses are already part of not only a pluralist provision of services (co-production), but also of a pluralist process for policy design and implementation. Three provisos are key when taking this approach:

1. The leading role in determining the strategy of the public policy for addictions should always be in public sector hands to enhance societal well-being

2. An evolved co-production system has to find ways of avoiding co-optation by both industry and NGOs dependent on public budgets

3. Transparency, checks, and balances should be ensured as the drivers to increase evidence-based impact in decision-making.

Nevertheless, reconciling the different stakeholder perspectives is challenging and consultation processes often struggle to achieve this (Roberts, 2014, and see Chapters 9 and 10 of this book). In recent years, the profile and importance of advocacy organizations in the drugs area has increased, and an exploratory mapping from EMCDDA (2013) identified 218 drug policy advocacy organizations in Europe. The most common tool used by these organizations to influence drug discourses and disseminate information is some form of awareness raising activity (used by 82% of the organizations), such as participating in media debates, providing commentary, or using social media such as blogs, Facebook, and Twitter. More than half (52%) of the advocacy organizations focused on lobbying at a national or EU–UN level, using policy submissions, petitions, and participation in policy forums to bring attention to their issues of concern. Lobbying was used by organizations with divergent

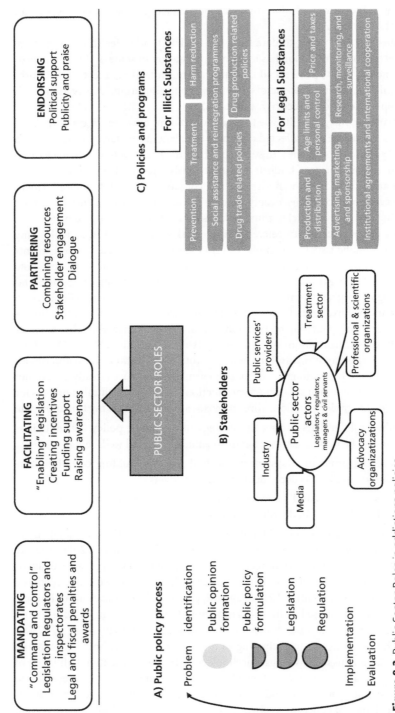

Figure 8.2 Public Sector Roles in addictions policies.

objectives. Education and training tools, such as seminars and conferences, were used by nearly half (45%) of the advocacy organizations to share and disseminate information on their viewpoints. Almost a third (31%) of the organizations sought to build and disseminate an evidence base through research and publications. Activist strategies, such as demonstrations and marches, were employed by a small proportion of advocacy organizations (11%). A further small proportion of the drug policy advocacy organizations used legal advocacy to promote a human rights-based approach to drug policy (4%).

Box 8.8 and Table 8.4 provide, in a nutshell, a map of stakeholders, the stages in the policy process they could participate in, and the different strategies they might adopt in the governance of addictions.

The creation of forums and participatory platforms is not a guarantee of an enriching involvement of civil society and corporations into the policy-making and implementation processes. Research shows that governance might have some limitations in addictions policy (Edwards and Galla, 2014; MacGregor et al., 2014), especially regarding illegal drugs, where the state and the formal institutions of government remain dominant. Futhermore, long-standing and more recent developments indicate high levels of industry influence on alcohol policy (Babor and Robaina, 2013; McCambridge et al., 2014), which reveal a conflict of interest between the common good and business interests.

Even if the industry uses the strategies shown in Table 8.4 (e.g. including commissioning research projects, corporate social responsibility activities to hone their reputation, access to policy-makers to foster policy in favour of their interests), it might be relevant to bear in mind the WHO's (2007: 48) recommendation that (alcohol)

Box 8.8 Actors involved in the governance of addictions

Public sector actors: policy-makers, civil servants, career bureaucrats, politicians.

Advocacy organizations: interest/pressure groups, SAPROs (social aspects/public relations organizations), drug-user organizations, family/career organizations, includes local residents ('not in my back yard' situations), charities, trade unions, social movements.

Professional and/or scientific associations

Treatment sector (providers): public–private, non-statutory/statutory, and mutual aid.

Researchers/scientists: universities, institutes, science-based initiatives, and think tanks.

Economic stakeholders: includes businesses associations, (pharmaceutical) industry, social enterprises, business with primarily social objectives

Media

Table 8.4 Political activity strategies

Approaches to political strategies	Transactional	Short-term exchange relationship; specific, salient issues (reactive), issue-by-issue; based on the substance
	Relational	Denotes a long-term relationship (build relations across issues); structures and processes are of key importance; long-term aims; contacts already in place (proactive); trust develops between suppliers and demanders of public policy
Participation levels	Individual	Organizational level
	Collective	Industry level
Type of strategies	Information	Lobbying (by internal or external professionals and executives)
		Reporting research and survey results
		Commissioning research projects
		Testifying as experts in hearings or before government bodies
		Supplying position papers
	Financial incentive	Financial support: direct contributions to a political decision maker or political party
		Political Action Committee contributions in US
		Honoraria for speaking
		Paid travel expenses
		Personal services (having a representative in a political position)
	Constituency-building	Grassroots mobilization of employees, customers, suppliers, retirees
		Advocacy advertising
		Public image or public relations advertising
		Press conferences on policy issues
		Economic or political education

Source: data from Hillman A and Hitt M. Corporate Political Strategy Formulation: A Model of Approach, Participation, and Strategy Decisions, *Academy of Management Review*, Volume 24, Issue 4, pp. 825–842, Copyright © 1999 Academy of Management; Bonardi JP, Hillman A, and Keim G. The attractiveness of Political Markets: Implications for Firm Strategy, *Academy of Management Review*, Volume 30 Issue 2, pp. 397–413, Copyright © 2005 Academy of Management; Miller D and Harkins C. Corporate strategy, corporate capture: Food and alcohol industry lobbying and public health. *Critical Social Policy*, Volume 30 Issue 4, pp. 564–589, Copyright © 2010 Critical Social Policy Ltd.; EMCDDA (2013) *Drug policy advocacy organisations in Europe*, EMCDDA Papers, Publications Office of the European Union, Luxembourg, Copyright © 2013 EMCDDA; McCambridge J, Kypri K, Miller P, Hawkins B and Hastings G. Be aware of Drinkaware, *Addiction*, Volume 109, Issue 4, pp. 519–524, Copyright © 2014 The Society for the Study of Addiction; Roberts M. Making drug policy together: Reflections on evidence, engagement and politics. *International Journal of Drug Policy*, Volume 25, pp. 952–956, Copyright © 2014 Elsevier, Inc.

industry bodies only be engaged in their roles as producers, distributors, and retailers: 'The Committee recommends that WHO continue its practice of no collaboration with the various sectors of the alcohol industry. Any interaction should be confined to discussion of the contribution the alcohol industry can make to the reduction of alcohol-related harm only in the context of their roles as producers, distributors and marketers of alcohol, and not in terms of alcohol policy development or health promotion'. Legality does not always equal legitimacy.

However, although the WHO cautioned that the private sector should not be trying to do the work of governments, which are properly the guardians of the public interest, it also considers in the same document that the industry has a particular role to play in the implementation of some specific policies and programmes. This can include providing server training to all involved in the sales chain to ensure responsibility in adhering to the law, and in reducing hazardous drinking and in ensuring that alcohol is not available to those under the legal drinking age.

If we would like to move addictions governance in Europe from this grey area to a well-being and 'whole-of-government' and society approach, the relation with stakeholders should establish rules regarding which phase of the policy cycle and which typologies of stakeholders contribute to the public good, as well as simultaneously to their own interests (see Box 8.9).

8.8 **Conclusions**

The main contributions from this chapter are that there are different historical factors that have contributed to the current consumerist model of drugs and alcohol. Western societies have been forced to find new forms of governance and renewed policies to counteract and better adapt to these realities. In our time, the pathways towards European public policies on addiction are characterized by three trends: decriminalization of drug use, wider introduction of harm reduction for both illegal and legal substances, and a shift from repression to regulation.

The complexity of addictions and drug issues leaves no doubt that this is a wicked problem that must be tackled by different levels of governments in collaboration with stakeholders. EU countries plus Norway involve, at least to some extent, non-profit organizations in the decision-making and, especially, in the implementation process. And its governance is influenced by many stakeholders, public, private, and non-profit, coming from different fields: health, justice, public order, safety, economy, trade, and so on. This wide range of stakeholders, and also the international domain related to drug trafficking and the EU, makes the governance of addictions more complex.

Four models of governance of addictions coexist in Europe (trendsetters in illegal substances, regulation of legal substances, transitioning model, and traditional approach). However, none of the four has yet been able to maximize results both for legal and illegal substances, while pursuing societal well-being. The challenge is now how to bring the best from the different models into one governance model when there are so many variables and stakeholders involved.

> ### Box 8.9 Main challenges for a whole-of-government governance
>
> - The leading role in determining the strategy of the public policy for addictions should always be in public sector hands to enhance societal well-being.
> - An evolved co-production system has to find ways of avoiding co-optation by both industry and NGOs dependent on public budgets.
> - Transparency, and checks and balances should be ensured as the drivers to increase evidence-based impact in decision-making.

To tackle addiction issues effectively, a whole-of-government approach is needed, moving from single-purpose organizations towards a more integrated approach to public service delivery (networked governance). Governments should provide leadership for whole-of-society approaches to be able to deliver broad solutions to both individuals and society, and not only reactive partial programmes.

To aim for this framework in Europe, two main governance challenges have to be taken into account: the effects of the economic crisis, and the contested role of the private sector in addictions policies. If we would like to move addictions governance in Europe from its current status to a well-being and whole of government approach, the relation with stakeholders should establish the rules regarding which phase of the policy cycle and which typologies of stakeholders can provide a contribution for the public good along with their own interests.

References

Arif A (1981). 'Los problemas de la droga en el mundo y las estrategias de la OMS'. In: Edwards G and Arif A (eds) *Los problemas de la droga en el contexto sociocultural. Una base para la formulación de políticas y la planificación de programas.* Ginebra: OMS, pp. 22–35.

Babor TF and Robaina K (2013) Public health, academic medicine, and the alcohol industry's corporate social responsibility activities. *Am J Public Health* **103**: 206–14.

Bonardi JP, Hillman A, and Keim G (2005) The attractiveness of political markets: implications for firm strategy. *Acad Manage Rev* **30**: 397–413.

Bovaird T (2004) Public private partnerships: from contested concepts to prevalent practice. *Int Rev Admin Sci* 70: 199–215.

Christensen T and Laegreid P (2007) The whole-of-government approach to public sector reform. *Publ Admin Rev* November/December: 1059–66.

Comas D (1985). *El uso de las drogas en la juventud.* Madrid: Instituto de la Juventud.

Council of the European Union (2012) EU drugs strategy (2013–2020). *CORDROGUE* **101**: doc. 17547/12.

Díaz A (1998) *Hoja, pasta, polvo, roca. El consumo de los derivados de la coca.* Bellaterra: Servei de Publicacions de la UAB.

Díaz A, Pallarés J, Barruti M, and Canales G (2004) *Observatori de nous consums de drogues en l'àmbit juvenil.* Barcelona: Institut Genus.

Edwards C and Galla M (2014) Governance in EU illicit drugs policy. *Int J Drug Policy* 25: 942–7.

EMCDDA (2013) *Drug Policy Advocacy Organisations in Europe, EMCDDA Papers.* Luxembourg: Publications Office of the European Union.

EMCDDA (2014) *Estimating Public Expenditure on Drug-Law Offenders in Prison in Europe, EMCDDA Papers.* Luxembourg: Publications Office of the European Union.

EMCDDA (2015) *European Drug Report 2015.* Luxembourg: Office for Official Publications of the European Communities.

Emerson K, Nabatchi T, and Balogh S (2012) An integrative framework for collaborative governance. *J Publ Adm Res Theory* 22: 1–31.

Esping-Andersen G (1990) *The Three Worlds of Welfare Capitalism.* Oxford: Polity Press.

European Commission (2006) Report on the results of the open consultation. Green paper on the role of civil society in drugs policy in the European Union. COM (2006) 316 final. Brussels, Commission of the European Communities.

Ferrera M (1996) The 'Southern' Model of Welfare in Social Europe. *J Eur Soc Policy* 6: 17–37.

Foucault M (1963) *El nacimiento de la clínica.* México: Siglo XXI.

Hellman M, Berridge V, Duke K, and Mold A (eds) (2015) *Concepts of Addictive Substances and Behaviours Across Time and Place.* Oxford: Oxford University Press.

Hillman A and Hitt M (1999) Corporate political strategy formulation: a model of approach, participation, and strategy decisions. *Acad Manage Rev* 24: 825–42.

Joossens L and Raw M (2010) *The Tobacco Control Scale 2010 in Europe.* Brussels: Association of the European Cancer Leagues.

Kickert W, Klijn EH, and Koppenjan J (1997) *Managing Complex Networks: Strategies for the Public Sector.* London: Sage Publications.

Lozano JM, Albareda L, Ysa T, Roscher H, and Marcuccio M (2008) *Governments and Corporate Social Responsibility: Public Policies Beyond Regulation and Voluntary Compliance.* Basingstoke: Palgrave.

MacGregor S, Singleton N, and Trautmann F (2014) Towards good governance in drug policy: evidence, stakeholders and politics. *Int J Drug Policy* 25: 931–4.

McCambridge J, Kypri K, Miller P, Hawkins B, and Hastings G (2014) Be aware of Drinkaware. *Addiction* 109: 519–24.

Mendoza X and Vernis A (2008) The changing role of governments and the emergence of the relational state. *Corp Govern* 8: 389–96.

Miller D and Harkins C (2010) Corporate strategy, corporate capture: food and alcohol industry lobbying and public health. *Crit Soc Policy* 30: 564–89.

NIDA (2005) Substance abuse and drug policy: strategies and national priorities in the U.S.A. and in Russia (comparative approach). Available at: http://www.drugabuse.gov/international/abstracts/substance-abuse-drug-policy-strategies-national-priorities-in-usa-in-russia-comparative-approach (accessed 2 July 2015).

NIDA (2012) Principles of drug addiction treatment: a research-based guide (third edition). Available at: http://www.drugabuse.gov/publications/principles-drug-addiction-treatment-research-based-guide-third-edition/frequently-asked-questions/drug-addiction-treatment-worth-its-cost (accessed 2 July 2015).

NIDA (2015) Trends and statistics. Available at: http://www.drugabuse.gov/related-topics/trends-statistics (accessed 2 July 2015).

Olivera J (2013) The impact of the economic recession on public expenditure on drug policy in the EU. Available at: www.emcdda.europa.eu/publications/emcdda-papers/recession-and-drug-related-public-expenditure (accessed 2 July 2015).

Österberg E and Karlsson T (1998) *Alcohol Policies in EU Member States and Norway. A Collection of Country Reports.* Brussels, European Commission DG Health.

O'Gorman A and Moore M (2012) *Mapping Study of Drug Policy Advocacy Organisations in Europe (Final Report).* Lisbon: EMCDDA.

O'Toole LJ (1997) Treating networks seriously: practical and research-based agendas in public administration. *Publ Admin Rev* **57**: 45–52.

Reuter P and Trautmann F (2009) *A Report on Global Illicit Drugs Markets 1998–2007 Full Report.* Brussels, European Commission, RAND Europe, Trimbos Institute.

Rittel H and Webber M (1973) Dilemmas in a general theory of planning. *Policy Sci* **4**: 155–69.

Ritter A and Bammer G (2010) Models of policy making and their relevance for drug research. *Drug Alcohol Rev* **29**: 352–7.

Roberts M (2014) Making drug policy together: reflections on evidence, engagement and politics. *Int J Drug Policy* **25**: 952–6.

Stoker G (1998) Governance as theory: five propositions. *Int Soc Sci J* **50**: 17–28.

Trautmann F (2013) Key trends of the illicit drugs market and drug policy in the EU: what do experts anticipate for the coming years? In: Trautmann F, Kilmer B, and Turnbull P (eds) *Further Insights into Aspects of the EU Illicit Drugs Markets.* Luxembourg: Publications Office of the European Union, pp. 447–501.

United Nations (2004) *U.N. 2004 World Drug Report. Office on Drugs and Crime (UNODC).* ISBN 92-1-148185-6. Available at http://www.unodc.org/pdf/WDR_2004/volume_1.pdf (accessed 2 July 2015).

World Health Organization (2007) *Who Expert Committee on Problems Related to Alcohol Consumption. Second Report WHO Technical Report Series.* Geneva: World Health Organization.

World Health Organization (2011) *Impact of the Economic Crisis on Mental Health.* Copenhagen: WHO Regional Office Europe.

Ysa T, Colom J, Albareda A, Ramon A, Carrión M, and Segura L (2014) *Governance of Addictions. European Public Policies.* Oxford: Oxford University Press.

Chapter 9

Private sector impact on the harm done by addictive substances

9.1 Introduction

In this chapter, we will outline the role of private businesses, both legal and illegal, in contributing to the harm done by addictive substances. The chapter will cover the alcohol and tobacco businesses, and will include businesses involved in the production and sale of illegal drugs. The chapter will describe how the businesses operate and their influence on governments, science, civil society, and the policy processes. The chapter will review the difficulties of engaging with such private companies in reducing the harm done by addictive substances, including transparency, conflict resolution, and negotiation.

9.2 How business operates

The first rule of business is that it aims for profit maximization—but business is not just a matter of economics. It is a matter of politics, too. This is important as—by necessity—those who run business corporations do so in particular political circumstances and they take decisions in what they judge to be the best interests of the corporation. However, these decisions involve both economic and political assessments by business leaders, as opposed to (just) the abstract laws of economics. As a result, business engages directly in politics and business decisions that reflect the information available to corporate executives, as well as their assessment of what is politically possible at a particular level or scale, and what is desirable. This has potential effects on addictions that can be both negative and positive in terms of public health.

The second key argument is that the historical epoch in which we currently live—neoliberalism—provides a master context for business action in politics. Neoliberalism has been usefully defined by David Harvey (2005) as 'the doctrine that market exchange is an ethic in itself, capable of acting as a guide for all human action'. It is important to stress that it is a doctrine and not a type of society. Neoliberalism affects societies unevenly and sometimes unpredictably. Often neoliberal reforms do not result in the claimed cuts to public spending or improvements in the 'efficiency' of public services. The gap between the claims of the doctrine and the results is perhaps produced, in part, because mistakes were made or the theory was inadequate, but most importantly it is because the doctrine is a means of pursuing—we might say masking—certain interests. It is, in other words, ideological (Miller, 2015).

For our purposes it is useful to think of how neoliberalism affects the policy environment in two ways: (1) that neoliberalism systematically advantages corporate, and especially transnational corporate, interests in relation to particular policy decisions; and (2) that it alters the policy architecture so that the practical decision-making regime that applies in relation to a range of decisions is altered to become more corporate friendly. This distinction is important as it not only draws attention to both the specific way in which particular policy decisions are made, but also the way in which the general regime of policy-making changes. For our purposes, this is important as there are a number of architectural decisions which, although apparently far distant from the concerns of tobacco, alcohol, or food companies, are actually implicated in systematically advantaging those corporations downstream in the discussion of specific policy measures. Furthermore, as we will see later, the industrial sectors thus advantaged can be shown to be active in lobbying on these 'architectural' issues—for example, better regulation, impact assessment, or the precautionary principle.

The organizations that manufacture and promote addictive products play an important but often poorly understood role in the field of addictions (Lee et al., 2004; Baggott, 2006; Miller and Harkins, 2010). These significant stakeholders are involved in a complex network of relationships with organizations in corporate, state, and non-governmental spheres (Connolly, 1995; Hastings and Angus, 2009). To examine the role played by economic actors in supporting and attenuating addictive behaviours we focus on corporate tactics in relation to public health. The growth of partnership modes of governance invites a range of stakeholders formally into the policy process. As modes of governance become increasingly reliant on these partnerships, and, indeed, these partners, it is important to have a full understanding of how economic and non-economic actors interact, and what implications this has for policy and related practices. Corporate actors form networks that are active across multiple domains. Thus, it is necessary to undertake a comparative analysis of regulatory and self-regulatory frameworks and practices; complemented by examination of the role of economic actors in public discourses on addictions, as well as expert and policy-related discourse (Babor et al., 1996; Barnoya and Glantz, 2006).

Recent research has suggested commonalities between the corporate strategy of the tobacco industry in the USA over the latter half of the twentieth century, and the current behaviour of elements within the food industry (Chopra and Darnton-Hill, 2004; Brownell and Warner, 2009). Do such comparisons work for other 'substance' addictions?

Corporations are units of economic and political decision-making that are legally and organizationally distinct units of activity. They both compete and act together with other firms via—most obviously—trade associations. However, they also collaborate with, create, or pass funding to non-economic actors such as lobby organizations; policy-planning groups, consulting, public relations (PR), and legal firms; think tanks; foundations; and non-governmental organizations. The establishment of a European single market and the emergence of a European public sphere (Fossum and Schilesinger, 2007; Michel, 2007) have prompted companies to reorient towards European Union (EU) policy-makers (Eising, 2009; Greenwood, 2011). Corporations engage in strategic decisions about how to pursue influence and in order to understand that influence we need to trace the routes that industrial actors take to pursue their interests. In practice, we find that multiple routes are taken across the various levels of policy engagement and thus we describe our approach as a 'multiple routes to influence' model.

Corporations adopt coordinated strategies that involve multiple organizations and channels of communication. For this reason, we argue that this research should start with the corporate actors themselves, before considering the arenas in which they mobilize and their relationship to institutions of governance. Arenas are defined as specific spaces of strategic action and contest, and we focus here on science, the political arena, civil society, and the public sphere. As a result, we need to conceive of corporate action in a number of domains. Thus, as Compston (2013) notes, 'If we take the view that business power is something to be established empirically, one factor to consider is the degree of business unity. The extent to which business is united, if at all, is one of the main issues dividing pluralists from elitists, but both assume that unity does or would enable business to exert more influence on public policy'.

Thus, we examine the extent of unity and the way in which corporate actors cohere or divide over particular issues.

9.3 **Networks**

Corporations form a variety of networks, with other firms in and between industries and with lobby groups. As Heemskerk et al. remind us:

> Ever since the birth of the modern corporation, interfirm relations that tie firms together in networks of ownership and control have been in place. At the level of corporate governance, corporations are connected through shared board members (interlocking directorates), shared owners, and direct stock-holdings between firms. Although often depicted as atomic, individualistic disconnected market actors, corporations are in fact deeply embedded in such networks. And in our days of ongoing financial, economic and cultural globalization it may come as no surprise that recent findings reveal that in the global network of corporate ownership a small group of corporations dominate. Forty per cent of the control over economic value of Trans National Corporations (TNCs) in the world is held, through complicated ownership structures, by a group of 147 of these corporations (Heemskerk et al. 2013: 1).

The number '147' is from a ground-breaking study that examined the extent to which there is a global network of global corporate control that exerts influence over global business (Vitali et al., 2011). The authors note that a quantitative study is 'not a trivial task' because firms 'may exert control over other firms via a web of direct and indirect ownership relations which extends over many countries. Therefore, a complex network analysis is needed' (Vitali et al., 2011). The authors performed this analysis by examining share ownership data on the total population of 43,060 TNCs identified in a business database. The resulting TNC network included 600,508 nodes and 1,006,987 ownership ties. When analysed, the data showed a small group of core corporations which 'despite its small size . . . holds collectively . . . nearly 4/10 of the control over the economic value of TNCs in the world'. It can be noted that three-quarters of the core are financial institutions. This is a hugely significant finding, which is only beginning to be understood. One early response is from Compston (2013: 359), who proposes to use the data in the study to test the hypothesis that 'the capacity of TNCs to influence public policy is greater than previously thought because TNC ownership and control is not only extremely concentrated but also extremely centralized'.

This shows the importance of analysing industry structure and interlocks, as well as following through the practical content of the views and activities pursued by firms in relation to policy and other domains. Other work has shown that network density of corporate board interlocks has been increasing notably in Europe.

Carroll (2009: 289) notes that 'overall, despite modest accretions in participation from the semi-periphery, and with the decline of the Japanese corporate network, the elite become centered even more strongly on the North Atlantic. With its growing regional cohesiveness, corporate Europe gains prominence within that heartland.' Furthermore, we can see that the integration of EU business notably tightens in a period of increasing political ambivalence.

'The process of European Unification', writes Compston (2013: 10) 'has always been strongly supported by large industrial conglomerates and business interests'. The common market and later the monetary union were seen as in the interest of European business in general. Over the last decade, however, the project of European unification has received more and more critique. In the light of the political turmoil about the Union's future, it is telling that European corporations increasingly link with each other across European borders.

Recent work has shown that the corporate board interlocks are a relatively weak element in the integration of the inner circle of the corporate community. By comparison, interlocking memberships of elite policy-planning groups are central to the web of connections between politically active corporate leaders. A study of 11 leading elite policy-planning groups gave the following results:

> In 2006, the 11 policy boards shared on average nearly 3.5 members; in the same year, European corporate boards shared a mean of 0.0362 members. In this sense, the policy-board network provides a *hard core* of politically active and socially cohesive cadre to the global corporate elite. This hard core is primarily active within European corporate capitalism. When we consider the firms with more than five interlocks with policy boards, we find that in 1996, 76% were based in Europe, with the rest in North America. By 2006, 80% were European, the other 20% North American by domicile (Carroll and Sapinski, 2010: 522).

This work provides the top level context in understanding corporate actions in relation to addictions. We focus on the elite policy planning groups and how they intersect with the industrial sectors we are examining. It is important, however, to understand that the model of interaction and webs of influence that we propose examines not just membership and funding relationships between corporations and policy intermediaries. The notion of the web of influence requires not only financial and personal relationships, but also actions and crucially communications. We thus conceive of the interlocking networks as networks of policy communications, (Philo et al., 2015) which take place in the context of wider circuits of communication (Miller et al., 1998).

Once we conceive of corporate action in terms of networks and circuits of action and communication, the empirical task is to construct a picture of the networks and follow them wherever they lead. This means following the networks in time and space, both vertically and horizontally. In the current case that means following the specific networks associated with the corporate actors in three ways:

1. In terms of the collective characteristics of each industry in which we are interested: tobacco and alcohol. We then follow this through to examine each industry.

2. Vertically, in relation to levels of governance; from national to regional and EU levels.

3. Horizontally, in terms of the domains with which they engage at any specific level of governance.

This allows us to examine the extent to which each industry adopts the same strategies or exhibits differentiation of both organization and action and the extent to which each corporation collaborates with others in their industry and, indeed, with other industrial sectors.

9.4 Levels of governance and domains of action

Corporate and other actors take decisions in time and (social) space. So we need to understand how historical processes and actors outside business provide the context in which corporate strategy is planned and executed. The historical context of governance in the EU discloses two tendencies—the first is the process of transnationalization (often called globalization), which, in the case of the EU, has moved the locus of decision-making up to the supranational level (Europeanization) along with other transnational tendencies associated with global governance. At the same time there has been a widespread tendency towards subsidiarity—meaning that decision-making is passed down to the lowest practical regional, national or local level. This can be seen in the huge increase in the number of states in the period after 1989, as well as in tendencies towards devolution of some powers—both of which are in addition to 'subsidiarity' proper as encoded in European policy documents and agreements.

9.5 Supranational governance in focus

Supranational governance is relevant to the study of addictive industries, because many issues related to the regulation, and governance of addictive products are influenced by levels of authority beyond the nation state. The World Health Organization (WHO), and the World Trade Organization (WTO) are important institutions and as such networks cluster around them and interact with them in multiple ways. The WHO is a target for corporate activity and a platform where economic actors make attempts to influence research and dissemination activities. The WTO is a trade platform that excludes contributions from the public health community and aims to liberalize trade laws and reduce trade barriers in order to facilitate economic growth. Often regulatory arrangements that seek to protect health in relation to addiction require specific restrictions, for example on the price and availability of alcohol, that are at odds with the interests of trade. In the case of Europe, the European polity is an important level of authority. The outcome of Scotland's efforts to introduce a minimum unit price for alcohol will be decided at the European level of authority; alcohol industry activity on this issue has been intense at European and member state levels of authority. The liberalization of Swedish alcohol policy is seen by some as a consequence of trade relationships between Sweden and the European polity. Economic stakeholders and their representatives engage in action at every level of governance authority. In order to provide fully an accurate representation of the shape and nature of corporate activity, multiple levels of governance authority should be considered in the analysis.

9.6 **Legal vs. illegal products**

It is important to recognize that the legal status of a substance has significant effects on how it is traded and regulated. Indeed, the legal status of the substance is itself one way in which substances are regulated. Furthermore, the way in which substances are defined as legal/illegal is a socially and politically constructed and historically variable process. What is defined as illegal in a society creates crime in a straightforward way. This is important because what does and what 'should' count as crime in relation to addictive industries is subject to a continual struggle.

The legal status of substances, and indeed the question of addiction itself, are subject to both scientific and policy debate and dispute. The history of the changing conceptualization of addiction as a notion and the particular attachment of the notion to specific substances—cocaine, heroin, alcohol, tobacco, so-called 'legal highs'—illustrates this very well (Anderson et al., 2010). Debates over whether sugar is addictive or whether obesity is a consequence of addiction illustrate the difficulties of defining addiction. Indeed, some argue that sugar and added sweeteners are addictive and should be subject to control in the same way as alcohol (Lustig et al., 2012). Alternatively, it has been argued that 'since the human body does not become physically dependent on sugar the way it does on opiates like morphine and heroin, sugar is not addictive'(Duchene, 2006). Ziauddeen et al. (2012) challenge the view that obesity and overeating can be described as addiction, suggesting that the application of a single model, in this case the model of addiction, is unhelpful at best.

These examples illustrate the contest over definitions of addiction across disciplines, substances, and behaviours. The concept of addiction is fluid and contestable and changes over time and as a result of increased knowledge and the level of political or policy debate.

We can think of the impact of the outcomes of these debates in two ways— definitional and material. Defining any substance as having particularly addictive or harmful effects to individuals or society is part of the process of delineating whether a 'crime' is committed in possessing, using, or trading in it. To put it most simply, policy and legal processes create criminality merely by enacting laws that define existing conduct as criminal. Thus—in a recent example—users of mephedrone one day were indulging in a behaviour that was entirely legal, while the next day they were vulnerable to being defined as criminals by virtue of a change in the law (BBC

News, 2010; Nutt, 2010). This is to say nothing of the effects that such a declaration has on existing conduct. This is a second and important way in which definitions produce changes in material circumstances including behaviours. Thus, prohibition of alcohol in the USA in 1920 created a whole new class of criminals, but the bootleg-ging industry that grew up in response transformed the way in which alcohol was produced, traded, and consumed. The involvement of organized crime is well known in that case. It is also clear that the creation of a 'black market' in alcohol resulted in a very significant infrastructure for the manufacture, distribution, and sale of illicit alcohol, even if this did not account for the majority of alcohol production or con-sumption in most areas of the USA, with exceptions such as Chicago (Levine and Reinarman, 1991). Such infrastructure, can, in principle, be adapted for the manu-facture, distribution, and sale of other illicit products. Thus, some of the bootleggers were also implicated in the organized distribution of heroin and cocaine in the USA from the 1920s onwards.

This example reminds us that there is both an economics and a politics to black markets and to attempts to regulate them. Looking back at the history of 'illegal' substances also reminds us that regulatory decisions intended to limit or eliminate markets in addictive substances can all too easily and in some cases foreseeably do the opposite. They can end in encouraging the expansion of the market.

We can see these processes in relation especially to the global market in opium and heroin, although similar issues are found in all other examples of substance use, and indeed in relation to other behaviours that might be subject to discussion as 'addic-tions' or 'crimes', such as gambling.

9.7 **Business and government: illegal drugs**

The analytical separation between business and government used in almost all inter-est group studies (Truman, 1971; Kingdon and Thurber, 1984; Marsh and Rhodes, 1992) is not always replicated clearly in reality. In situations of unstable government or great conflict in society, such as in some regions which produce illegal drugs—for example, Afghanistan—the distinction between those in charge of government min-istries and those engaged in the (illegal) drug trade is not always clear. Not only does this challenge our analytical distinctions, but also implicates those nations that are engaged in military intervention or other support to governments or particular fac-tions in those countries. We can examine this issue in relation especially to the role of the UK and the USA in the heroin trade, although similar points could be made about the USA and the cocaine trade (McCoy, 2003). It is also important to be clear that even where clear analytical distinctions can be made, one of the fundamental roles of the nation state is to pursue the 'national interest'. In practice, that usually includes the economic health of the corporate sector. This is perhaps the most impor-tant lesson of history in relation to drugs, which, currently, are illegal in almost every Western nation.

In some ways there is a sharp distinction between legal and illegal substances in terms of those who trade in them. The alcohol and tobacco industries are not at the centre, nor even on the periphery of, the Medellin cartel, which has played a central role in the cocaine industry. Nor have they been in any obvious or structural way in the heroin trade (going back to the historically leading role of South East Asia in the 1970s or to Afghanistan today). But we can make two caveats to this general proposition. First, historically, there have been connections between those who traded in heroin or cocaine and other substances or, indeed, other sorts of (legal) business and second the state has often been implicated in fostering both legal and illegal drugs trades.

Two well-known examples—the heroin trade in the period up to 1920 and the prohibition of alcohol in the early twentieth century—illustrate that this has depended primarily on the contested legal status of the substances involved. Of the first example, the heroin trade which was the subject of the opium wars, Hanes and Sanello (2004: xi) write:

> Imagine this scenario: the Medellin cocaine cartel ... mounts a successful military offensive against the United States, then forces the U.S. to legalize cocaine and allow the cartel to import the drug ... plus the U.S. has to pay war reparations of $100 billion—the Colombians' cost of waging the war to import cocaine into America.

They point out how seemingly preposterous and incredible this scenario seems, and yet that such a situation occurred not once but twice during the nineteenth century, with the UK forcing very comparable conditions on China.

Of course, this account leaves out a number of things, such as the role of two British companies, the British East India Company and Jardine, Matheson and Co., China's biggest opium importer. As the conglomerate, Jardine Matheson Holdings, the latter company still exists today (*Scotsman*, 2005).

Hanes and Sanello's account also neglects the role of trade interests in addition to (as a motivator of) state interests and involvement. As Chen and Winder (1990: 660) note, by the middle of the seventeenth century, Chinese tea and silk imports to the UK resulted in 'a balance of trade favourable to the Chinese government'. This was part of the impetus for the British East India Company 'with the aid of the British government' to 'greatly expand' the importation of opium to China. Although the Chinese banned importation they were not able to enforce the ban. When, in 1838, the Chinese moved against the trade, the British escalated matters, sending an 'expeditionary force' in the summer of 1840. Chinese defeat in 1842 led to the treaty of Nanking, which ceded Hong Kong to the UK, thus allowing the opium trade to flourish. The second opium war (1856–60) resulted in the final defeat of the Chinese and the legalization of the opium trade.

Looked at from this distance in the context of the contemporary demonization of heroin, even compared with tobacco, the opium wars can look like an example from a forgotten and long surpassed world, but the connection between corporations and the nations that house and sponsor them is an enduring feature of our global political economy. It is not too surprising therefore to find authors such as Chen and Winder (1990) describing the role of the US government in forcing open South East Asian markets for tobacco in the 1980s and 1990s as reminiscent of the opium wars.

The second example is the era of prohibition in the USA. This came at the end of the period of free trade in opium production, which was increasingly legally circumscribed following moves by the League of Nations in 1925 and 1931 (McCoy, 2003). These measures had a significant impact on cutting global production by more than half between 1907 and 1934 (McCoy, 2003: 10). From 1919 to 1933 the USA introduced prohibition on alcohol and this coincidence of legal status meant that the alcohol and heroin 'industry' became partially integrated. As McCoy puts it: 'prohibition drove the vast alcohol and narcotics trades into a new vice economy, organized crime expanded correspondingly from localized gangs into nationwide syndicates that won political power in cities such as New York and Chicago' (2003: 11).[1] This latter point is of significance as it points to a clear, if obscured, relation between the 'industry' involved in illegal drink and drug production and relations and networks of corruption in politics, a set of relations that, as we will see, are still present in the global political economy of illegal drugs (Owens, 2011).

While prohibition of alcohol was repealed in 1933 the illegal networks set up in the 1920s remained as 'narcotics were driven from legal commerce to the illicit traffic, acquiring a distinctive politics and elusive economics'. After 1945 prohibition would 'foster a global illicit economy that funded criminals, warlords, rebels, terrorists and covert operations' (McCoy, 2003: 11). The inclusion of the last term in that list is a reference pre-eminently to the covert operations of the US state, which McCoy describes in relentless detail.

9.8 Business and government: legal drugs

Our analytical distinctions are also challenged in EU member states and at the EU level where business is increasingly internal to the state. We examine, therefore, cases of the interpenetration of government and business, including the revolving door, party funding, and new forms of institutional corruption (Miller and Dinan, 2009; Miller, 2015).There is acknowledgement in various theoretical accounts of governance that its changing modes of have resulted in the creation of a space for non-state actors within policy circles. However, thereafter, the role of corporate actors is habitually underestimated or even overlooked all together.

The neoliberal era ushers in a new political geography of governance. This does not necessarily mean that the nation state has 'lost' power, but rather that the venues of decision making have diversified (Rhodes, 1997; Kooiman, 1999). Consequently, it is no longer enough to take the nation state as the primary or only unit of analysis. We need to pay close attention to the vertical differentiation of corporate agency at the local, national, and supranational level. Stratification occurs horizontally as well, so that decision-making and power flow out from the state to private actors. In turn, private actors (and some others) are invited into the state to make policy. It is no longer enough to think about corporations only as attempting to influence policy. In reality, much decision-making power has been directly devolved to them, while corporations are increasingly 'internal' to the state.

At each level of governance, lobbyists attempt to influence decisions by capturing policy processes and outcomes. This is a sort of 'institutional corruption' described, for example, as 'market-driven politics' or as 'post-democracy' (Leys, 2001; Crouch, 2004; Miller, 2015). The lobbyists make sure to secure and capitalize on favourable assumptions by offering incentives in the form of travel and hospitality, paid and unpaid advisory positions, and—the big prize—board memberships once politicians and senior civil servants leave public service. This phenomenon is so well known that a term has been invented to describe it—the revolving door (Makkai and Braithwaite, 1992)

9.8.1 **Upstream and downstream strategies**

Institutional corruption is not the term used by theorists of governance, although they do discuss the rise of the 'unelected' in policy making—a development of which writers such as Vibert (2007) approve. We see this as symptomatic of what Janine Wedel has called 'flex networks', a new development whereby the entanglement of public and private sectors leads to the breakdown of notions of ethical behaviour and the collapse of the ability to police such standards as exist (Wedel, 2009). This leads, so it can be argued, to institutionalized corruption (Miller, 2015). The network of influence that corporate actors attempt to construct reaches into every area of public life and does not simply focus on policy as is assumed in much work on lobbying (Marsh and Rhodes 1992; Mazey and Richardson 1993; van Schendelen, 1993). Furthermore, the empirical picture of corporate lobbying activities is that corporations engage with the full range of issues that could affect them, even if these seem, on the face of it, to be distant from their apparent concerns (Miller, 2009).

The context within which policy-making in addiction issues takes place is of high importance. *Neoliberalism* systematically if unevenly strengthens the hand of politically active, organized, transnationally operating business. Within this context we can also identify both upstream and downstream engagement. Downstream is the most widely understood and refers to most of the policy measures that directly affect addictive industries, including marketing and health policies and all polices explicitly concerned with the substances or behaviours relevant to addictions. Corporate engagement with the content of policy or the outcome of particular policy discussions (or on policy implementation) is extensive.

Upstream engagement that has effects on how policy issues should be handled in general are a very significant and poorly understood area of engagement. This has potential effects on the policy architecture. It might, for example, involve creating or shaping the rules and practices by which particular policies will be judged in the future. Examples include the governance of risk, precaution, better regulation, and partnership governance (Smith et al., 2010a, 2010b; Fooks et al., 2011, 2013) All of these can have very important implications for corporations, which are not always immediately apparent from the outside.

In both upstream and downstream engagement corporations use a very wide variety of vehicles or agents, most notably including multi-client lobbyists and similar for-hire policy professionals, as well as their own 'in-house' lobby departments (ALTER-EU, 2010).

9.9 **Domains of action: business influence on policy—civil society, science, and the media**

9.9.1 **The multiple voices of the corporation**

Business attempts to influence policy take traditional forms of coalition and alliance building (via Trade Associations, elite policy planning groups, issue-specific lobby groups, on the one hand that represent business directly and by, lobbying/

PR, legal, financial, and other consultancies. We refer to these consultants as 'policy intermediaries'. Their defining characteristic is that they are available for hire, and although they may not formally be private corporations themselves (law or accountancy firms often have partnership structures), they are, as a result, distinctive.

By contrast we identify civil society as composed of groups that are separate from the state and political parties on the one hand and business on the other, which engage in voluntary action on particular issues. There is some debate about the precise limits of civil society (Edwards, 2005); however, we include all those not-for-profit groups that organize around a particular cause or issue. Organizations that claim some form of independence from those with which they work are included, such as think tanks, policy institutes, and lobby groups that coalesce around particular interests or issues. Also part of civil society are pressure groups, trade unions, and a whole host of other similar bodies.

This definition makes it easier to examine both the direct and indirect (or covert and opaque) role of corporations. This is important as one of the oldest corporate techniques is the creation of front groups—organizations claiming to be independent but actually controlled or influenced by corporations (Miller and Dinan, 2008a). However, it is important not simply to reduce civil society groups with some corporate involvement to mere instruments of corporate power.

As well as 'front groups' (Megalli and Friedman, 1991; Apollonio and Bero, 2007; Laurens, 2015), there are a range of tactics including 'astroturf' (Beder, 1998; Lyon and Maxwell, 2004; Kohler-Koch 2010), 'sock puppets'(Cook et al., 2014; Monbiot, 2013), think tanks (Miller and Mooney, 2010; Hawkins and McCambridge, 2014), corporate social responsibility (Sklair and Miller, 2010), and others that are seen as 'force multipliers' by business strategists, providing them with a range of additional voices intended to appear to be independent of or unrelated to business. In this section we briefly review some examples of corporate attempts to manage or capture civil society, science, and the media, each of which is an important domain in itself. It is important to recognize, however, that influencing one domain is often only part of a wider strategy to influence policy by indirect means. The sheer variety of voices employed by corporate actors and the varying routes to influence are an important element of corporate strategy. The fact that many of the voices and routes used strategically involve attempts to disguise the corporate interest is an additional complexity in assessing corporate influence and power.

9.9.2 Policy, lobbying, and civil society

In practice, much work on civil society leaves out the inconvenient case of corporate involvement in civil society (Lipschutz, 1992; Salamon et al., 1999) This, however, is central to understanding as—empirically speaking—corporate strategy has multiple routes in and out of civil society.

What seems apparent is that, seen from the perspective of the corporations, the distinction between a lobby group, a policy discussion forum, a think tank, and a 'front group' is more a question of targeting and strategy than location at some point on the scale of 'independence'.

9.9.3 **Lobby groups**

By these means corporations are able to populate the policy environment with a wide variety of seemingly independent and unconnected organizations that have the advantage of uttering messages consonant with corporate interests. Lobby groups join together to form groups or coalitions to undertake action when their aims are shared. We list some key types of policy intermediaries, as well as civil society groups, which are either influenced or created by corporate interests. First are groups that are open about their role as advocates for corporate interests, even if they seek to emphasize the quality of their research or their orientation towards general interests. We identify these as policy intermediaries or lobby groups. Then we examine those groups that are less transparent about their links with the corporations.

9.9.4 **Policy planning groups**

These are elite lobbying organizations bringing together senior business executives and often senior figures from policy, academia/science, and the media/entertainment industries. They operate at the global level (e.g. World Economic Forum (WEF)—made up of 1000 leading global companies) or at the EU level (European Roundtable of Industrialists), as well as in relation to industry sectors or on specific issues such as human rights, business responsibility, and similar issues (Peschek, 1987). For some the WEF and other similar organizations are superceding elected parliaments (Rothkopf, 2008), although others have rightly cautioned against overestimating the specific power of particular elite groups (Graz, 2003). Policy-planning groups aim to promote intra-elite debate, foster unity, and collaborate on the development of policy proposals in common (elite) interests (Pigman 2007; Rothkopf, 2008: 266–76). According to Garsten and Sörbom's (2014: 161) study, the WEF attempts to 'coordinate, structure and shape global markets'. Giesler and Veresiu (University of Chicago Press, 2015; See also Giesler and Veresiu, 2014) go further, saying it 'actively shifts the burden for the solution of problems from governments and corporations to individual consumers, with significant personal and societal costs'. This role is very much aligned with the strategies of the global tobacco, alcohol, and food industries, some of which are members, including Coca Cola, Nestlé, PepsiCo, SABMiller and Unilever (see Box 9.1).

When we consider the key elite policy planning groups together in terms of interlocking memberships and connections over time we find, as Carroll and Sapinski (2010: 522) show, that 'the policy-board network provides a *hard core* of politically active and socially cohesive cadre to the global corporate elite. This hard core is primarily active within European corporate capitalism' (see Table 9.1).

9.9.5 **Front groups**

Front groups are campaign groups that claim to be working towards citizen or public interest goals but which can be contrasted with genuine campaign groups such as environmental and social movements or trade unions. A key analytical distinction is that the latter groups generally operate as social movements from below, whereas front groups always have a link of some sort with social movement from 'above',

Box 9.1 European Roundtable of Industrialists

The European Roundtable of Industrialists (ERT) is a peak business association or policy planning group for over 50 EU CEOs, who are 'Chairmen and Chief Executives of large multinational companies, representing all sectors of industry, which have their headquarters in Europe and also significant manufacturing and technological presence worldwide'. Membership is by invitation only. Almost all observers agree that the ERT is an immensely powerful body, which is well integrated into the EU machinery and has a key role in framing EU policies and directives (Apeldoorn, 2000a, 2000b; Nollert and Fielder, 2000; Balanya et al., 2000; Cowles, 1995; Pageaut, 2010; Corporate Europe Observatory, 2012a).

The ERT was founded in Paris in 1983 as a group of 17 European industrialists with encouragement from key figures in the European Commission. ERT 'advocates policies at both national and European levels, with the goal of improving European competitiveness, growth and employment' (European Roundtable of Industrialists, 2015). Its work covers a wide range of subjects, from education to liberalization of the economies of developing countries. ERT Members meet in Plenary Session twice a year. The Plenary Session determines the ERT work programme, sets priorities, votes budgets, and decides on the publication of ERT reports and proposals. The decisions are taken by consensus (ERT, 2015). The ERT claims to have been a significant actor in the creation of the Single Market, the Maastricht Treaty, and the Lisbon Agenda (Corporate Europe Observatory, 2014). The ERT also supports the activity of the Trans Atlantic Business Dialogue and the Transatlantic Policy Network (TPN). The TPN was a key element in 'preparing the ground' for negotiations on the Transatlantic Trade and Investment Partnership (Transatlantic Policy Network, 2015). All of these are measures favoured by transnational companies in addiction-related industries.

defined as 'the collective agency of dominant groups to reproduce or extend their power and hegemonic positions'(Cox and Nilsen, 2014). We can identify specific types of such groups, including Astroturf groups—meaning fake grassroots groups (Lyon and Maxwell, 2004; Jacobson, 2005; Kohler-Koch, 2010). These are organizations set up or significantly influenced by corporate funding or direction but which deny or conceal such connections. A more recent term referring to deceptive personas on the Internet is the 'sock puppet' (Cook et al., 2014).

9.9.6 Think tanks

Think tanks are policy-related bodies in civil society that conduct research and focus on particular issues. Some are narrowly focused, such as the International Center for Alcohol Policies—a Washington-based think tank funded by the alcohol

Table 9.1 List of members of the European Roundtable of Industrialists from alcohol, tobacco, or food companies 1983–2015

Helmut Maucher—Nestlé	1983–1999
Antoine Riboud—Danone (BSN)	1983–1985
Kenneth Durham—Unilever	1983–1985
Patrick Sheehy—B.A.T Industries	1986–1995
Poul J. Svanholm—Carlsberg	1986–1996
Floris Maljers—Unilever	1988–1994
Morris Tabaksblat—Reed Elsevier (Unilever)	1994–2003
Simon Cairns—B.A.T. Industries	1996–1998
Flemming Lindeløv—Carlsberg	1997–2001
Franck Riboud—Danone	1998–2000
Antony Burgmans—Unilever	1999–2007
Peter Brabeck-Letmathe—Nestlé	1999–2012
Nils S. Andersen—Carlsberg	2001–2011
Martin Broughton—British Airways (British American Tobacco)	2001–2010
Paul Walsh—Diageo	2003–2006
Anthony Ruys—Heineken	2004–2005
Paul Adams—British American Tobacco	2005–2010
Jean-François van Boxmeer—Heineken	2005–2015
Patrick Cescau—Unilever	2007–2008
Paul Polman—Unilever	2009–2011
Paul Bulcke—Nestlé	2013–2015

Source: data from Wayback Machine Internet Archive, 'ERT (European Roundtable of Industrialists): All members since 1983', https://web.archive.org/web/20070828121334/http://www.ert.eu/all_members_since_1983.aspx, accessed 28 Aug. 2007; Wayback Machine Internet Archive, 'ERT (European Roundtable of Industrialists): All members since 1983', https://web.archive.org/web/20111011033811/http://www.ert.be/all_members_since_1983.aspx, accessed 11 Oct. 2011.

industry. Others have a broader remit, such as the Brussels based European Policy Centre (see Box 9.2).

The rise of think tanks is a key way in which corporate money is channelled into research and advocacy organizations that are said to provide a bridge between knowledge and policy (Stone, 2007; Silverstein, 2014). Latest research estimates that EU think tanks number 150 (Boucher and Hobbs, 2004). However, European think tank networks such as the new European party foundations and European Policy Institutes Network (EPIN) have a membership of at least 500 (Plehwe, 2010). Think tank networks play a fundamental role in the politics of expertise in Brussels (Sherrington, 2000; Stone and Denham, 2004; Anheier, 2010) (see Box 9.3).

Box 9.2 International Center for Alcohol Policies

The International Center for Alcohol Policies (ICAP) was established in 1995 and is funded by large global alcohol producers. It produces a 'voluminous output of scientific conferences, book-length collections of articles, issue reports and briefing papers, and other written products' (Jernighan, 2012: 83).

ICAP made initial 'efforts to recruit current WHO staffers working on alcohol issues' but were unsuccessful, 'so it relied on employees in other sectors . . . employees in WHO regional offices, and retired WHO officials' (Jernighan, 2012: 83).

The think tank has been criticized for commissioning reports from scientists that resembled WHO documents. ICAP has also 'performed "literature reviews" that were incomplete, not subject to traditional peer review, and either supportive of industry positions or emphasizing high levels of disagreement among scientists' (Jernighan, 2012: 83). One reviewer of an ICAP publication has reported in *Addiction* that the 'peer review' process was inadequate: 'The comments I made were generally critical of the substance of the ICAP report . . . I drew particular attention to the inappropriate use of evidence. Yet [in] the final report . . . there are some mainly cosmetic changes . . . The specific comments I made . . . were substantial and ran to four typed sides of A4 paper' (Foxcroft, 2005: 1066).

ICAP has acted as a lobbyist in influencing alcohol strategy in four African countries (Bakke and Endal, 2010), including by providing 'model national and global alcohol policies based on the least effective strategies, and offered technical assistance in how to adopt and implement these policies. These publications were distinguished not by what was in them . . . but by what was not: they excluded or attempted to refute evidence regarding the most effective strategies to reduce and prevent alcohol-related harm' (Jernighan, 2012: 83). Instead ICAP follows the industry strategy of 'consistently' emphasizing alcohol education. (Jernighan, 2012: 86). 'Industry arguments must', writes Jernighan (2012: 86), 'be "science-based" and clothed in research credentials, as the ICAP has done with its many briefing papers and policy reviews'. McCreanor et al. (2000: 180) refer to the 'efforts' or ICAP 'to establish 'partnership' between the alcohol industry and public health' which is preferred over 'direct confrontation with public health' (Jernighan, 2012: 86).

This orientation provides a clue to the use of policy intermediaries like ICAP— they are used as entitites that can be perceived as distanced from the industry and which puruse apparently research- and science-based strategies. This indicates the important of the management of science in industry efforts to colonize civil society.

9.9.7 Science and the insecurity of the evidence base

Business attempts to influence, divert, evade, or otherwise tamper with the evidence base in science are widely recognized as both significant and difficult to quantify or evaluate properly. It is also important to recognize that attamptes to influence civil

Box 9.3 The European Policy Centre

The European Policy Centre (EPC) was founded in 1991 as the Belmont European Policy Centre. The EPC defines its mission as 'contributing to the construction of Europe', and to achieve this it 'encourages a debate among all significant interest groups and channels the results to policy-makers'. The EPC is one of the most prominent EU think tanks; it relies on both corporate funding and public money. It makes no secret of placing 'special emphasis on strengthening the interface of government with business'. 'We are action oriented', it notes, 'and we believe that business must be more involved in public policies'(cited in Powerbase, 2015). The EPC does, however, present itself as a neutral venue for discussion and as independent from any specific vested interests. This is quite routine for think tanks as a means to shore up credibility and also indicate *sotto voce* that they are for hire. US think tank scholar Tom Medvetz (2012: 18) notes that think tanks must carry out 'a delicate balancing act that involves signaling their cognitive autonomy to a general audience while at the same time signaling their heteronomy—or willingness to subordinate their production to the demands of clients—to a more restricted audience'.

Among the funders of the EPC are a range of lobbying consultancies many of which also work for addiction-related companies. In addition, direct corporate members of note are BAT, Ferrero Group—Soremartec, Nestlé, and Philip Morris International. In addition, trade association members include the Confederation of European Community Cigarette Manufacturers, The Brewers of Europe, and the Union of EU Soft Drinks Associations. This funding contributes to a range of activities that include the following activities pursued by the tobacco and alcohol industries.

Roundtable on alcohol-related harm

The European Commission began developing an alcohol strategy for Europe in 2001 and introduced it in 2006. Just before the introduction of the strategy, DG Sanco asked the EPC to host four meetings between the alcohol industry and health-focused non-governmental organizations (NGOs). These round tables on 'Alcohol related harm: ways forward' aimed to reach consensus on policy interventions and to 'identify areas of agreement between the stakeholders as to actions that can contribute effectively to the reduction of alcohol-related harm and indicate where and why there is disagreement, and in so doing help create confidence between stakeholders' (cited in Anderson and Baumberg 2007). According to the bulletin of the Institute of Alcohol Studies these meetings were 'At the behest of the Industry, DG SANCO officials organised roundtable discussion through the aegis of the European Policy Centre, between representatives of the Commission, Member States, Industry and NGOs to discuss the draft proposals for a European Alcohol Policy Strategy' (Rutherford, 2006).

The meetings involved working through 78 issues or policy proposals related to alcohol harm reduction that were presented by the European Commission in an informal draft of their communication on alcohol. Participants graded each item using a traffic lights system: green issues were broadly agreeable to all present, amber a possibility, and red a clear no. Sixty-eight of the measures were marked green; seven were amber, indicating no overall agreement but that some compromises might be reached. Three were categorized as red issues where the industry simply refused to negotiate.

Anderson and Baumberg (2007: 335) note that although the EPC describes itself as independent 'its prime corporate members and sponsors include InBev, the world's largest brewer and Philip Morris International'. The final outcome of this process, and other consultations resulted in the launch of the European Alcohol and Health Forum, from which health NGOs resigned in June 2015 expressing 'deep concern' at the lack of a comprehensive EU alcohol strategy (Jacobs, 2015).

Tobacco industry work

Noting that the EPC is 'well respected', Action on Smoking and Heatlh (2010) has described it as 'the key consultancy group, sometimes alongside the Weinberg Group to help with lobbying to ensure policy makers are legally obliged to include tobacco companies' opinions in European policymaking development and decision making processes'. The EPC had the 'particular advantage that it had developed a broad profile and received funding from the European Commission allowing it to acquire insider status in policy making circles'.

The EPC were part of a policy network used by British American Tobacco (BAT) to make changes to EU treaties in order to minimize legislative burdens on business. From 1995 BAT organized other corporate actors, including the EPC, Shell, Zeneca, Tesco, SmithKline Beecham, Bayer, and Unilever, to mount a multiyear lobby campaign aimed at shaping the EU's impact assessment regime, with the result that regime undermined public health and protected business interests (Smith et al., 2010a, 2010b).

BAT's use of a policy network distanced the tobacco industry from the lobbying efforts and obscured the tobacco industry's involvement. BAT were also helped by a UK lobby firm, Charles Barker, which warned BAT that they would need to tread carefully, lobbying through a 'front' organization and enlisting other 'big industry names' in support. The EPC provided the front. David Byrne, Commissioner for Health and Consumer Protection 1999–2004 was reportedly shocked: 'I would be absolutely astonished and would find it very difficult to believe if there was any available information which tended to indicate that the European Policy Centre was advocating on behalf of the tobacco industry—that would be shocking' (Smith et al., 2010b).

Shocking or not, the EPC was so engaged. It continues to take money from the tobacco industry and to present it self as a neutral and independent actor. This illustrates the opaque nature of corporate political activities at the EU level.

society and the media also represent attemtps to influence the information environment on which the public and policy-makers draw in their assessments of addiction-related information.

Science is a key domain in addiction-related corporate strategy. Industries engage in a wide range of science-related activities. Corporations are involved in commissioning, production, and the dissemination of scientific research. They are also strongly involved in the science policy arena and in the use of science in policy discussion. Thus, it is of interest to examine (in the list below) the funding of science policy-related bodies, as well as connections between corporations and expert groups convened by the European Commission. In this respect the issue of conflict of interest is increasingly important (Horel and CEO, 2013; Oreskes and Conway, 2010; Stenius and Babor, 2010; Miller and Harkins, 2015;).

- ◆ Funding of science. Corporate funding of science is potentially influential in two ways, both of which relate to decisions about which science to fund. First, corporations almost exclusively fund research relevant to their interests in developing or sustaining markets, as opposed to basic curiosity-driven science. This by itself can distort the evidence base, especially where the products produced by the corporation are known to be harmful to health. This is true even where, as is often the case, the science is the best that can be found. Second, corporations can fund science that they think is going to turn up the results that they want. This is more likely to be the case where the science relates to safety concerns about products than about the technical development of future products.

- ◆ Manipulation of science. When results are not expected and there is a potential regulatory context corporations can attempt to manipulate the results or the reporting of science in the scientific literature. This can be done by suppressing inconvenient results, meaning that the results are not published. It can also be done by direct manipulation of data in particular studies or by massaging how the results are presented in scientific journal articles.

- ◆ Refusing, curtailing funding. This also performs a demonstration effect to those scientists tempted to put the interests of science above those of the sponsor.

- ◆ Manipulating the evidence base, discrediting 'dissident' science. Where particular results are not conducive to corporate interests, action can be taken. This can involve campaigns to have inconvenient papers retracted, threats of legal action, and threats to the institution housing the researchers who published inconvenient results.

All of these activities are known to have been engaged with by the alcohol, tobacco, and food industries (see Box 9.4).

9.9.8 Media

The media are important as they provide opportunities to connect with popular opinion, as well as elite opinion. The relation with elite opinion (and therefore policy) is important because the media can play a direct role in lobbying and policy-making, while also mediating popular concerns.

Box 9.4 International Life Sciences Institute

The International Life Sciences Institute (ILSI) is an industry-funded organization that specializes in engaging with scientists and national and international agencies such as the European Food Safety Authority or the WHO. Its members include many big food, chemical, pharmaceutical, and genetically modified crop companies. The ILSI is headquartered in Washington, DC, but ILSI Europe has an office in Brussels, opened in 1986. ILSI says that it creates 'neutral fora' by bringing scientists together from government, industry, and academia to 'jointly provide the best available fact-based, objective science on key public health issues'. It has been alleged, however, that its activities are 'a vehicle to promote business-friendly "scientific" concepts and methodologies' (Corporate Europe Observatory, 2012b). As part of these activities ILSI is recognized as a NGO by the WHO and has specialized consultative status with the Food and Agriculture Organization. However, the activities of the ILSI resulted in a WHO decision in 2006 that ILSI 'can no longer take part in WHO activities setting microbiological or chemical standards for food and water, the UN health agency's executive board decided Friday in Geneva, Switzerland'. The ILSI was barred 'from helping set global standards for protecting food and water supplies because of its funding sources' (Heilprin, 2006). However, it remained one of the NGOs with accreditation as an observer at WHO meetings.

The downgrading of ILSI's status followed a letter to the WHO protesting ILSI's role in setting standards from the Natural Resources Defense Council (NRDC), Environmental Working Group, United Steelworkers of America, and a coalition of other groups. In the letter, NRDC senior scientist Jennifer Sass wrote that ILSI has a demonstrated history of putting the interests of its exclusively corporate membership ahead of science and health concerns, and that ILSI's special status with the WHO provides a back door to influence WHO activities (cited in Heilprin, 2006)

Research on conflicts of interest among experts advising the European Food Safety Authority shows that at least half of the experts have at least one conflict of interest and that connections with ILSI are manifold (Corporate Europe Observatory, 2011; CEO and Earth Open Source, 2012; Horel and CEO 2013). We can conclude from this that one significant result of the activities of groups such as the ILSI is that experts on EU agencies or expert groups owe something to the ILSI.

The full range of mechanisms by which the media are 'captured' by the corporations is well known in academic work on media institutions and processes. Any such account includes the influence of media ownership, advertising, public relations and spin, attacking critics, and—at least in some models—the question of ideology. We do not dissent from these models which—Marxist or liberal—are largely agreed on the mechanisms, if varying in their emphasis and theoretical frameworks (McChesney,

2008). It is well known that the mainstream media find it much easier to discuss addiction issues in relation to the notion of personal responsibility as opposed to societal or corporate responsibility for addiction (Wallack and Dorfman, 1996; Kim and Willis 2007). This by itself is a major advantage for the corporations. There is, however, some evidence that print media coverage of alcohol issues has historically increased its emphasis on environmental/societal factors in alcohol problems and that the proportion of coverage on personal responsibility has declined (Lemmens et al., 1999).

To the more general models of media performance we would add the use and role of the media in securing policy capture, and, in particular, the sophisticated use of seemingly independent organizations that perform a public relations role for industry at one remove (Miller and Dinan, 2008a) (see Box 9.5).

Capturing the media is done by both traditional means such as the use of apparently independent organizations set up to target the media, as well as newer attempts to take over the means of communication directly. It is important for the corporations to try to exert maximum message control while at the same time appearing to be subject to the vagaries of 'independent' media. As a result, in recent years the media and the Internet have become important resources in lobbying campaigns.

So much so that one US PR and lobbying firm has invented what has been called 'journo-lobbying' (Confessore, 2003). This blurring of the line between journalism and lobbying is central to the contemporary use of the traditional media, but is obviously given a significant boost by the birth of the Internet and especially Web 2.0 techniques. Thus, it is important to examine the use of the media and of groups targeting the media in assessing corporate strategies.

9.9.9 Policy partnership and self-regulation

As well as following the corporate routes to policy vertically and horizontally we need to pay close attention to the comparatively recent innovation of policy partnership and industry self-regulation. Such novel approaches to governance can also be conceptualized in relation to corporate political agency.

In the EU, alcohol policy has been taken forward by the European Alcohol and Health Forum (EAHF), composed of non-governmenal organizations and the alcohol, advertising, and sponsorship industries, although it is dominated by commercial interests (Eurocare, 2007). We have suggested that corporations adopt multiple voices in the policy realm and the EAHF is a good example of this. Established in 2007, it provides a platform for a range of stakeholders to make commitments to support the agreed areas for action through voluntary commitments. In 2014, it had 65 members, including nine alcohol corporations, ten alcohol trade associations, and six allied trade associations, a total of 25 members. Of these members several alcohol companies have multiple memberships. For example Diageo is a direct member but also owns 17 of the 41 Scotch Whisky manufacturers in the Scotch Whisky Association—another member of the Forum. Diageo also influences the EAHF via membership of the European Sponsorship Association and the European Travel Retail Council. Another group the European Transport Safety Council receives sponsorship from the Brewers of Europe; Diageo is involved as a member of one

Box 9.5 The Social Issues Research Centre and the Science Media Centre

The Social Issues Research Centre (SIRC) is an 'independent, non-profit organisation' that says it carries out 'balanced, calm and thoughtful' research on lifestyle issues such as drinking, diet, and pharmaceuticals (www.sirc.org).[2] However, it may be perceived that the organization acts more like a PR agency for the corporations that fund its activities. These include Diageo, Flora, CocaCola, GlaxoSmithKline, and Roche, among others. Although SIRC does publish this partial list of funders, it is not immediately apparent which company has sponsored which study. And in some instances this information is not included in media reports.

Although SIRC's publicity material regularly uses the term 'social scientists' to refer to its own staff, it uses the same personnel and office as a commercial market research company, MCM Research. SIRC's co-directors, Peter Marsh and Kate Fox, work for both organizations. The MCM website used to ask: 'Do your PR initiatives sometimes look too much like PR initiatives? MCM conducts social/psychological research on the positive aspects of your business. The results do not read like PR literature, or like market research data. Our reports are credible, interesting and entertaining in their own right. This is why they capture the imagination of the media and your customers'.

SIRC was taken seriously enough by government for it to be commissioned to produce two independent reviews for an investigation by the UK Department for Children, Schools and Families of the commercialization of childhood. The reports, published in late 2009, oppose a public-health approach that is based on population-level measures, including the restriction of advertising or marketing. The conclusion that SIRC reached is that 'the issues involved are very much more complex'—a position consistent with that advanced by elements of the food and advertising industries.

Its guidelines on science and health communication were produced in partnership with the Royal Society and the Royal Institution, two important learned societies (Social Issues Research Centre, 2001). Both were involved shortly after the production of the guidelines in the creation of the Science Media Centre in the UK. This is an organization that claims to be 'independent'. 'We do not have any specific agenda', it notes, 'other than to promote the reporting of evidence-based science' (Science Media Centre, nd). Among its funders are companies from the food and drink, chemical, pharma, and biotech industries. Studies of its activities have shown, however, that it adopts a 'line' on certain topics, on which there is significant scientific debate (Haran, 2012; Williams and Gajevic 2013; Rödder, 2015).

of its national members, the British Beer and Pub Association. Finally, Diageo also funds several think tanks that are members of the forum, including the International Center on Alcohol Policies (discussed above). In total, there are 38 members with some connection to or funding from industry of the total 65.

9.10 **How to manage big business: problems of engaging with private companies**

9.10.1 **Managing the private sector**

The private sector is a major driver of harm. Managing private actors requires transparency and skills of conflict resolution and negotiation. There may be circumstances in which partnership with industry is appropriate, but such circumstances will be rare and will depend on a wide variety of factors, including wider policy trajectories.

In most cases managing the private sector will require binding regulation. However, the trend in contemporary governance structures is to engage directly with business and to develop 'voluntary' approaches to governance. We will review some key examples of this approach showing the limitations in principle or practice and drawing on the existing evidence base.

9.10.2 **Partnership governance, social responsibility, and self-regulation**

The dominant trend in governance in the EU and most member states is towards partnership governance, including strategies of 'nudge', self regulation, 'better regulation', and corporate social responsibility. All of these aim to persuade business to improve their performance in relation to specific goals. In the field of addictions and public health we can see examples at the EU level in the EAHF or the EU Platform on Diet Physical Activity and Health. In the UK similar examples include Change for Life (Miller and Harkins, 2010) and the various responsibility deals (in relation to food, alcohol, and health at work) From the public health point of view each of these approaches is flawed first of all because they are ineffective. Any gains that they do make are used by the companies in their lobbying strategies to avoid meaninful progress and in many cases alleged gains of the relevant programmes are either matters of representational sleight of hand, commitments that have already been made in other contexts, or simply reflect pre-existing trends in market decline (Keenan et al., 2009; Sustain , 2010, 2011; Gilmore et al., 2011; House of Lords Science and Technology Select Committee, 2011; Panjwani and Caraher, 2014).

Although the tobacco and alcohol industries are at the forefront of pushing for further concessions via Better Regulation and indeed via the Transatlantic Trade and Investment Partnership(Corporate Europe Observatory, 2015), it is also the case that some progress has been made, especially in the regulation of tobacco. We can briefly refer to the Framework Convention on Tobacco Control to illustrate why it is necessary to adopt a firm hand with addictive industries (see Box 9.6).

9.11 **Conclusions**

The conclusions we can draw from this review of the evidence on corporate strategies on addictions are that corporations are constituiontally bound to pursue profit but that they pursue such goals not only by economic means, but also by the conscious planning and pursuit of political strategies. These are designed to influence civil society, science, and the media and to capitalize on such influence in their

Box 9.6 The Framework Convention on Tobacco Control

The most advanced international instrument for managing the relations between an addiction-related industry and policy is the WHO Framework Convention on Tobacco Control. The legally binding Convention came into force in 2005. By December 2014, 180 of the United Nation's 193 member states were Parties to the Treaty. As Gilmore et al. (2015) note, 'Given overwhelming evidence of the tobacco industry's efforts to subvert public health policy making, the treaty includes Article 5.3, which requires parties to protect their public health policies from the "vested interests of the tobacco industry"'. Gilmore et al. (2015) note, however, that 'implementation has been slow and uneven in large part because of tobacco industry efforts to subvert progress in tobacco control'. The evidence suggests that tackling the public health effects of addiction-related products like tobacco, and also alcohol and food, is more complex than simply enacting laws or, indeed, a global convention.

Gilmore et al. (2015) outline 'three mechanisms' used by tobacco companies to stymie progress on tobacco control—'the use of international economic agreements, litigation and the illicit trade in tobacco'. These are enhanced by exploiting the rhetoric of harm reduction and pushing for business-friendly changes in the regulatory architecture, such as Better Regulation. These have been highly successful as 'successful implementation of Article 5.3 is almost non-existent'.

This is, in part, because of successful industry tactics, but the conclusion that can be drawn from the experience of countering tobacco industry influence is that it must be based on up-to-date and ongoing research on tobacco industry tactics and strategies and that the responsibility cannot rest with government or regulatory agencies alone. When faced with concerted action the industry typically tries to find another way around by using third parties, indirect lobbying, and the range of tactics noted in this chapter. Thus, counteracting industry influence requires concerted action across society, including investigative research, protection of the evidence base/science, and civil society action, as well as governmental measures. This requires 'civil society to actively monitor and publicise industry misconduct ... and for ministries of health to help disseminate these findings within government and beyond'. 'It is no coincidence', note Gilmore et al. (2015) that, 'the countries (in all income groups) with the most successful tobacco control policies also have the most active programmes of industry monitoring'. The specific measures needed include 'limiting interactions with industry and ensuring their transparency, rejecting partnerships with industry, avoiding conflicts of interest for officials, denormalising activities industry describes as "socially responsible")'.

Such measures must be complemented by more general transparency measures (Miller and Harkins, 2015) and by 'ensuring greater public health involvement in trade and investment agreement negotiations would help' (Gilmore et al., 2015).

The obvious lesson of the case of tobacco is that similar measures will be needed if public health measures are ever to be effectively introduced in relation to alcohol and food and perhaps other substances and behaviours.

direct policy-related lobbying. When it comes to lobbying corporations certainly pursue certain (downstream) policies that directly relate to their products, but they also expend considerable energy in designing and redesigning the (upstream) policy architecture that determines the general way in which specific decisions are taken, as we saw with the example of Better Regulation.

9.11.1 Regulation is the first watchword

Although they have differing ways of operating the answer to the problem of harms from legal and illegal drugs is regulation. Illegal drugs can be regulated by managing processes of decriminalization and legalization. This will reduce harm by (1) improving quality and purity, and (2) undermining organized crime and associated intrinsic harms of the illegal market, as well as the perverse outcomes of attempts at suppression—such as via successive iterations of the 'war on drugs'. It will also have additional benefits of raising revenue through tax that could and should be channelled to health and social care for the most disadvantaged communities.

Legal substances should also be regulated. The evidence of this book suggests a move to stricter regulation of harmful substances. In particular, there is a need to move beyond the individual approach to a whole-society approach. This should include—specifically—a recognition that business regulation is one of the most significant cutting-edge policies to building a society-wide coalition to tackle addiction harms. This should not stop at policies that regulate how products are sold, for example via marketing or advertising, but impose direct controls on business where these are the most effective means for minimizing harm.

9.11.2 Negotiation, partnership, and coalition building

Very little will be achieved if we wait for government to act. Instead key public-health tasks must include building society wide coalitions for improving public health and reducing harm. Not only will these be useful in themselves, but they will also encourage government action and make it harder for the private sector to resist positive moves.

Notes

1. Tyrrell (1997: 1406) questions the extent that this was new, noting 'widespread political corruption, gang warfare and the existence of crime syndicates in the cities of America's north prior to 1910'. Quite so, but Tyrrell agrees that prohibition allowed 'the consolidation of these forces, albeit augmented by the possibility of illicit gains in alcohol'.

2. Material on SIRC draws on Miller and de Andrade (2010).

References

Action on Smoking and Health (2010) The smoke filled room. Available at: http://www.ash.org.uk/SmokeFilledRoom (accessed 7 October 2015).

Alter EU (2010) *Bursting the Brussels Bubble. The Battle to Expose Corporate Lobbying at the Heart of the EU.* Brussels: Alliance for Lobbying Transparency and Ethics

Regulation in the EU (ALTER-EU). Available at: http://www.alter-eu.org/book/bursting-the-brussels-bubble

Anderson, P., & Baumberg, B. E. N. (2007). Alcohol policy: who should sit at the table?. *Addiction, 102*(2), 335-336.

Anderson T, Swan H, and Lane D (2010) Institutional fads and the medicalization of drug addiction. *Sociol Compass* 4: 476–94.

Anheier H (2010) *Social Science Research Outside the Ivory Tower: The Role of Think-tanks and Civil Society.* Paris: UNESCO.

Apeldoorn BV (2000a) Transnational class agency and European governance: the case of the European Round Table of Industrialists. *New Polit Econ* 5: 157–81.

Apeldoorn BV (2000b) Transnationale Klassen und europäisches Regieren: Der European Round Table of Industrialists. In: *Die Konfiguration Europas: Dimensionen einer kritischen Integrationstheorie.* Münster: Westfälisches Dampfboot, pp. 189–221.

Apollonio DE and Bero LA (2007) The creation of industry front groups: the tobacco industry and 'get government off our back'. *Am J Public Health* 97: 419.

Babor T, Edwards G, and Stockwell T (1996) Science and the drinks industry: cause for concern. *Addiction* 91: 5–9.

Baggott R (2006) *Alcohol Strategy and the Drinks Industry: A Partnership for Prevention?* York : Joseph Rowntree Foundation.

Balanya B, Doherty A, Hoedeman O, Ma'anit A, and Wesselius E (2000) *Europe Inc.* London: Pluto Press.

Barnoya J and Glantz S (2006) The tobacco industry's worldwide ETS consultants project: European and Asian components. *Eur J Public Health* 16: 69–77.

BBC News (2010) Mephedrone to be made Class B drug within days. Available at: http://news.bbc.co.uk/2/hi/uk_news/8616758.stm (accessed 1 September 2016).

Beder S (1998) Public relations' role in manufacturing artificial grass roots coalitions. *Public Relations Q* 43: 21–3.

Boucher S and Hobbs B (2004) *Europe and Its Think Tanks: A Promise to Be Fulfilled.* Brussels: Norte Europe, Studies & Research No. 35.

Brownell K and Warner K (2009) The perils of ignoring history: big tobacco played dirty and millions died. How similar is big food? *Milbank Q* 87: 259–94.

Carroll W (2009) Transnationalists and national networkers in the global corporate elite. *Global Networks* 9: 289–314.

Carroll B and Sapinski J (2010) The global corporate elite and the transnational policy-planning network, 1996–2006: a structural analysis. *Int Sociol* 25: 501–38.

Chen TT and Winder AE (1990) The opium wars revisited as US forces tobacco exports in Asia. *Am J Public Health* 80: 659–62.

Chopra M and Darnton-Hill I (2004) Tobacco and obesity epidemics: not so different after all? *BMJ* 328: 1558–60.

Compston H (2013) The global network of corporate control: implications for public policy. *Business Politics* 15: 357–79.

Confessore N (2003) Meet the press: how James Glassman reinvented journalism as lobbying. *Washington Monthly* 35: 32–9.

Connolly G (1995) The marketing of nicotine addiction by one oral snuff manufacturer. *Tob Control* 4: 73–9.

Cook DM, Waugh B, Abdipanah M, Hashemi O, and Abdul Rahman S (2014) Twitter deception and influence: issues of identity, slacktivism, and puppetry. *J Inform Warfare* 13: 58–71.

Corporate Europe Observatory (2011) Serial conflicts of interest on EFSA's management board. Available at: http://corporateeurope.org/sites/default/files/2011-02-23_mb_report. pdf (accessed 8 October 2015).

Corporate Europe Observatory (2012a) The Roundtable goes for full conquest. Available at: http://corporateeurope.org/news/roundtable-goes-full-conquest (accessed 1 September 2016).

Corporate Europe Observatory (2012b) The International Life Sciences Institute (ILSI) a corporate lobby group. Available at: http://corporateeurope.org/sites/default/files/ilsi-article-final.pdf (accessed 1 October 2015).

Corporate Europe Observatory (2014) The 'permanent liaison': how ERT and BusinessEurope set the agenda for the EU Summit. Available at: http://corporateeurope. org/lobbycracy/2014/03/permanent-liaison-how-ert-and-businesseurope-set-agenda-eu-summit (accessed 1 September 2016).

Corporate Europe Observatory (2015) Black-out on tobacco's access to EU trade talks an eerie indication of TTIP threat. 26 August. Available at: http://corporateeurope.org/ international-trade/2015/08/black-out-tobaccos-access-eu-trade-talks-eerie-indication-ttip-threat (accessed 1 September 2016).

Corporate Europe Observatory and Earth Open Source (2012) Conflicts on the menu: a decade of industry influence at the European Food Safety Authority. Available at: http:// corporateeurope.org/sites/default/files/publications/conflicts_on_the_menu_final_0.pdf (accessed 7 October 2015).

Cowles MG (1995) The European round table of industrialists: the strategic player in European affairs. In: Greenwood J (ed.) *European Casebook on Business Alliances*. London: Prentice Hall, pp. 225–36.

Cox L and Nilsen AG (2014) *We Make Our Own History: Marxism and Social Movements in the Twilight of Neoliberalism*. London: Pluto.

Crouch C (2004) *Post-Democracy*. Cambridge: Polity Press.

Duchene L (2006) Probing question: is sugar addictive? Available at: http://news.psu.edu/ story/141336/2006/01/16/research/probing-question-sugar-addictive (accessed 1 September 2016).

Edwards M (2005) *Civil Society*. Cambridge: Polity Press.

Eising R (2009) *The Political Economy of State–Business Relations in Europe*. London: Routledge.

Eurocare (2007) Eurocare and members to join the EC's Alcohol and Health Forum. Press Available at: http://www.eurocare.org/press/eurocare_ press_releases/eurocare_and_members_to_join_the_ec_s_alcohol_and_health_forum (accessed 3 July 2009).

European Roundtable of Industrialists (2015) About ERT. Available at: http://www.ert.eu/ about-us (accessed 1 October 2015).

Fooks GJ and Gilmore AB (2013) Corporate philanthropy, political influence, and health policy. *PLOS ONE* 8: e8086.

Fooks GJ, Gilmore AB, Smith KE, Collin J, Holden C, and Lee K (2011) Corporate social responsibility and access to policy élites: an analysis of tobacco industry documents. *PLOS Med* 8: e1001076.

Fooks G, Gilmore A, Collin J, Holden C, and Lee K (2013) The limits of corporate social responsibility: techniques of neutralization, stakeholder management and political CSR. *J Business Ethics* 112: 283–99.

Fossum J and Schilesinger P (eds) (2007) *The European Union and the Public Sphere: A Communicative Space in the Making?* London: Routledge.

Foxcroft D (2005) International Center for Alcohol Policies (ICAP)'s latest report on alcohol education: a flawed peer review process. *Addiction* 100: 1066–8.

Garsten C and Sörbom A (2014) Values aligned: the organization of conflicting values within the World Economic Forum. In: Alexius S and Hallström KT (eds) *Configuring Value Conflicts in Markets*. Cheltenham: Edward Elgar Publishing, pp. 159–77.

Giesler M and Veresiu E (2014) Creating the responsible consumer: moralistic governance regimes and consumer subjectivity. *J Consum Res* 41: 840–57.

Gilmore A, Savell E and Collin J (2011) Public health, corporations and the New Responsibility Deal: promoting partnerships with vectors of disease? *J Public Health* 33: 2–4.

Gilmore AB, Fooks G, Drope J, Bialous SA, and Jackson RR (2015) Exposing and addressing tobacco industry conduct in low-income and middle-income countries. *Lancet* 385: 1029–43.

Graz JC (2003) How powerful are transnational elite clubs? The social myth of the World Economic Forum. *New Polit Econ* 8: 321–40.

Greenwood J (2011) *Interest Representation in the European Union*. Basingstoke: Palgrave.

Hanes WT and Sanello F (2004) *Opium Wars: The Addiction of One Empire and the Corruption of Another*. Naperviller, IL: Sourcebooks, Inc.

Haran J (2012) Campaigns and coalitions: governance by media. In: Rödder S, Franzen M, and Weingart P (eds) *The Sciences' Media Connection–Public Communication and its Repercussions*. Sociology of the Sciences Yearbook, Volume 28. Amsterdam: Springer, pp. 241–56.

Harvey D (2005) *A Brief History of Neoliberalism*. Oxford: Oxford University Press.

Hastings G and Angus K (2009) *Under the Influence The Damaging Effect of Alcohol Marketing on Young People Available*. London: British Medical Association.

Hawkins B and McCambridge J (2014) Industry actors, think tanks, and alcohol policy in the United Kingdom. *Am J Public Health* 104: 1363–9.

Heemskerk E, Daolio F, and Tomassini M (2013) The community structure of the European network of interlocking directorates 2005-2010. *PLOS ONE* 8: e68581.

Heilprin J (2006) WHO to rely less on U.S. Research. Available at: http://www.trwnews.net/Documents/News/2006/ap012706.htm (accessed 1 September 2016).

House of Lords Science and Technology Select Committee (2011) Behaviour Change Report: The Government Approach to Changing Behaviour (Chapter 5). Available at: http://www.publications.parliament.uk/pa/ld201012/ldselect/ldsctech/179/17908.htm#n125 (accessed 21 September 2011).

Horel S and CEO (2013) Unhappy meal. The European food safety authority's independence problem. Available at: http://corporateeurope.org/sites/default/files/attachments/unhappy_meal_report_23_10_2013.pdf (accessed 1 September 2016).

Jacobs H (2015) Health NGOs walk out of EU alcohol forum. Available at: http://www.euractiv.com/sections/health-consumers/health-ngos-walk-out-eu-alcohol-forum-315075 (accessed 2 October 2015).

Jacobson MF (2005) Lifting the veil of secrecy from industry funding of nonprofit health organizations. *Int J Occup Environ Health* **11**: 349–55.

Jernigan DH (2012) Global alcohol producers, science, and policy: the case of the International Center for Alcohol Policies. *Am J Public Health* **102**: 80–9.

Keenan SJ, Lawler H, Monadajemi F, and Jewell K (2009) Monitoring implementation of alcohol labelling regime (including advice to women on alcohol and pregnancy). London: Department of Health.

Kim SH and Willis AL (2007) Talking about obesity: news framing of who is responsible for causing and fixing the problem. *J Health Commun* **12**: 359–76.

Kingdon JW and Thurber JA (1984) *Agendas, Alternatives, and Public Policies*, Vol. **45**. Boston, MA: Little, Brown.

Kohler-Koch B (2010) Civil society and EU democracy: 'astroturf' representation? *J Eur Public Policy* **17**: 100–16.

Kooiman J (1999) Social-political governance: overview, reflections and design. *Public Manage* **1**: 67–92.

Laurens S (2015) *Les courtiers du capitalisme. Milieux d'affaires et bureaucrates à Bruxelles*. Paris: Agone.

Lee K, Gilmore A, and Collin J (2004) Looking inside the tobacco industry: revealing insights from the Guildford Depository. *Addiction* **99**: 394–7.

Lemmens PH, Vaeth PA, and Greenfield TK (1999) Coverage of beverage alcohol issues in the print media in the United States, 1985–1991. *Am J Public Health* **89**: 1555–60.

Levine HG and Reinarman C (1991) From prohibition to regulation: lessons from alcohol policy for drug policy. *Milbank Q* **69**: 461–94.

Leys C (2001) *Market-driven Politics: Neoliberal Democracy and the Public Interest*. London: Verso.

Lipschutz RD (1992) Reconstructing world politics: the emergence of global civil society. *Millenn J Int Stud* **21**: 389–420.

Lustig R, Schmidt L, and Brindis C (2012) Public health: the toxic truth about sugar. *Nature* **482**: 27–9.

Lyon TP and Maxwell JW (2004) Astroturf: Interest group lobbying and corporate strategy. *J Econ Manage Strat* **13**: 561–97.

McChesney RW (2008) *The Political Economy of Media: Enduring Issues, Emerging Dilemmas*. New York: Monthly Review Press.

McCoy A (2003) *The Politics of Heroin: CIA Complicity in the Global Drug Trade, Afghanistan, Southeast Asia, Central America*. Chicago, IL: Chicago Review Press.

McCreanor T, Casswell S and Hill L (2000) ICAP and the perils of partnership. *Addiction* **95**:179–85.

Makkai T and Braithwaite J (1992) In and out of the revolving door: making sense of regulatory capture. *J Public Policy* **12**: 61–78.

Marsh D and Rhodes RAW (1992) *Policy Networks in British Government*. Oxford: Clarendon Press.

Mazey S and Richardson J (eds) (1993) *Lobbying in the European Community*. Oxford: Oxford University Press.

Medvetz T (2012) *Think Tanks in America*. Chicago, IL: University of Chicago Press.

Megalli M and Friedman A (1991) *Masks of Deception: Corporate Front Groups in America*. Washington, DC: Essential Information.

Michel H (2007) 'La société civile' dans la 'gouvernance européenne'. *Actes de la recherche en sciences sociale* **166**: 144.

Miller D (2009) Corporate lobbying's new frontier: from influencing policy-making to shaping public debate. In: Zinnbauer D (ed.) *Global Corruption Report*. Cambridge: Cambridge University Press in association with Transparency International, pp. 39–41.

Miller D (2015) Neoliberalism, politics and institutional corruption: against the 'institutional malaise' hypothesis. In: Whyte D (ed.) *How Corrupt is Britain?* London: Pluto Press, pp. 59–70.

Miller D and De Andrade M (2010) The Social Issues Research Centre. *BMJ* **340**: 10.1136/bmj.c484.

Miller D and Dinan W (2009) *Revolving Doors, Accountability and Transparency: Emerging Regulatory Concerns and Policy Solutions in the Financial Crisis*. Paris: OECD.

Miller D and Dinan W (2008a) *A Century of Spin*. London: Pluto Press.

Miller D and Dinan W (2008b) Corridors of power: lobbying in the UK' in 'Les Coulisses du Pouvoir' sous la direction de Susan Trouve-Finding. *L'Observatoire de la Societe Britannique* **6**: 25–46.

Miller D and Harkins C (2010) Corporate strategy, corporate capture: food and alcohol industry lobbying and public health. *Crit Soc Policy* **30**: 564–89.

Miller D and Harkins C (2015) Addictive substances and behaviours and corruption, transparency and governance. In: Anderson P, Rehm J and Room R (eds) *Impact of Addictive Substances and Behaviours on Individual and Societal Well-being*. Oxford: Oxford University Press, pp. 215–37.

Miller D and Mooney G (2010) Introduction to the themed issue. Corporate power: agency, communication, influence and social policy. *Crit Soc Policy* **30**: 459–71.

Miller D, Kitzinger J, Williams K, and Beharrell P (1998) *The Circuit of Mass Communication: Media Strategies, Representation and Audience Reception in the AIDS Crisis*. London: Sage.

Monbiot G (2013) The educational charities that do PR for the rightwing ultra-rich. Guardian, 18 February. Available at: https://www.theguardian.com/commentisfree/2013/feb/18/charities-pr-rightwing-ultra-rich.

Nollert M and Fielder N (2000) Lobbying for a Europe of big business: the European Roundtable of Industrialists. In: Bornschier V (ed.) *State-building in Europe: The Revitalization of Western European Integration*. Cambridge: CUP, pp. 187–209.

Nutt D (2010) Lessons from the mephedrone ban. Available at: http://www.theguardian.com/commentisfree/2010/may/28/mephedrone-ban-drug-classification (accessed 1 September 2016).

Oreskes N and Conway EM (2010) *Merchants of Doubt*. New York: Bloomsbury Press.

Owens EG (2011) The birth of the organized crime? The American temperance movement and market-based violence. Available at: http://ssrn.com/abstract=1865347 or http://dx.doi.org/10.2139/ssrn.1865347 (accessed 1 September 2016).

Pageaut A (2010) The current members of the European Round Table: a transnational club of economic elites. *French Politics* **8**: 275–93.

Peschek JG (1987) *Policy Planning Organizations: Elite Agendas and America's Rightward Turn*. Philadelphia, PA: Temple University Press.

Philo G, Miller D, and Happer C (2015) Circuits of communication and structures of power: the sociology of the mass media. In: Holborn M (ed), *Contemporary Sociology*. London: Polity Press, pp. 444–71.

Pigman GA (2007) *The World Economic Forum: A Multi-stakeholder Approach to Global Governance*. London: Routledge.

Plehwe D (2010) Im Dickicht der Beratung. Es mangelt nicht an EuropaThink Tanks, wohl aber an Transparenz. *WZB-Mitteilungen* **130**(S): 22–5.

Powerbase (2015) European Policy Centre. Available at: http://powerbase.info/index.php/European_Policy_Centre (accessed 8 October 2015).

Rhodes R (1997) *Understanding Governance: Policy Networks, Governance, Reflexivity and Accountability*. Philidelphia, PA: Open University Press.

Rödder S (2015) Science media centres and public policy. *Sci Public Policy* **42**: 387–400.

Rutherford D (2006) Editorial, The Globe, Issue 3. Available at: http://www.ias.org.uk/What-we-do/Publication-archive/The-Globe/Issue-3-2006/Editorial.aspx (accessed 15 September 2016).

Salamon LM, Anheier HK, List R, Toepler S, and Sokolowski SW (1999) *Global Civil Society. Dimensions of the Nonprofit Sector*. Baltimore, MD: The Johns Hopkins Comparative Nonprofit Sector Project.

Science Media Centre (nd) About us. Available at: http://www.sciencemediacentre.org/about-us/ (accessed 1 October 2015).

Scotsman (2005) The opium wars: how Scottish traders fed the habit. Available at: http://www.scotsman.com/news/the-opium-wars-how-scottish-traders-fed-the-habit-1-465743 (accessed 1 September 2016).

Sherrington P (2000) Shaping the policy agenda: think tank activity in the European Union. *Global Society* **14**: 173–90.

Silverstein K (2014) *Pay to Play: Think Tanks: Institutional Corruption and the Industry of Ideas*.
Cambridge, MA: Edmund J. Safta Institute for Ethics, Harvard University.

Smith K, Fooks G, Collin J, Weishaar H, and Gilmore A (2010a) Is the increasing policy use of Impact Assessment in Europe likely to undermine efforts to achieve healthy public policy? *J Epidemiol Commun Health* **64**: 478–87.

Smith K, Fooks G, Collin J, Weishaar H, Mandal S, and Gilmore A (2010b) 'Working the System'—British American tobacco's influence on the European Union Treaty and its implications for policy: an analysis of internal tobacco industry documents. *PLOS MED* **7**: e1000202.

Social Issues Research Centre (2001) Guidelines on science and health communication. Available at: http://www.sirc.org/publik/revised_guidelines.shtml (accessed 1 September 2016).

Stenius K and Babor TF (2010) The alcohol industry and public interest science. *Addiction* **105**: 191–8.

Stone D (2007) Recycling bins, garbage cans or think tanks? Three myths regarding policy analysis institutes. *Public Admin* **85**: 259–78.

Stone D and Denham A (2004) *Think Tank Traditions: Policy Research and the Politics of Ideas*. Manchester: Manchester University Press.

Sustain (2010) Yet more hospital food failure Good Food for Our Money Campaign'. Available at: http://www.sustainweb.org/pdf/GFFOM_Hospital_Food_Second_Report.pdf (accessed 14 September 2016).

Sustain (2011) The irresponsibility deal why the government's responsibility deal is better for the food industry than public health . Available at: http://www.sustainweb.org/resources/files/reports/The_Irresponsiblity_Deal.pdf (accessed 15 September 2016).

Transatlantic Policy Network (2015) TTIP Negotiations: contributing to global trade rules. Available at: http://www.tpnonline.org/ttip-negotiations/ (accessed 1 October 2015).

Truman DB (1971) *The Governmental Process.* New York: Alfred A. Knopf.

Tyrrell I (1997) The US prohibition experiment: myths, history and implications. *Addiction* **92**: 1405–9.

University of Chicago Press (2015) What Does Davos Really Do? Analyzing the World Economic Forum. 27 January. Available at: http://www.press.uchicago.edu/pressReleases/2015/January/150127_JCR_world_economic_forum.html (accessed 1 October 2015).

van Schendelen MPCM (ed.) (1993) *National Public and Private EC Lobbying.* Aldershot: Dartmouth Publishing Company.

Vibert F (2007) *The Rise of the Unelected: Democracy and the New Separation of Powers* New York: Cambridge University Press.

Vitali S, Glattfelder J, and Battiston S (2011) The Network of Global Corporate Control. *PLOS ONE* **6**: e25995.

Wallack L and Dorfman L (1996) Media advocacy: a strategy for advancing policy and promoting health. *Health Educ Behav* **3**: 293–317.

Wedel JR (2009) *Shadow Elite: How the World's New Power Brokers Undermine Democracy, Government, and the Free Market.* New York: Basic Books.

Williams A and Gajevic S (2013) Selling science? Source struggles, public relations, and UK press coverage of animal–human hybrid embryos. *Journalism Stud* **14**: 507–22.

Ziauddeen H, Farooqi I, and Fletcher P (2012) Obesity and the brain: how convincing is the addiction model? *Nat Rev Neurosci* **13**: 279–86.

Chapter 10

Civil society approaches to reducing the harm done by addictive substances

10.1 The role of civil society

In today's saturated and individualized societies, citizens are increasingly separated from traditional bases of social and political solidarity mobilization. Instead, they tend to engage with multiple causes that are filtered in relevance to personal lifestyles. Lifestyle issues have so become a thematic field with great relevance for civic engagement. Meanings assigned to lifestyles constitute impetus and personal contact surfaces for activism in overarching political issues, such as climate change, sexual rights, and quality of food. In this chapter we will show that these circumstances provide both opportunities and challenges for civil society (CS) approaches to reduce harm caused by 'addictive' substances.

Throughout history, CS has played a tremendous role in identifying substance use problems and setting agendas for dealing with the same. Underpinning the temperance movement's rise in the early nineteenth century was an articulated civic concern regarding the social, health, and economic harm that alcohol caused in work and family life, and to social order. Throughout the nineteenth and early twentieth centuries, temperance movements provided a nexus of grassroots activism along with the suffragist and labour movements throughout Europe and North America. These concerns were intimately connected with other issues of modernity: inclusive citizenship, social hygiene, 'living wage', and individual autonomy (Sulkunen and Warpenius, 2000; Schrad, 2014). Labour unions, associations of the medical profession, and singular medical doctors have often been the ones to first raise concerns, such as in the question of infant opium doping in the nineteenth century (Berridge and Edwards, 1982: 97–105), or the correlations between tobacco use and cancer a century later (Parascandola et al., 2006).

Broadly speaking, two capital challenges to the common good are identified by Sievers (2010), both of which can be viewed as tied to overall strategies to engage CS. The first one is *value pluralism* in terms of radically different concepts of human ends, as defined by diverse community members and ideologies. The definition of collective purpose becomes a matter of dispute and subject to competition between heterogeneous and inharmonious visions of the good life. In the addiction field, the freedom of the autonomous individual to enjoy life according to one's own preferences, and for entrepreneurs to produce commodities that make everyday life more social, enjoyable, or comfortable for citizens, are values that are typically opposed to restrictions on availability or promotion of products and limitations on behaviours.

The second fundamental challenge for the pursuit of the common good is the rather complicated generic problem of *collective action*. Individuals can pursue a common goal, while at the same time being guided by self-interested behaviour: the individual rationality is simply often not sufficient enough to cover the span of collective rationality. The flipside of how public good is to be collectively achieved—that is, who is to pay for and enjoy the public good—involves public 'bads', situations in which individuals can treat the common elements as an economic externality without having to pay for the consequences of excessive consumption of their damaging acts, as in the case of ocean fisheries, or air pollution. In addition to these larger bulks of concerns surrounding the kind of common good to strive for, and the definition of the good of collective action, collective civic political action and engagement has changed shape with information and communication technologies. In a digitalized networked society, government control over many issues has become both complex and dispersed (Bennett and Segerberg, 2011; Couldry, 2012).

The role of CS organizations (CSOs) was expected to become weaker with the consolidation of the modern welfare states after the Second World War. Many believed that the functions of CS associations would be taken over by the public sector (Alexander, 2006). However, CSOs play fundamental roles in the mixed economy welfare, as well as the new public management governance of lifestyles and public health, that has spread in post-'Iron Curtain' Europe.

Theories of modernity have emphasized that, in individualized societies, the body and the 'Self' as identity projects have, in particular, become fields of negotiation— both in a political and private sense. In the 1990s people were thought to be increasingly oriented inwards and act in line with internalized beliefs and truths. The concept of *life politics* was coined by Anthony Giddens, describing political issues that flow from processes of self-actualization in post-traditional contexts (Giddens, 1991). Life politics was juxtaposed to the solid and interest-based emancipatory politics of earlier times, which strived for elimination of exploitation, inequality, and oppression. In this chapter, we will account for the characteristics of CS in the addiction field by presenting recent shifts and introducing some topical and relevant new trends and possibilities for future work in the area. We suggest that the primary discrepancy to be made is perhaps not the one between identity-shaping, self-reflexive content vs earlier solidarity ethics of justice and equality. Rather, there are some interesting conclusions to be drawn when comparing the modes in which civil activism takes place in today's world and the level of influence the initiatives will have in both existing and new political structures (see, e.g., Kaun, 2015).

10.2 **Recent shifts in civil society responsibility**

Owing to the rather similar aims of the state sector and CS, the boundaries between the two have typically been blurred in the policy field of addictive behaviours. The picture has become even more intricate in contemporary times, when, first, government increasingly forms contracts with both CSOs and private sector in a 'from patron to partner' trend. Government as patron sets conditions on public funding, and as partner develops the action together with the concerned institutions (e.g. Rosenblum and Post, 2002; Rosenblum and Lesch, 2012). In addition to their traditional representational and advocacy function in complex social and ethical issues, non-governmental organizations (NGOs) or CSOs have gained an increasingly important role as service providers in many European states. They are expected to know and reflect the special needs of their clients, as they often employ people recruited from their ranks or from among their near ones, such as in patient associations. As such, CS has become an important part of strategies to enforce what sometimes is called 'the involving public sector' (e.g. Newman, 2011).

Another partly related trend that has weakened the very constituents of autonomous CS and added a great deal of workload to NGOs in the field of addictive substances, is the intra-national and international multi-stakeholder decision-making forums and roundtable hearings that aim to combine representatives of for-profit interests with non-profit NGOs to achieve consensus on health and lifestyle policies (see Hellman, 2012). This model of cooperation is sometimes—and even inevitably so—heavily weighted in favour of profit interests. An example of ideology clashes reaching insurmountable levels was when in 2013 European NGOs in the alcohol field saw themselves forced to withdraw from the European Forum for Alcohol and Health owing to the dubious objectives of their industry peers (see eucam.info, 2013; IOGT-NTO, 2013).

Both of the abovementioned trends—the CS receiving a larger role in service provision and also in policy-making contexts competing increasingly with the private sector—reflect a political climate that Sulkunen has referred to as an 'ethics of not taking a stand' (Sulkunen, 2009), which he claims disengages governmental decision-making procedures from moral responsibility. CS, which often represent values pertaining to social inclusion, long-term health and welfare are, by governments and intra-national governance bodies, positioned in line with companies who gain economically from the same service provision or from the selling of products that causes the problems in the first place. When CS are heard in a policy matter, so are the producers, retailers, and other commercial forces concerned with the issue. Both trends also relate to Sievers' dilemmas of value pluralism and the generic problem of collective action: the organization representing citizens's interests are defined as, and presupposed to be, clients of the preventive and promotional work, rather than democratically engaged subjects and beneficiaries of control policy.

In a longer perspective, a reason for the increased CSO participation in service provision has been the proven success of peer support and self-help during the twentieth century, where Alcoholics Anonymous (AA) has been an especially influential model. The strong position of the self-help and 12-step movements has also contributed to fuzzy boundaries between the private sphere and the common good. The *Oxford Handbook of Civil Society* explains why AA cannot be clearly grouped as a CSO:

> An association such as AA, which is frequently cited as an example of a group that is formal, voluntary, and grassroots, benefits society by helping individuals to stay alcohol-free, create networks of support, and become productive members of society, but does participation necessarily translate into involvement beyond the group itself? Does AA build civil society outside of its own private spaces? Does the organization work for the public good above and beyond the needs of its individual participants? (Edwards, 2011: 57)

The AA movement and other mutual self-help groups have come to produce competing narratives to the traditional collective emancipatory tasks of CS. A cultivation of 'habits of the heart' like the one of the AA movement can easily be seen as something in between 'civil society' and democratic governance (Foley and Edwards, 1996). Regarding independence and detachment from state interference, a recent study by Hellman and Room (2015) shows that the AA recovery narratives have a good fit in residual welfare states such as the USA, where the involvement of NGOs and interest groups is a natural part of a primarily non-public social policy. It is frequently the case that the commercial treatment industry—the so-called 'business of recovery'—borrows models from the AA movement's recovery programme and benefits from its advantageous status in popular opinion. Some economic operators have been heavily criticized by investigators who have compared the knowledge base underpinning treatment interventions in relation to the fees paid by clients.

Some stakeholders have long struggled to be represented in the public debates and policy processes. A still rather weak, but important, stakeholder-based CS movement in the addiction field, is that of drug-user organizations (DUOs). The first advocacy/activist user group was founded in 1977 in the Netherlands and was called the Rotterdam Junkie Union. In the same year, a medical–social service for heroin users was initiated in Amsterdam (see Bröring and Schatz, 2008). Humane approaches that pay attention to the user's perspective when striving to heighten the well-being of intravenous drug addicts—such as substitution treatment, practices of harm reduction, and HIV prevention—have run parallel with, and been crucial for, the birth and maintenance of users' organizations. Priorities of DUOs include advocacy, harm reduction, peer support, training, service providing programmes, detoxification and treatment, community empowerment, education, and networking; and their main activities concern peer support and education (Bröring and Schatz, 2008) (see Box 10.1).

Box 10.1 Summary of roles, possibilities, and challenges for civil society

- Lifestyle questions hold great relevance for new personalized civil engagement.
- CS has played a crucial role in recognizing, articulating, and addressing problems associated with substance use and addictive behaviours.
- The service provision role of CSOs has grown and become more varied in late-modern European states with mixed welfare models.
- Business interests have gained ground in areas that have traditionally been covered by CS.
- Dilemmas pertaining to the common good especially concern radically different definitions of what is to be considered public good; the ways in which the public good is to be achieved; and who is to gain from it.

10.3 **Transnational civil society**

One characteristic of CS activism in questions of addictive substances has been its highly synchronized global character. Events leading up to The Hague Opium Convention (1912), the struggles to reform society, temperance groups, and missionaries for the international prohibition of alcohol followed a similar course (Keane, 2003). Although approaches to substances vary between religions (Room, 2013), religion and spirituality have been important globalizing forces; a common trait in many religions being some sort of programme for addiction counselling (Edwards, 2011).

Research has shown that there is great added value of CS interacting with global health initiatives (GHIs) to strengthen countries' health and welfare systems (Cohn et al., 2011). Some of the major international CS operators today are, for example, the NGO network Global Alcohol Policy Alliance (GAPA), which strives to be 'a strong voice for evidence based alcohol policy' (http://www.globalgapa.org/) and provides an advocacy network at global, regional and national levels. The GAPA, founded in 2000, emerged from the concern of the alcohol industry's intrusion into policy matters. On the drug policy side, The Global Initiative for Drug Policy Reform, coordinated by The Beckley Foundation, promotes health-oriented, cost-effective drug policies based on scientific evidence and human rights. It hopes to achieve this by bringing together (1) The Global Commission on Drug Policy; (2) countries that have implemented progressive drug policies; and (3) countries interested in drug policy reform, in order to present new evidence and debate ways forward (http://reformdrugpolicy.com/). The initiative has commissioned and published the first cost–benefit analysis of a regulated and taxed cannabis market in the UK; and the Rewriting the UN Drug Conventions report. In the tobacco field, the Framework Convention Alliance is made up of over 350 organizations from more than 100 countries working on the development, ratification, and implementation of the World Health Organization's (WHO) Framework Convention on Tobacco Control.

Often, the global NGO networks in the addiction field are concerned with the agendas and frame conventions of the WHO or the United Nations (UN), aiming for these to become, partly or fully, integrated in policy and praxis all over the world. The transnational NGOs have therefore been referred to as 'the citizen sector' and agents of accountability. It is no coincidence, but rather a well-established successful strategy, that the civil sector gathers its forces internationally (Florini, 2000). O'Gorman et al. (2014) have reviewed and mapped over 200 European Union (EU)-based drug policy advocacy organizations and show that NGOs and large-scale CS organizations in Europe have greater capacity to access and engage in governance spaces at the national, EU, and UN levels. The problematic side of global epistemic governance pertains to risk assessment, tensions, and political responsibility (Jordan and van Tuijl, 2000), as well as simplified definitions/views on problems; identification of actors and norms that underpin the work conducted (e.g. Alasuutari and Qadir, 2014, on epistemic governance).

The relationship of influence between transnational governmental agreement organisations and CS is interactive in character, and, naturally, most transnational bodies would not exist without long and solid preparatory work, support, and advocacy by CS. A concrete example of a value-based global campaign directly leading to targeted action is that of baby foods and pro-breastfeeding, including a boycott of Nestlé in 1970s, which led to the introduction of the International Code of Marketing of Breastmilk Substitutes by the World Health Assembly in 1981 (Van Esterik, 1997). Civic opposition directed by the International Organization of Consumers Unions expanded in the 1980s and came to include export not only of hazardous products, but also of hazardous *production*, and, later on, to waste disposal, as seen in transnational campaigns against toxic waste dumping, incineration technology, and shipbreaking (Sheoin, 2015). Although the boundaries between civic society and the market have often been contested, when it comes to reducing the harm caused by addictive substances these two fields have competing interests and expectations from the political system to the extent that they can be treated as clearly distinct entities.

10.4 Civil society vs industry

At the same time as NGOs becoming more globally organized, so are the industry conglomerates that benefit economically from addictive substances. Government controls over many issues have become more diffused and complex, reflecting a need for social pressure to be applied to diverse national and transnational governing institutions, as well as to corporations that have used global business models to gain autonomy from government regulation (Bennett and Segerberg, 2011). The influence over governments by business are generally seen as increasing in areas, such as alcohol policy (Hawkins et al., 2012) and food policy (Pivato et al., 2008). Multinational corporations (MNCs) are striving to influence the same transnational bodies as CS, and claiming to be aiding the work conducted by the transnational political and governmental bodies. Nevertheless, as pointed out in the Organisation for Economic Co-operation and Development Guidelines for Poverty Reduction (OECD, 2001), the lack of interest in long-term commitment to development, and the political and economic muscle of MNCs are the main corporate influences on poverty. In response, guidelines have been drawn up to promote more foreign direct investment and to build linkages with local economies (Kolk and Van Tulder, 2006).

In the 1990s, corporate campaigns began increasingly mixing moral and financial bases: clean business was good business and would bring economic gains. Others argued that embracing clean technology would give MNCs an advantage over their competitors. Sheoin (2015) describes how this change in framing brought some corporate campaigns, especially those embracing shareholder activism, into line with the reformist corporate social responsibility (CSR) movement. The growth of CSR led corporate firms working in the fields of accountancy, consultancy, and public relations to move into this area. By the turn of the millennium, there were signs that another approach was gaining ground, one that involved new campaigns for corporate accountability and legalistic regulation. Utting (2005) has shown how this changed the contours of contestation and CS–business relations. He identifies two sets of conditions that are driving the contemporary 'corporate accountability movement': transformations occurring in the nature of capitalism that connect transnational corporations with global inequality and injustice; and the failures and limitations of the general, mainstream CSR agenda.

Box 10.2 Characteristics of civil society in the field of addictive substances.

- ◆ CS in the addiction field has an international character.
- ◆ CS has a strong interdependent relationship with transnational governmental and political bodies.
- ◆ Today, more than ever, CS is in a double defensive and offensive position vs industry stakeholders. The biggest battle globally and locally is with agents of the for-profit sector.

The most advanced attempts to counteract a 'globalization from above' by a 'globalization from below' might so far have been achieved by the so-called anti-corporate global NGO movement (Sheoin, 2015). Typically, transnational anti-corporate campaigns are based on sophisticated and thorough on-going research on corporations, which is used to target vulnerable corporate activities and stakeholders: corporate campaigns seek to alter the company's behaviour by attacking those relationships that appear most vulnerable. Campaign tactics include boycotts, networking, publicity, lobbying, litigation, public hearings, exposure, blockades, barricades, seizures, and closures, and so on (Sheoin, 2015, referring to Tuodolo, 2009).

Anti-corporate campaigns have been especially important in the geographic periphery to the actual companies under scrutiny. In addition to the Nestlé boycott mentioned already, other examples of such campaigns are those that have kicked out Coca-Cola from India (Hills and Welford, 2005) and attempts to counteract McDonalds in the Third World (Friedmann, 1992). The NGOs' targeting of the palm oil industry is an example of a campaign where there is no return to 'business as usual', as Khor (2011) puts it. A campaign that started with the spread of health consideration in the 1980s is still actively affecting the palm oil industry, for example in Indonesia and Malaysia, where European NGOs continue to be influential. A powerful tactic in the anti-palm oil campaign has involved film clips and campaign messages spread on the Internet through social media and popular websites. This is a form of CS advocacy, awareness raising, and concrete power influence that constitutes a so called 'uninvited branding' (Fournier and Avery, 2011) (see Box 10.2).

10.5 New technology, new modes of activism

New media provides a 'new space of the social' (Couldry, 2012), in which citizens can partake in political conversations, express opinions, and organize political movements. The very idea of the Internet as a provider of a free and open space for CS to flourish has brought much debate (Himelboim, 2011). Analyses of contemporary CS have stressed its novelty, its mode of transnational action in relation to innovative use of information and communication technology (Bray, 2000). But is the Internet generation 'engaged citizens or political dropouts' (Milner, 2010)? For engagement in the age of technological transformation, modes of political socialization and engagement in collective aims is tightly connected to Siever's second challenge on the public good: who will engage, why, and on whose behalf? For CS involved in questions related to addictive substances, the possibilities for reaching out to the general public with politically relevant messages in a personalized format have shown great potential to engage citizens in questions that are constantly morally contested from different angles. This demands use of the Internet in new and dynamic ways (Kingston and Stam, 2013).

Authority concepts are becoming more ambivalent in the age of the Internet as people are, on the one hand, becoming fixated with scientific explanations and actively searching for answers on the web, and yet, on the other hand, feeling increasingly suspicious as the amount of knowledge is growing (Brossard, 2013). Movements that have an agenda of epistemic claims that contradict established truths and beliefs can become rather well organized through Internet platforms. A telling example of how alternative movements can appear, organize themselves, and contradict normative institutionalized epistemic messages is one of the Swedish movements that follows the ketogenic diet principle: Low carbohydrates and high fat (LCHF).

The LCHF movement has provided possibilities of social organization and mobilization by new media. During the last ten years an enormous online movement has grown around LCHF: blogs, receipt books, experts, legitimized LCHF nutritional advice education programmes, and lifestyle magazines (Holmberg, 2015; Jauho, 2016). Today it is believed that one in every four Swedes follows some sort of variation of the LCHF diet (Demoskop, 2013). What, then, has made the movement so efficient? Both Huhta (2014) and Gunnarsson and Elam (2012) show that the LCHF movement has efficiently debunked established dietary advice for failing to live up to idealized standards of 'sound science'.

The diets of most people in modern Western nations contain large amounts of starches, including refined flours, and substantial amounts of sugars, including fructose. The LCHF movement has been able to convince and engage people in an alternative epistemic claim, making them eat butter, cream, and coconut oil—dietary advice that would not have received any followers during times of greater consensus regarding the relationship between level of cholesterol, hard fats, and cardiovascular diseases. And one can see that it competes not only with the balanced plate and calorie model of official dietary advice, but also with the epistemic claims, for example, of a powerful global sugar industry (see, e.g., Bes-Rastrollo et al., 2013; Bolton, 2015; Kearns et al., 2015)

Digitalized civil action involves communication and interaction that allow for personalized engagement through questions that can tie in narratives with relevance for citizens' self-understanding and a desire for authenticity (Yerbury, 2010). This circumstance has been suggested to contribute to a public experience of the self, rather than one of collective solidarity (McDonald, 2002). As such, it creates demands on NGOs in the addiction field to present narratives that feel relevant and specific enough for citizens to engage with and take action. A good example of such an effort is the animated explainer 'Drugs and the Brain', available in 15 languages, by the Dutch addiction resource centre Jellinek (available at: http://www.jellinek.nl/

brain/). The presentation shows in an easily comprehended manner how the brain is affected by ecstasy, speed, cocaine, cannabis, heroin, alcohol, and nicotine. In addition, the presentation contains a short comprehensive general presentation of how the brain works. This can be seen as representing a personalized neuro-politics that lead to great increase of interest in the general public, but may only engage collectives in a secondary sense in work which may have an actual political impact to reduce harmful outcomes from addictive substances.

The right types of strategies in digital technologies are increasingly central to the organization and collective action of NGOs. A potential problem is that this sort of communication seems to be at odds with the emphasis on unity and alignment conventionally associated with the communication processes of effective collective action, and which the concrete modus operandi of policy change that the CSO needs to aim for.

Protest networks in digitalized milieus not only offer possibilities for CSO, but are also simultaneously platforms in which work against health-promoting and harm-reduction aims can take place. In the autumn of 2014, a mobilization of a protest movement against restrictions in the public display of alcoholic beverage brands at the National Beer Expo flooded social media in Finland with unprecedented speed (Hellman and Katainen, 2015). This event also demonstrated the more prominent role played by personal networks in protest movements, and the ridiculing stance that anti-moralism campaigns have to their advantage in the age of social media punchlines. The roles of NGOs and social movement organizations become increasingly those of facilitators and with expertise and know-how on research and the evidence-base, and who react with alternative stories after the initial media storm has settled. The rapid spread of messages situates the different stakeholders in competing positions to get their version of the story out first, as this is the one that tends to stick in the collective memory.

One example of the huge possibilities offered to CSO by the online speed of mobilization, scope of issues, and the ability to focus public attention in the short-term is the simple rule of thumb adopted by the 2015 Estonian campaign 'Joome Poole vähem' ('Let's drink half as much', see http://www.poolevähem.ee/), which spread quickly and was disseminated in different online formats. However, the short-term possibilities of enlightening people with cogent messages may not be the most efficient way to achieve the conventional political goals that remain important for CS. NGOs need to ask themselves what role they want to give personalized communication (modes and content), and whether large-scale concentrated efforts in this direction will, in the long run, lead organizations to compromise their articulated goals (e.g. by underspecifying them in political action), and whether the personalized messages result in incoherent noise which fails to travel well or at all in the mass media (Bennett and Segerberg, 2011).

The most continuous and static online modes of service provision by CSOs in the addiction area are those, for example, which provide help for citizens with problems—providing advice on ways to help themselves, or opportunities to interact in forums and discussion threads about their problems. Online watchdogs and information platforms like the Dutch EUCAM (http://eucam.info/) or the American

Alcohol Justice industry watchdog (https://alcoholjustice.org/) mix data banks, campaigns, and news, and are used globally by CS, researchers, and policy-makers. A typical problem related to online campaigns is that it sometimes remains unclear for the reader who the sender/creator is. A good example of this is the large-scale anti-smoking campaign group 'truth' with their multimodality web campaigns such as the 'Left swap dat' music video. Nowhere on the truth website can a sender or creator of the campaign be found (http://www.thetruth.com/). Another example of this is the 'campaign against alcohol and drug abuse', or CAADA, which appears on the social media platform Facebook (https://www.facebook.com/CAADA.com.gh/photos_stream), with no indication of the country of origin.

The dilemma of using personalized lifestyle messages to find contact surfaces with citizens who can be engaged in the issues, yet recruiting the relevant and solid long-term engagement needed for political change, is closely tied to the complicated question of ethics and morals in a world (online) where liberalism dominates—and often negatively articulated liberalism (defending intimate spheres from governance intrusion). Although the appeal of the message may be personalized, the engaged citizen may not be willing to formulate themselves as part of the political project identifying themselves in an active position which may influence their profile and identity as a person (Yerbury, 2010). Engaging questions are often those where the citizen is able to take a stand representing interests of a weaker part: the new H2O ('harms to others') movement in the 2010s is a good example of a way of detaching the responsible, 'normal' substance user from those who cause harm to others (Laslett et al., 2010). Another pressing and conveniently 'detached' question for civil engagement relates to low-income countries, which may supply a meaningful way of engagement without having to politically—morally and ethically—ascribe oneself a direct role in the actual problem.

10.6 Reducing harm in low-income countries

Non-institutionalized socioeconomic and political bodies in low-income countries can be locally and regionally established, but often they have either head offices, donors, or just close connections to high-income country NGOs, transnational institutions, governments, and private funds. CSO have played a crucial role in advocacy and implementation of the GHIs that have strengthened and improved health systems in low-income countries. Also, NGOs are often the most neutral and competent actors to identify shortcomings and system errors in the same processes. Cohn et al. (2011) interviewed a range of health-system stakeholders in Kenya, Malawi, Uganda, and Zambia; in total, 2910 CS participants provided information reporting that GHIs have contributed to dramatic health benefits within and outside of a disease-specific focus, including health systems strengthening efforts. However, the informants reported that certain opportunities for synergy between GHIs and health systems had typically been missed, and GHIs had not worked sufficiently to close capacity gaps of grassroots CSOs. Despite some governance innovations, the opportunities of CS to participate meaningfully in GHI priority-setting efforts were thought to be limited. Cohn et al. (2011) end their analysis with the formulation of some recommendations for how to best use GHIs to strengthen health systems by partnering with CS.

In low-income countries, for-profit actors may see potential for getting involved in policy processes that they hope will lead to profitable circumstances for their own business activities. Countries with non-institutionalized or non-democratized governance and decision-making processes, or high levels of corruption, are especially vulnerable to global industry 'activism'.

Zhang and Monteiro (2013) have studied the practices and tactics of the alcohol industry in Latin America, focusing on industry globalization and consolidation, implementation of research studies, marketing, and corporate responsibility initiatives, and discuss how these areas of influence may have an impact on alcohol policy development in this region. They conclude that effective alcohol-control policies are unlikely to succeed if the influence of the alcohol industry and its actions cannot be reined in by policy makers in Latin American countries. They highlight:

> a need to increase knowledge of the alcohol industry's role and actions and of its conflicts of interest with public health, and to build capacity across various sectors of government to implement effective policies, using clear rules for engagement (Zhang and Monteiro, 2013: 75).

They also point out a pressing need for research on alcohol industry practices in emerging markets, particularly in Latin America and the Caribbean, spanning marketing, CSR practices, and the industry's influence on policy.

A comparison between four draft National Alcohol Policy documents from Lesotho, Malawi, Uganda, and Botswana showed almost identical wording and structure to the degree that they are likely to originate from the same source, likely alcohol producer SAB-Miller and the industry-funded Center for Alcohol Policies. The comparison, conducted by Bakke and Endal (2010), provides insights into the methods and strategic political objectives of the multinational drinks industry. The study demonstrates how the industry policy vision chooses selectively from the international evidence base on alcohol prevention and disregards or minimizes a public health approach to alcohol problems. The policies reviewed maintain a narrow focus on the economic benefits from the trade in alcohol. In terms of alcohol problems (and their remediation) the documents focus upon individual drinkers, ignoring effective environmental interventions. The proposed policies serve the industry's interests at the expense of public health by attempting to enshrine 'active participation of all levels of the beverage alcohol industry as a key partner in the policy formulation and implementation process', concludes Bakke and Endal (2010).

Some examples of CSOs in the field of addictive substances in Africa are South African National Council on Alcoholism and Drug Dependence (SANCA), Central and Southern Africa; Zanzibar Association of Information Against Drug and Alcohol (ZAIADA) Eastern Africa; and Zambia Alcohol and Drug Programme (ZADP). In addition, non-CS actors cooperate in singular campaigns and ventures, such as the Rwanda national police's anti-crime awareness campaign in 2014 where students of the Lycée de Kigali in Nyarugenge district were empowered to work actively against crimes, especially gender-based violence and drug abuse (http://www.police.gov. rw/news-detail/?tx_ttnews[tt_news]=1147&cHash=44f82cf3655fc3756193e79591 80f678) (see Box 10.3).

> ## Box 10.3 Summary of some overall contemporary trends in global civil society in the field of addictive substances and behaviours
>
> ◆ Today, a big challenge for CSOs is how to mobilize and engage citizens.
>
> ◆ The adoption of digital media has led to a shift in mobilization from organization to individuals.
>
> ◆ Demands of flexibility may challenge the standard models for achieving effective collective action.
>
> ◆ The personalized engaging formats for the common good may make it more difficult to achieve conventional political goals, sustaining a certain level of formal and centralized organization.
>
> ◆ There is a need for the CS to evaluate commitment and mobilization capacity; agenda strength; and network strength and political capacity.
>
> ◆ The most pressing front for CS to oppose industry interests have been shown to be in low-income countries.

10.7 Conclusions

In Europe, a number of crucial changes in welfare and service provision have led to a situation where service systems and service units, rather than being part of a clear-cut sector, have increasingly become hybrids, combining varying balances of resources and mixes of governance principles associated with the market, the state, and CS (Evers, 2005).

The trend of giving goal-oriented and value-oriented political aims the same starting point and role in political negotiations is especially well preserved through the austerity argument of prosperous states, with small-state sectors and well-oiled business life being better prepared to take care of citizens' health and welfare provision. Business interests are also presented as welfare interests. In addition, the increased emphasis on agency of citizens in new consumerist governance trends constitutes another challenging circumstance when dealing with addiction-related problems—issues that, by definition, signify a lack of agency by the people with the problems (Hellman, 2012).

Other typical contemporary challenges and possibilities for CS approaches to reducing the harm done by addictive substances involve new modes of individualized, yet public, engagement and empowerment, as well as an ongoing struggle with for-profit operators on many fronts. The latter challenge is especially pressing in low-income countries.

CS has no monopoly on claiming ethical accountability regarding improvement of citizens' well-being. Besides the struggle of dealing with forces of the for-profit sector that benefit financially from the addictive activities, a continuous parallel struggle has been to deal with overlapping claims of responsible action made by these actors. Almost all alcohol producers have formulated declarations of missions to deal with 'alcohol misuse' and self-restriction of different sorts (age limits, marketing restrictions). Also, business operators have declared intentions to support member states in implementing the WHO global strategy to reduce the harmful use of alcohol (e.g. Diageo, 2015). The work involved for CSO to claim their own role and profile– and often, defend their views on efficient action—in relation to industry actors is a tough task in Europe today.

The potential of NGOs to influence preventive policies has been very strong historically, and they are still a necessary voice representing large subpopulations and their concerns about health, social issues, the environment, and lifestyle.

In hearings and policy consultations, at the EU level, as well as nationally, NGOs compete for influence with representatives of for-profit interests, with an in-built bias against them. They have more chances for success in parliamentary representative processes than through executive channels, but this will depend on their potential for effective coalitions, which is, at the moment, very difficult to foresee.

References

Alasuutari P and Qadir A (2014) Epistemic governance: an approach to the politics of policy-making. *Eur J Cultur Polit Sociol* 1: 67–84.

Alexander JC (2006) *The Civil Sphere*. Oxford: Oxford University Press.

Bakke Ø and Endal D (2010) Vested interests in addiction research and policy alcohol policies out of context: drinks industry supplanting government role in alcohol policies in sub-Saharan Africa. *Addiction* 105: 22–8.

Bennett WL and Segerberg A (2011) Digital media and the personalization of collective action: social technology and the organization of protests against the global economic crisis. *Inform Commun Soc* 14: 770–9.

Berridge V and Edwards G (1982) *Opium and the People*. ABC. London and New York: St Martin's Press.

Bes-Rastrollo M, Schulze MB, Ruiz-Canela M, and Martinez-Gonzalez MA (2013) Financial conflicts of interest and reporting bias regarding the association between sugar-sweetened beverages and weight gain: a systematic review of systematic reviews. *PLoS Med* 10(12): e1001578. Available at: http://journals.plos.org/plosmedicine/article?id=10.1371/journal.pmed.1001578 (accessed 26 October 2016).

Bolton D (2015) Coca-Cola caught funding scientists who deflect blame for obesity away from sugary drinks. Available at: http://www.independent.co.uk/life-style/health-and-families/health-news/cocacola-caught-funding-scientists-who-deflect-blame-for-obesity-away-from-sugary-drinks-10448986.html (accessed 25 August 2016).

Bray J (2000) Web wars: NGOs, companies and governments in an Internet-connected world. *Terms for Endearment: Business, NGOs and Sustainable Development* 49: 49–63.

Brossard D (2013) New media landscapes and the science information consumer. *Proc Natl Acad Sci U S A* 110(Suppl. 3): 14096–101.

Bröring G and Schatz E (eds) (2008) *Empowerment and Self-organisations of Drug Users: Experiences and Lessons Learnt*. Amsterdam: Foundations Regenboog.

Cohn J, Russell A, Baker B, Kayongo A, Wanjiku E, and Davis P (2011) Using global health initiatives to strengthen health systems: a civil society perspective. *Global Public Health* 6: 687–702.

Couldry N (2012) *Media, Society, World: Social Theory and Digital Media Practice.* Cambridge: Polity.

Demoskop (2013) Livsmedelsföretagen. Julmat och dieter. Utgivningsort: Stockholm. 2013. Available at: http://www.livsmedelsforetagen.se/wp-content/uploads/2013/11/Julmat-och-dieter.pdf (accessed 18 September 2015).

Diageo (2015) Alcohol in society. Available at: http://www.diageo.com/en-row/csr/alcoholinsociety/Pages/default.aspx (accessed 25 August 2016).

Edwards M (ed) (2011) *The Oxford Handbook of Civil Society.* Oxford: Oxford University Press.

eucam.info (2013) European civil society organizations decide to leave the European Alcohol and Health Forum. Available at: http://eucam.info/2013/11/30/european-civil-society-organizations-decide-to-leave-the-european-alcohol-and-health-forum/ (accessed 25 August 2016).

Evers A (2005) Mixed welfare systems and hybrid organizations: changes in the governance and provision of social services. *Int J Public Admin* 28: 737–48.

Florini AM (2000) *Third Force, The; The Rise of Transnational Civil Society.* Tokyo and Washington: Japan Center for International Exchange and the Carnegie Endowment for International Peace.

Foley MW and Edwards B (1996) The paradox of civil society. *J Democ* 7: 38–52.

Fournier S and Avery J (2011) The uninvited brand. *Bus Horizons* 54: 193–207.

Friedmann H (1992) Distance and durability: shaky foundations of the world food economy. *Third World Q* 13: 371–83.

Giddens A (1991) Modernity and self-identity: self and society in the late modern age. Palo Alto: Stanford University Press.

Gunnarsson A and Elam M (2012) Food fight! The Swedish low-carb/high fat (LCHF) movement and the turning of science popularisation against the scientists. *Sci Culture* 21: 315–34.

Hawkins B, Holden C, and McCambridge J (2012) Alcohol industry influence on UK alcohol policy: a new research agenda for public health. *Crit Public Health* 22: 297–305.

Hellman M (2012) Multistakeholder alcohol policy: goal-based and value-based rationalities in an alcohol marketing task force In: Hellman M, Roos G, and von Wright J (eds) *A Welfare Policy Patchwork: Negotiating the Public Good in Times of Transition.* Helsinki: Nordens välfärdscenter, Stockholm, pp 143–62.

Hellman M and Katainen A (2015) #Viski – The autonomous man against the nanny state in the age of online outrage. *Sosiologia* 4: 334–49

Hellman M and Room R (2015) What's the story on addiction? Popular myths in the USA and Finland. *Crit Public Health* 25: 582–98.

Hills J and Welford R (2005) Coca-Cola and water in India. *Corp Soc Responsib Environ Manage* 12: 168–77.

Himelboim I (2011) Civil society and online political discourse. the network structure of unrestricted discussions. *Commun Res* 38: 634–59.

Holmberg C (2015) Politicization of the low-carb high-fat diet in Sweden, promoted on social media by non-conventional experts. *IJEP* 6: 27–42.

Huhta AM (2014) Internetin karppauskeskustelut virallisia ravitsemussuosituksia haastamassa. [The Internet's low carbohydrate discussions challenge public nutritional guidelines]. Available at: http://ojs.tsv.fi/index.php/inf/article/download/48050/13883 (accessed 25 August 2016).

IOGT-NTO (2013) Civil society organizations to leave the European Alcohol and Health Forum: we call for a revised structure and a renewed EU Alcohol Strategy. Available at: http://iogt.se/pressmeddelanden/civil-society-organizations-to-leave-the-european-alcohol-and-health-forum-we-call-for-a-revised-structure-and-a-renewed-eu-alcohol-strategy/ (accessed 25 August 2016).

Jauho M (2016) The social construction of competence: conceptions of science and expertise among proponents of the low-carbohydrate high-fat diet in Finland. *Public Underst Sci* 25: 332–45.

Jordan L and Van Tuijl P (2000) Political responsibility in transnational NGO advocacy. *World Develop* **28.12**: 2051–65.

Kaun A (2015) Regimes of time: media practices of the dispossessed. *Time Soc* **(24)2**: 221–43.

Keane J (2003) *Global Civil Society?* Cambridge: Cambridge University Press.

Kearns CE, Glantz SA, and Schmidt LA (2015) Sugar industry influence on the scientific agenda of the National Institute of Dental Research's 1971 National Caries Program: a historical analysis of internal documents. *PLOS MED* **12**: e1001798.

Khor YL (2011) The oil palm industry bows to NGO campaigns. *Lipid Technol* **23**: 102–4.

Kingston LN and Stam KR (2013) Online advocacy: analysis of human rights NGO websites. *J Hum Rights Pract* **5**: 75–95.

Kolk A and Van Tulder R (2006) Poverty alleviation as business strategy? Evaluating commitments of frontrunner multinational corporations. *World Develop* **34**: 789–801.

Laslett A-M, Catalano P, Chikritzhs T, Dale C, Doran C, Ferris J, et al. (2010) The range and magnitude of alcohol's harm to others. Available at: https://melbourneinstitute.com/downloads/hilda/Bibliography/Other_Publications/pre2010/Laslett_etal_Alcohol%27s_Harm_to_Others.pdf (accessed 25 August 2016).

McDonald K (2002) From solidarity to fluidiarity: social movements beyond 'collective identity'—the case of globalization conflicts. *Soc Mov Stud* **1**: 109–28.

Milner H (2010) *The Internet Generation: Engaged Citizens or Political Dropouts*. Lebanon, NH: UPNE.

Newman J (2011) The involving public sector. *Distinktion* **12**: 331–41.

OECD (2001) *The DAC Guidelines. Poverty Reduction*. Paris: Development Assistance Committee.

O'Gorman A, Quigley E, Zobel F, and Moore K (2014) Peer, professional, and public: An analysis of the drugs policy advocacy community in Europe. *Int J Drug Policy* **25**: 1001–8.

Parascandola M, Weed DL, and Dasgupta A (2006) Two surgeon general's reports on smoking and cancer: a historical investigation of the practice of causal inference. *Emerg Themes Epidemiol* **3**: 1–11.

Pivato S, Misani N, and Tencati A (2008) The impact of corporate social responsibility on consumer trust: the case of organic food. *Bus Ethics* **17**: 3–12.

Room R. (2013) Spirituality, intoxication and addiction: six forms of relationship. *Substance Use and Misuse* **48**:1109–1113.

Rosenblum NL and Post RC (eds) (2002) *Civil Society and Government*. Princeton, NJ: Princeton University Press.

Rosenblum N and Lesch C (2012) *Civil Society and Government*. Available at: http://www.oxfordhandbooks.com/view/10.1093/oxfordhb/9780195398571.001.0001/oxfordhb-9780195398571-e-23 (accessed 25 August 2016).

Schrad M (2014) *Vodka Politics: Alcohol, Autocracy, and the Secret History of the Russian State*. Oxford: Oxford University Press.

Sheoin TM (2015) Transnational Anti-Corporate Campaigns: Fail Often, Fail Better. *Soc Just* **41**: 198.

Sievers BR (2010) *Civil Society, Philanthropy, and the Fate of the Commons*. Lebanon, NH: UPNE, Tufts University Press.

Sulkunen P (2009) *Saturated Society*. Los Angeles, London, New Delhi, Singapore, Washington: SAGE.

Sulkunen P and Warpenius K (2000) Reforming the self and the other: the temperance movement and the duality of modern subjectivity. *Crtic Public Health* **10**: 423–38.

Tuodolo F (2009) Corporate social responsibility: between civil society and the oil industry in the developing world. *ACME* **8**: 530–41.

Utting P (2005) Corporate responsibility and the movement of business. *Develop Pract* **15**: 375–88.

Van Esterik P (1997) The politics of breastfeeding. *Food Culture* 370–82.

Yerbury H (2010) Who to be? Generations X and Y in civil society online. Available at: https://opus.lib.uts.edu.au/bitstream/10453/15919/1/2010002903.pdf (accessed 30 October 2016).

Zhang C and Monteiro M (2013) Tactics and practices of the alcohol industry in Latin America: what can policy makers do? *Int J Alcohol Drug Res* **2**: 75–81.

Chapter 11

Conclusions

11.1 Introduction

We started this book by noting that illegal drugs were responsible for 1.4 per cent of all years lost due to ill health and premature death in the European Union (EU) in 2010, alcohol for 5.3 per cent, and tobacco for 11.4 per cent, imposing economic burdens in excess of 2.5 per cent of gross domestic product (Shield and Rehm, 2015; see Chapter 1). These are not the full impacts of drugs on society, as, to any great extent, they do not take into account the harms to people other than drug users for alcohol and illegal drugs. Also, they do not take into account the harms that drugs can impose on other aspects of individual and societal well-being, including, for example, poorer educational achievement, impaired civic engagement, and diminished personal security (Stoll and Anderson, 2015; see Chapter 3). We also noted that no one European country has been fully successful in implementing effective and sustainable drug policies in a coherent way (Ysa et al., 2014; see Chapter 8), and that sometimes as much harm can result from a policy itself (its adverse side effects) and from stigma as from the drugs themselves (Moskalewicz and Klingemann, 2015; see Chapter 3).

In this final chapter, we bring together much of the substance of this book and draw on all of the work of the ALICE RAP project (www.alicerap.eu) to propose 12 points for policy that can be considered in redesigning governance approaches to reduce the individual and societal harm done by alcohol, illegal drugs, and tobacco (hereafter referred to as 'drugs').

11.2 Heavy use over time should be the replacement descriptor for concepts and terms such as 'addiction' or 'dependence'

As we argued in Chapter 2, heavy use over time (HUOT) is the determinant and predictor of the health and social sequelae normally captured by concepts and terms such as addiction and dependence. HUOT is a more accurate description, and one that recognizes that use and harm exist within continua with no natural cut-off points. As a continuous rather than categorical concept, HUOT helps reduce the stigma associated with dichotomous labelling (e.g. addict vs non-addict). Heavy use of drugs over time is responsible for: the changes in the brain, and other physiological characteristics of 'addictive' disorders; intoxication, and for the loss of control characterizing current definitions of addiction; the main social consequences of addiction, such as problems in fulfilling social roles; and, the majority of addiction-attributable burden of disease and mortality (Rehm et al., 2013a). As a descriptor, HUOT eliminates many of the historical and political uncertainties and current problems with definitions and operationalization, which vary a great deal between different countries (see Hellman et al., 2016).

The concepts of HUOT have best been worked out for heavy drinking and smoking (Rehm et al., 2013a, 2014a). This unpacking of understanding needs further development for illegal drugs. HUOT should be captured in epidemiological studies, and it should be the core concept for future research of the drivers and determinants of harm. Reducing HUOT should be a defined outcome for the impact of policy and for the impact of prevention programmes and clinical advice and treatment.

11.3 Policies should address and reduce the social stigma linked to drug use

As we pointed out in Chapters 3 and 6, heavy use of drugs is one of the most stigmatized behaviours over time and place, and 'substance use disorders' are the most stigmatized of all the mental and behavioural disorders (Bjerge et al., 2016). This moralistic approach helps to maintain policies that are ineffective, and is a barrier to the normalization of advice and treatment for heavy drug use that meets the same standards of care as for any other chronic condition, such as diabetes or high blood pressure.

We still have a lot to learn on how best to reduce stigma (Rüsch et al., 2005; Pinto-Foltz and Logsdon, 2009; Dalky, 2012). Certainly, widespread adoption of the concept of HUOT, a continuum rather than dichotomous classification ('addict' vs 'non-addict'), is likely to reduce stigma, according to Social Identity Theory (Tajfel and Turner, 1986; Schomerus et al., 2013). Sympathetic portrayal of heavy users who have run into problems, and sympathetic portrayal of successful help and treatment may also reduce stigma (McGinty et al., 2015). A European coordinated and continued action, involving both public and private sectors, should be mobilized to reduce the stigma associated with heavy drug use.

11.4 Policies should be based on a sound understanding of evolutionary behaviour

Understanding human evolutionary behaviour and the common mismatch between the way we run our lives in present times and the way our lives were run in the environment in which we evolved can provide better pointers as to what needs to be done to reduce ill health and premature death, in particular from non-communicable diseases (Lieberman, 2013).

As we mentioned in Chapter 4 (and further explored in Dudley (2014) and Sullivan and Hagen (2015)), ecological analyses find that humans have evolved to be active and functional, rather than passive and vulnerable with respect to the drugs that we take. Many drugs (other than alcohol) are neurotoxins, developed by plants as defence mechanisms against being eaten by animals. Ethanol results from fermenting fruit, as a defence mechanism to avoid premature rotting. Humans, as many other plant-eating animals, have counter-exploited plant neurotoxins for advantage. Nicotine is used for its anti-parasitic properties, with, for example people living in high intestinal worm-burden areas, titrating cigarettes smoked with burden (the heavier the smoker, the lower the worm burden) (Roulette et al., 2014). Moreover, treating the worm burden with anthelmintic drugs treats the heavy use of tobacco—the number of cigarettes smoked drops. Ethanol vapour is used for olfactory location of ripe fruit, and thus giving nutritional advantage (Dudley, 2014).

An understanding of evolutionary behaviour has at least two implications for drug policy: first, policies that prohibit the use of drugs are unlikely to succeed because people are biologically programmed to seek these chemicals; and, second, high modern drug potency (as opposed to the lower potency in habitats in which humans first evolved) is likely to be a core driver of harm, with potency largely determined by producer organizations operating in suboptimally managed markets (Schmidt, 2015).

11.5 Policies should be assessed for their impact on a range of societal well-being outcomes beyond physical and mental health

In Chapter 3, we brought forward the importance of assessing drug policies for their impact on a range of societal well-being outcomes beyond physical and mental health (see also Stoll and Anderson, 2015), and noted that at the international level, the Organisation for Economic Co-operation and Development's societal well-being frame is a useful benchmark (see OECD, 2011, 2015a). With a well-being frame, we found that while drug policies can reduce health harms and bring co-benefits across different sectors, they can also have adverse side effects, including criminalization and violence, and social stigma and social exclusion, which detract from individual and societal well-being. Thus, as we argued in Chapter 8 (see Ysa et al., 2014), drug policies should be based on a well-being and relational management strategy combined with a comprehensive structure that involves different stakeholders; balance decriminalization of illegal substances with innovative harm reduction policies; and effectively regulate the legal drugs, nicotine, and alcohol, and their drug delivery systems. In Chapter 3, (see Figure 3.2), we concluded that regulation of all drugs, not an unfettered free market at one extreme, or prohibition with its attendant criminalization at the other extreme, should be the central approach of all drug policies.

11.6 Policies should be guided by standardized assessment procedures such as the toxicology-based margins of exposure analyses

In Chapter 4, we introduced margins of exposure (MOEs), a toxicological approach to assessing drug-related harms (see also Lachenmeier and Rehm, 2015).

In our daily life, we are exposed (voluntarily or not) to a whole range of chemicals that are potentially toxic or carcinogenic. Legal and illegal 'addictive' drugs are a subset of these toxic substances, with adverse outcomes for individuals and society. The science of toxicology has developed a methodology to estimate and guide exposure levels in relation to risk for toxic substances, called the MOE.

The MOE gives us, for any substance, an indication of whether populations are exposed to (or use) a substance at an agreed level of risk or not; and the methodology adopts a standard level of highest acceptable risk, which can be applied to any legal or illegal drug, enabling comparisons of MOEs between drugs, which can indicate which drug requires a policy shift or amendment.

The MOE is a ratio between a benchmark toxic dose, and level of exposure, so that an MOE of 1 means that one is consuming or exposed to the benchmark toxic dose; an MOE of 100 means that one is consuming at one-hundredth the benchmark toxic dose—the higher the MOE, the lower the level of risk. We propose that all drug policies, notwithstanding all their other needs (promoting societal well-being, reducing stigma, and closing treatment gaps) should adopt a target that the MOE for individual daily use of any drug does not fall below 10.

In toxicology, MOE analyses use a measure called the BMDL10 (benchmark dose lethal 10%), meaning that a benchmark toxic dose is set at that which is 95 per cent certain to cause 10 per cent of lethal outcomes in animal studies (or human epidemiological studies). However, instead of considering only physiological toxicity and lethal doses, MOEs for drugs can be calculated taking into account a range of harm outcomes, in health and other well-being domains. Further research is needed to identify the data needed to calculate the MOEs of drugs using these broader definitions of harm, beyond mortality.

MOE analyses can also be used to define cut-off points for clinical interventions in the continua of HUOT, with MOE analyses based on health and well-being outcomes due to sustained heavy use rather than BMDL10 data based on LD_{50} data (see Chapter 4).

11.7 Policies should ensure that they reduce heavy drug use

We argued in Chapter 5 that policies should aim to find a balance in addressing not only the whole population, but also heavy users, and, in Chapter 6, we outlined a swathe of approaches at the population and individual level that have evidence in reducing drug use, heavy drug use, and drug-related harm. In general, the risk of harm from drugs increases with the dose of the drug taken along a continuum of risk (Rehm et al., 2014b). The functions of the risk curves vary, depending on the drug, and the harm being measured, between linear risk curves and curvilinear risk curves, where risks increase faster at higher doses. The finding of a preponderance of curvilinear risk curves for more long-term health problems leads to the conclusion that the majority of individual and societal drug-related harms results from heavy use (see Rehm et al., 2012, 2013b). The consequence of this is that the same absolute reduction in heavier use brings greater individual and societal benefit than the same absolute reduction in lighter use (Rehm and Roerecke, 2013). Thus, policies and actions, including individually directed advice and treatment programmes, will bring greater health gain when they specifically aim to reduce heavy drug use than when they fail to affect heavy drug use.

11.8 Drug policies should recognize the vulnerability of the adolescent brain, particularly with respect to decision-making abilities

As we argued in Chapter 7, drug policies should not penalize or stigmatize underage drug users. Young people should be engaged in the development and implementation of drug policies. Youth-informed policies should focus on harm reduction, reducing early onset or heavy use, and reducing the use of high potency or unregulated harmful substances. Policies and actions should aim to reduce risk, build resilience, and promote physical and mental health. Drug policies focused on youth need to be embedded in whole-of-society and whole-of-government youth development policies that aim for security of education, employment, and full civic engagement. Policies that restrict access to these basic rights for underage users are expensive and can lead to greater risk of drug use and harmful use due to secondary effects of social exclusion.

Adolescence is a time of enormous biological and social change accompanied by increased risk taking, with evolutionary adaptation and benefit (Konner, 2010; Ellis et al., 2012). During adolescence, the brain undergoes profound structural change, a process not complete until about 25 years of age. During this time, young people have a well-developed reward system, but they do not have a good executive control centre, meaning that their skills in controlling impulses and planning behaviour are still being developed. Adolescent brain development itself might be impaired by drug use (Cservenka and Nagel, 2015; Spas and Weyandt, 2015), which, in turn, renders a young user at greater risk of longer-term drug use.

11.9 Smart drug policies require whole-of-society and whole-of-government approaches

In Chapter 8, we stressed the importance of government leadership for whole-of-society approaches to reducing the harm done by drug use (see also Ysa et al., 2014). Chapter 9 unpacked the role of the private sector, concluding that regulation is the watchword (see also Miller et al., 2016), and Chapter 10 examined the role of civil society, with the power of knowledge becoming a driving force for civil society activism.

Whole-of-society approaches are a form of collaborative governance that emphasizes coordination through normative values and building trust among various actors in society (Kickbusch and Behrendt, 2013). The whole-of society approach goes beyond institutions, and influences and mobilizes local and global culture and mass media, as well as all relevant public and private policy sectors, such as agriculture, education, transport, media and entertainment, justice, and urban design, in reducing harmful drug use. The whole-of-government approach, sometimes called joined-up government, represents the diffusion of governance vertically across levels of government and areas of governance, as well as horizontally throughout sectors (Kickbusch and Gleicher, 2012). This approach requires building trust, a common ethic, a cohesive culture, and new skills to reduce the harm done by drugs throughout all parts of government. The approach includes cabinet committees, interministerial or interagency units, intergovernmental councils, task forces, lead agency assignments, cross-sectoral programmes and projects, and mechanisms for overseeing drug policies and convincing agencies to work together.

As we touched on in several chapters (Chapters 5–7 and 10), smart, comprehensive drug policies also need to move with technological advances and cultural changes and make use of new technologies. These can be employed in improving health literacy (e.g. with Massive Open Online Courses or interactive learning programmes), to promote self- and co-management of advice and treatment, to deliver precisely tailored advice and treatment to specific populations and contexts (e.g. timed to coincide with greater risk periods), and to extend and support engagement in policy development and monitoring (for instance, with crowd sourcing and consultation platforms).

11.10 Government policy-making for drugs should be free of the influence of relevant producer companies, while recognizing producer company responsibilities for reducing harm

In Chapter 9, we stressed that producer companies generally wield a great deal of economic, political, and organizational power in the policy arena, often fostering common policy interests that are not conducive to health. There are many structural factors to counter private sector influence, one of which includes redesign of governance systems that shift away from the present short-term, fast-scale economic and political systems in favour of longer timescale systems that promote sustainable health and well-being (see Stoll and Anderson, 2015).

However, as we noted in Chapter 8, and as is the case with many other 'wicked' public issues, reducing the harm done by drugs cannot be brought about by governments alone (see also Kickbusch and Behrendt, 2013). Whole-of-government and whole-of-society approaches to drug policy should define the relation with private sector stakeholders and establish the rules of the game for stakeholder engagement in the policy cycle through accountability for the common good, where private sector stakeholders contribute to the public health good, simultaneously to their own interests. In order to ensure societal well-being is enhanced, rather than in the hands of commercial interests, the leading role in determining the strategy of public policy for drugs should be in public sector hands. Transparency systems, controls on the revolving door and enhanced conflict of interest policies should be put in place in government, science, civil society, and the media as drivers to increase the impact of evidence-based information on decision-making.

As a reflection of this, while the World Health Organization (WHO) has cautioned that the private sector should not be trying to do the work of governments, which are properly the guardians of the public interest (WHO, 2007), it has indicated, for example, that the alcohol industry has the capacity to prevent and reduce harmful use of alcohol within its core role as a developer, producer, distributor, marketer, and seller of alcoholic beverages (WHO, 2010). As pointed out in Chapter 4, one approach for producer companies to reduce harm is to change the potency of their products (e.g. reducing the alcohol concentration of existing products) and the toxicity of their drug-delivery systems (e.g. cigarette companies shifting to electronic nicotine delivery devices). Shifts towards less harmful products could be incentivized by smart government tax policies.

11.11 A health footprint should be used as the accountability tool to apportion the ill health and premature death imposed by the drivers of drug use and related harm

Chapter 4 and Figure 4.1 listed and described some of the drivers of drug-related harm. Structural drivers of harm include biological attributes and functions, population size and structure, and levels of wealth and income disparities within jurisdictions. Core drivers refer to the processes, mechanisms, and characteristics that influence harm, sometimes through the structural drivers, and sometimes not. Core drivers include drug potency and drug exposure and the technological developments that might influence them, as well as social influences and attitudes. Included in the policies and measures level are policies that reduce drug exposure, actions that promote research and development to reduce drug potency, co-benefits and adverse side-effects of policies and measures, incentivizing healthy individual behaviour, and defining and applying rules of engagement of the private sector to manage markets. Policies and measures affect the core drivers. The structural and core drivers may, in turn, influence policies and measures.

At the centre of the drivers, we placed the health footprint as the accounting system for identifying the determinants of drug-related harm and the management tool to evaluate opportunities by the public and private sectors and civil society to reduce harm. Modelled on the carbon footprint, we defined the health footprint as a measure of the total amount of risk factor attributable disability-adjusted life years (DALYs) of a specific population, sector, or action of interest, defined by specific spatial (e.g. jurisdiction) and temporal (e.g. stated year, such as 2014) boundaries. It can be calculated using standard risk factor-related DALY methodologies of the Global Burden of Disease Study and of the WHO. The health footprint (which is applicable across all health issues) can measure the impact of a range of structural and core drivers of impaired health and the policies and measures that impact upon them, thus, in this case, accounting for who and what causes the harm done by drugs. Drug-related health footprints should become standard components of annual reporting by relevant public and private sector bodies.

Eventually, once the science and methodology for using the health footprint in policy is established, and with parallel developments in research fields such as social costs of drug use and measurement of population well-being in different domains, the concept could be expanded to encompass aspects of well-being beyond health impacted by drug use, resulting in a well-being footprint for entities influencing the consumption of drugs.

11.12 Drug policies should ensure that programmes designed to prevent harm are assessed for their cost-effectiveness by agencies similar to those that assess pharmacological treatments

Programmes and actions designed to promote health and healthy lifestyles, and to prevent health problems and illnesses can improve individual and societal health and well-being, and give a good return on investment. Yet, many current prevention programmes are poorly evaluated or not evaluated at all. Some programmes actually do harm and should be withdrawn. Through mapping and systematic reviews of reviews, there is little evidence to support the majority of prevention approaches currently adopted and delivered by many European countries to address drug problems (Conrod et al., 2015). By contrast, prevention efforts can lead to substantial reductions in drug-related harm when evidence-based programmes are implemented (see Chapter 7). Considerable improvements in health and well-being could be gained from implementing, and only implementing, known evidence-based effective programmes.

Although some countries have bodies that review the impact of prevention and lifestyle programmes (e.g. the National Institute for Health and Care Excellence in the UK, https://www.nice.org.uk/), the existence of such institutions is not consistent or widespread across Europe. In contrast, all countries have mechanisms in place to assess the safety and effectiveness of pharmacological treatments. At the European level, the European Medicines Agency (EMA; http://www.ema.europa.eu/ema/) is responsible for the scientific evaluation of medicines developed by pharmaceutical companies for use in the EU.

Modelled on the EMA, prevention and health promotion programmes could be approved by national agencies or a European Prevention Agency, specifically set up for the purpose, and covering all health topics (Faggiano et al., 2014).

11.13 Drug policies should ensure that gaps between need and advice and treatment are overcome

United Nations Sustainable Development Goal 3 aims to ensure healthy lives and promote well-being for all ages (http://www.un.org/sustainabledevelopment/sustainable-development-goals/), with goal 3.5, strengthening the prevention and treatment of substance use problems, including narcotic drug use and harmful use of alcohol. The indicator to monitor achievement of the goal is coverage of treatment interventions (pharmacological, psychosocial, and rehabilitation and aftercare services) for substance use disorders.

As we pointed out in Chapter 6, across all drugs, there is an unacceptable treatment gap that leads to loss of life and societal well-being. Across Europe, fewer than 1 in 10 people with alcohol use disorders receive any treatment (Rehm et al., 2012). Over four-fifths of heavy drinkers in primary healthcare never received any advice (Rehm et al., 2015). In the USA, only 13.5 per cent of adults with a formal diagnosis of drug use disorder during the previous 12 months have received treatment, and only 24.6 per cent with a lifetime diagnosis of drug use disorder have received treatment (Grant et al., 2015). Further, there are also many lost years between the incidence of substance use disorders and receipt of treatment, often referred to as the 'decade of harm'. Closing the treatment gap brings health gains and reduces preventable deaths (OECD, 2015b), as well as improving social inclusion, and reducing stigma.

11.14 **Conclusions**

As we started out in Chapter 1, the complexity of drug issues leaves no doubt that drugs are wicked problems, ones that appear highly resistant to resolution. Drug issues are wrapped by emotion and compounded by stigma and social control. Moving forward to better governance is not an easy task, and one that will require incremental change and learning by trial and error. We cannot possibly have all the solutions; however, we conclude with three ways forward.

First, drug policy needs to recognize that the human evolutionary evidence suggests that humans are active and functional with respect to the drugs that we use, rather than passive and vulnerable, with the use of drugs infrequent and in relatively low doses in the environments in which we evolved. This contrasts with the present environment in which drugs are generally easily available, often in highly potent forms or packaging, and often delivered through highly risky delivery systems. The consequences of this assessment are that drug policies should move away from illegality to legality, as illegality is unlikely to succeed owing to our evolutionary basis to 'seek out' drugs; and that drug policies should better manage and incentivize lower-potency forms of drug packaging and safer delivery systems.

Second, drug policies can be driven and monitored with a number of objective tools that can be further developed, expanded, and operationalized. One such tool is to embed the impact of drugs and drug policy within a societal well-being frame, whereby all facets of life and their sustainability are taken into account when assessing the impact of drugs and drug policy, including health status, education and skills, social connections, civic engagement, personal security, and jobs and earnings. An overriding implication of the well-being frame is a move from drug illegality to drug legality, with effective regulation managed by whole-of-government and whole-of-society governance. Such a move to legality should be done incrementally, ensuring that the necessary infrastructures and resources are in place for effective governance. Another such tool is MOE analyses, which can provide a common and standard measure across drugs to define acceptable risk levels of individual and societal use. A start has been made using benchmark toxic doses based on risk of acute death. There is still a long way to go to develop benchmark toxic doses based on morbidity outcomes and on well-being outcomes.

And, *third*, a health footprint, with drug-related DALYs as the metric, can be used as a measure to apportion accountability for drug-related harm across drivers of harm, including drug producers and governments through their application or in-application of effective drug policy measures. Accountability requires reporting of the footprint by both private sector and public sector entities, as well as reporting proposals for future action to reduce the footprint.

References

Bjerge B, Duke K, Asmussen Frank V, Rolando S, and Eisenbach-Stangl I (2016) Exploring user groups as stakeholders in drug policy processes in four European countries. In: Hellman M, Berridge V, Duke K, and Mold A (eds) *Concepts of Addictive Substances and Behaviours Across Time and Place.* Oxford: Oxford University Press, pp. 107–28.

Conrod P, Brotherhood A, Sumnall H, Faggiano F, and Wiers R (2015) Drug and alcohol policy for European youth: current evidence and recommendations for integrated policies and research strategies. In: Anderson P, Rehm J, and Room R (eds) *Impact of Addictive Substances and Behaviours on Individual and Societal Well-being.* Oxford: Oxford University Press, pp. 119–42.

Cservenka A and Nagel BJ (2015) Neurocognition and brain abnormalities among adolescent alcohol and drug users. In: Wilson SJ (ed.) *The Wiley Handbook on the Cognitive Neuroscience of Addiction.* London, Wiley Blackwell, pp. 311–32.

Dalky HF (2012) Mental illness stigma reduction interventions review of intervention trials. *West J Nurs Res* 34: 520–47.

Dudley TR (2014) *The Drunken Monkey: Why We Drink and Abuse Alcohol.* Berkeley, CA: University of California Press.

Ellis BJ, Del Giudice M, Dishion TH, Figueredo AJ, Gray P, Griskevicius V, et al. (2012) The evolutionary basis of risky adolescent behaviour: implications for science, policy and practice. *Dev Psychol* 48: 598–623.

Faggiano F, Allara E, Giannotta F, Molinar R, Sumnall H, Wiers R, et al. (2014) Europe needs a central, transparent, and evidence-based approval process for behavioural prevention interventions. *PLOS MED* 11: e1001740.

Grant BF, Goldstein RB, Saha TD, Chou SP, Jung J, Zhang H, et al. (2015) Epidemiology of DSM-5 alcohol use disorder: results from the National Epidemiologic Survey on Alcohol and Related Conditions III. *JAMA Psychiatry* 72: 757–66.

Hellman M, Berridge V, Duke K, and Mold A (eds) (2016) *Concepts of Addictive Substances and Behaviours Across Time and Place.* Oxford: Oxford University Press.

Kickbusch I and Gleicher D (2012) *Governance for Health in the 21st Century.* Copenhagen: World Health Organization Regional Office for Europe.

Kickbusch I and Behrendt T (2013) *Implementing a Health 2020 Vision: Governance for Health in the 21st Century. Making it Happen.* Copenhagen: World Health Organization Regional Office for Europe.

Konner M (2010) *The Evolution of Childhood.* Cambridge, MA: Harvard University Press.

Lachenmeier DW and Rehm J (2015) Comparative risk assessment of alcohol, tobacco, cannabis and other illicit drugs using the margin of exposure approach. *Sci Rep* 5: 8126.

Lieberman D (2013) *The Story of the Human Body.* London: Allen Lane, Penguin Books Ltd.

McGinty EE, Goldman HH, Pescosolido B, and Barry CL (2015) Portraying mental illness and drug addiction as treatable health conditions: effects of a randomized experiment on stigma and discrimination. *Soc Sci Med* 126: 73–85.

Miller D, Harkins C, and Schlögl M (2016) *Impact of Market Forces on Addictive Substances and Behaviours.* Oxford: Oxford University Press.

Moskalewicz J and Klingemann JI (2015) Addictive substances and behaviours and social justice. In: Anderson P, Rehm J, and Room R (eds) *The Impact of Addictive Substances and Behaviours on Individual and Societal Well-being.* Oxford: Oxford University Press, pp. 143–60.

OECD (2011) *How's Life?: Measuring Well-being.* Paris: OECD Publishing.

OECD (2015a) *How's Life?* 2015 Paris: OECD.

OECD (2015b) *Tackling Harmful Alcohol Use.* Paris: OECD Publishing.

Pinto-Foltz MD ad Logsdon MC (2009) Reducing stigma related to mental disorders: initiatives, interventions, and recommendations for nursing. *Arch Psychiatr Nurs* 23: 32–40.

Rehm J and Roerecke M (2013) Reduction of drinking in problem drinkers and all-cause mortality. *Alcohol Alcohol* 48: 509–13.

Rehm J, Shield KD, Rehm MX, Gmel G, Jr, and Frick U (2012) *Alcohol Consumption, Alcohol Dependence, and Attributable Burden of Disease in Europe: Potential Gains from Effective Interventions for Alcohol Dependence.* Toronto: Centre for Addiction and Mental Health.

Rehm J, Marmet S, Anderson P, Gual A, Kraus L, Nutt DJ, et al. (2013a) Defining substance use disorders: do we really need more than heavy use? *Alcohol Alcohol* 48: 633–40.

Rehm J, Shield KD, Gmel G, Rehm MX, and Frick U (2013b) Modeling the impact of alcohol dependence on mortality burden and the effect of available treatment interventions in the European Union. *Eur Neuropsychopharmacol* 23: 89–97.

Rehm J, Anderson P, Gual A, Kraus L, Marmet S, Nutt DJ, et al. (2014a) The tangible common denominator of substance use disorders: a reply to commentaries to Rehm et al. (2013a). *Alcohol Alcohol* 49: 118–22.

Rehm J, Lachenmeier DW, and Room R (2014b) Why does society accept a higher risk for alcohol than for other voluntary or involuntary risks? *BMC Med* 12: 189.

Rehm J, Allamani A, Elekes Z, Jakubczyk A, Landsmane I, Manthey J, et al. (2015) General practitioners recognizing alcohol dependence: a large cross-sectional study in six European countries. *Ann Fam Med* 131: 28–32.

Roulette CJ, Mann H, Kemp B, Remiker M, Wilcox J, Hewlett B, et al. (2014) Tobacco vs. helminths in Congo basin hunter-gatherers: self medication in humans? *Evol Hum Behav* 35: 397–407.

Rüsch N, Angermeyer MC, and Corrigan PW (2005) Mental illness stigma: concepts, consequences, and initiatives to reduce stigma. *Eur Psychiatry* 20: 529–39.

Schmidt LA (2015) What are addictive substances and behaviours and how far do they extend? In: Anderson P, Rehm J, and Room R (eds) *Impact of Addictive Substances and Behaviours on Individual and Societal Well-being.* Oxford: Oxford University Press, pp. 37–52.

Schomerus G, Matschinger H, and Angermeyer MC (2013) Continuum beliefs and stigmatizing attitudes towards persons with schizophrenia, depression and alcohol dependence. *Psychiatry Res* 209: 665–9.

Shield KD and Rehm J (2015) The effects of addictive substances and addictive behaviours on physical and mental health. In: Anderson P, Rehm J, and Room R (eds) *The Impact of Addictive Substances and Behaviours on Individual and Societal Well-being.* Oxford: Oxford University Press, pp. 77–118.

Spas JJ and Weyandt L (2015) Alcohol and its effect on adolescent brain development and executive functioning: some results from neuroimaging. *J Alcohol Drug Depend* 3: 220.

Stoll L and Anderson P (2015) Well-being as a framework for understanding addictive substances. In: Anderson P, Rehm J, and Room R (eds) *The Impact of Addictive Substances and Behaviours on Individual and Societal Well-being.* Oxford: Oxford University Press, pp. 53–76.

Sullivan RJ and Hagen EH (2015) Passive vulnerability or active agency? An evolutionarily ecological perspective of human drug use. In: Anderson P, Rehm J, and Room R (eds) *The Impact of Addictive Substances and Behaviours on Individual and Societal Well-being.* Oxford: Oxford University Press, pp. 13–36

Tajfel H and Turner JC (1986) The social identity theory of intergroup behavior. In: Worchel S and Austin WG (eds.), *Psychology of Intergroup Relations*, Vol. 2. Chicago, IL: Nelson-Hall, pp. 7–24.

World Health Organization (2007) *WHO Expert Committee on Problems Related to Alcohol Consumption. Second Report WHO Technical Report Series.* Geneva: World Health Organization.

World Health Organization (2010) *Global Strategy to Reduce Harmful Use of Alcohol.* Geneva: World Health Organization.

Ysa T, Colom J, Albareda A, Ramon A, Carrión M, and Segura L (2014) *Governance of Addictions: European Public Policies.* Oxford: Oxford University Press.

Index